"An amazing resource for anyone and everyone that works with children, youth, and families in or out of school settings! The book tackles head-on the realities, challenges, disasters, and crisis situations of our times using an informative, hands-on, and practical approach. Whether you are a school principal, district or state administrator, school counselor, teacher, psychologist, therapist, or social worker, this will be your go-to book. Chapters include both broad approaches and specific steps and procedures for preventing, preparing for, and intervening in the aftermath of a crisis or disaster such as school violence, a natural disaster, or an incident of cyber bullying. In addition, each chapter also includes extremely helpful sections on multicultural considerations, specific challenges and their solutions, and sources for additional information."

Dale Fryxell, *PhD, Dean, School of Education and Behavioral Sciences, Professor of Psychology, Chaminade Uniiversity of Honolulu, Hawaii, United States*

"A world in crisis, disasters everywhere. Whether natural disasters or the result of human inability to live in peace and harmony, children and families around the world are faced with innumerable challenges to their mental health and optimal living conditions. School-based family counselling offers, with this compilation of 27 chapters from around the globe, a valuable resource for SBFC practitioners enabling resilience amongst those most affected by various kinds of crises and disasters. Focusing on both prevention and intervention, this book aims to assist schools, children, families, and communities to emerge with hope and courage to deal with disastrous situations wherever they are."

Gertina J. van Schalkwyk, *PhD, Emerita Professor of Psychology, University of Macau, Macau, China*

"With a list of international experts from a variety of disciplines, this book is very timely. Timely because so many children across the world are living in situations of man-made and natural disaster. Even more children are afflicted by mental health problems which will interfere with their ability to enjoy childhood and to function as mature adults who can contribute to their societies.

This book provides scholarly data on useful interventions and prevention strategies within families, in the classroom and in the broader community."

Professor Kim Oates, *AO, MD, DSc, MHP, FRACP, FRCP, FAFPHM, Emeritus Professor, Discipline of Child and Adolescent health, The University of Sydney, Sydney, New South Wales, Australia*

"This is a timely collection, coming as it does as we begin to contemplate the challenges that lay ahead of us in repairing the trauma left by a global pandemic. The book offers insights for practitioners in responding to this disaster as well as other and future crises. The book provides an introduction to readers unfamiliar with school-based family counselling, while offering specialist readers new insights direct from the field. It will satisfy readers seeking practical tips, as well as those seeking to advance theoretical and conceptual understandings. Notably, this book brings together a diverse group of international scholars who are leaders in their fields, at a time when global thinking and responses to disaster and crisis is much needed."

John Scott, *PhD, Head, School of Justice, Faculty of Creative Industries, Education and Social Justice, Queensland University of Technology, Brisbane, Queensland, Australia*

"In the midst of global warming, political polarization, environmental and economic crisis, domestic and school violence…, supporting families with school age children is most important. This is a great book on School-Based Family Counseling for Crisis and Disaster Global Perspectives with 30 distinguished contributors on 27 chapters from all over the world. A really timely book that can empower school counsellors and families."

Professor Cecilia L.W. Chan, *PhD, RSW, FHKPCA, FHKASW, FAOSW, J.P. Professor Emeritus, Department of Social Work and Social Administration, Founding Director and Associate Director, Centre on Behavioral Health, The University of Hong Kong, Hong Kong (SAR)*

"School Based Family Counselling for Crisis and Disaster is an extremely important book to support parents, children and teachers to cope with a range of disasters which occur in many societies with regular frequency. I was particularly impressed by the culturally sensitive chapters on immigrant and refugee children and parents and the promotion of resilience and pragmatic techniques to alleviate stress and mental health issues such as panic attacks and trauma. As such, it will be a valuable resource for all schools promoting teacher parent engagement, family solidarity, and the promotion of trauma sensitive interventions for students. This book can benefit school professionals on an international global basis as there is a global perspective and practical suggestions for school-based support."

Stephen Adams-Langley, *D Psych, MA, UKCP REG., MBACP (Snr. Accred), ADDIPExPsych, UKRC REG., Senior Clinical Consultant, Place2Be, London, United Kingdom*

"Young people globally are experiencing unprecedented rates of change although many are still fortunate to enjoy a constancy of support from their families and schools. This book, written by practitioners and academics from across the world, is dedicated to supporting those families and schools when attempting to nurture and keep young people safe at moments of greatest risk. I commend this timely contribution most warmly."

Tom Billington, *PhD, Emeritus Professor of Educational and Child Psychology, the School of Education, University of Sheffield, United Kingdom*

"Authors from every continent address global issues and articulate reality checks on what is happening today – from COVID global pandemic to mitigating destructive effects of disasters and crises on children, families, schools – and their communities. The extensive chapters written by international scholar-practitioners delve into necessary survival skills and guide us through crises and disaster intervention and prevention."

Walter H. Gmelch, *PhD, Professor, Department of Leadership Studies, School of Education, University of San Francisco*

"This book is being published at the right time. It covers the important areas, which is family counseling in the school setting and counselling related to crisis and disaster. Counseling the family members in school settings during crises, can prevent further escalation of mental health issues, increase resilience, and can reduce the treatment gap. The book covers important chapters that address different areas and settings that are written by eminent researchers and practitioners from across the globe. It gives a wide coverage of different domains, which will be highly beneficial not only for students, academicians, researchers, and practitioners in the area of mental health; but also for teachers, school counsellors and school administrators."

Dr. B. N. Roopesh, *MPhil, PhD, Additional Professor, Child and Adolescent Mental Health Unit; Adjunct Faculty: Dept of Psychosocial Support in Disaster Management, Dept of Clinical Psychology, National Institute of Mental Health and Neurosciece, Bengaluru, India*

"An invaluable must have resource book for educators, teachers, principals, school administrators and policymakers; as well as mental health clinicians. Written by experienced school-based family professionals from several countries, they underscore the importance of working with the two most powerful systems in a child/student's life; school and family, when mitigating crises and disasters in schools and communities.

The unique how to approach of this book provides the reader with a clear description of procedures, of how various research-based interventions and strategies are used when mediating an actual crisis or disaster in schools. As a clinical/educational child psychologist who worked with children and families for many years, I have found it uplifting to read this most useful, creative, and ready-made resource, that can be used immediately by so many professionals."

Teresita A. José, *PhD, Life member: Psychologists Association of Alberta, Canada*

"This book is easy to understand, informative, and helpful for any psychologist, counsellor or family therapist who works with clients who have experienced a major disaster and crisis. Each one of twenty seven chapters is of real benefit. I highly recommend it to mental health workers, principals, parents, and teachers from kindergarten to high school."

Quan Chaolu, *Professor, Department of Psychology,*
Shandong Normal University, China

"School-Based Family Counseling for Crisis and Disaster: Global Perspectives, is global-oriented and particularly benefits Asian families dealing with crisis and disaster for two reasons. First, family and school are both highly precious in Asian culture. Combining these two areas is a double-advantageous way to comfort Asian families. Second, Asians consider family as a private domain. The school-based family counseling approach will cultivate emotional wellness in the family with a subtle and respectful professionalism. This book is strongly recommended for mental health professionals and educators who work with Asian families."

Ming-Kuo Hung, *EdD, Chaoyang University*
of Technology, Taiwan

"This book, written by many Disastershock Global Response Team (DGRT) members, with a global perspective, addresses how to deal with the stress of major crises and disasters through school-based family counseling (SBFC). It contains chapters such as the chronic disaster described in the case of South Africa; responding to cyberbullying in school children; and preventing school violence through school engagement, to name a few. This book is another generous effort resulting from this wonderful momentum generated by the *Disastershock Global Volunteer Team. School-Based Family Counseling for Crisis and Disaster: Global Perspectives* is a mandatory practical book to make the most of in the post-covid era where the new pandemic is related to mental health problems."

Damián Gallegos-Lemos, *MD, Family Physician*
and Family Therapist, Senior Specialist ICT & Health,
Health Intelligence (Electronical Medical Record) at Spanish
Ministry of Health, Madrid, Spain

"There is little doubt that the book in this fast-developing area will become a seminal addition to the field of the Psychology of Education, specifically in School-based family counseling. This relevant book takes an in-depth look at how school personnel can prepare school communities (students, families, and school staff) to cope with the stress of major crises and disasters. This book will be consulted around the world, not only by academics, but also by teachers, students of education, and curriculum developers who are looking for practical and inspiring ideas about instruction in our age of global challenges. I am sure of the book's future success, both in distribution, reaching broad audiences, and being regularly used for reference and study."

Dr. Mirta Susana Ison, *Professor, Department of*
Psychology, Aconcagua University, Senior Researcher,
National Scientific and Technical Research Council
(CONICET), Argentina

"This is a most timely resource in the context of relentless crises and disasters worldwide. Drawing together leading experts from around the globe, this book provides strength-focused practical approaches (based on the cutting-edge School-Based Family Counselling model) to prevention, intervention, and recovery from the impact of severe adversity on young people. The great appeal of this book is the recognition of the capacity for resilience and the vital role that schools can play in harnessing the protective factors at the child, family, and school level. This is a wide-ranging resource that will benefit policy makers, school personnel, and caregivers all over the world."

Ian Shochet, *PhD, Professor of Clinical Psychology, Queensland University of Technology, Brisbane, Australia*

"While the School-Based Family Counseling for Crisis and Disaster book is written by top researchers from across the world- it has been intentionally designed as a practical 'how to' manual for school-based practitioners interested in fostering the success of their students. With a focus on purposeful partnerships across systems such as families and schools - the book provides robust yet accessible overviews, examples and interventions for a host of different challenges. The ultimate goal is to provide tools to prevent potential disruption and devastation to a child's life when they are faced with a catastrophe. This is exactly the kind of resource that makes a difference and I wish I had access to it as a new school-based counselor when I was beginning my own career!"

Joelle Powers, *PhD, MSW, Associate Dean, Interim Director, School of Social Work, College of Health Sciences, Boise State University, Boise, Idaho, United States*

"When crisis and disaster occur, vulnerable populations - especially children - are placed in difficult situations. We are more aware of such situations with the COVID-19 pandemic. At such times, a school-based family counseling (SBFC) approach can help children in difficult situations find psychological comfort and relief. This book presents a wealth of examples and concrete measures to address how to integrate family and school mental health interventions through SBFC. Therefore, this book should be read not only by SBFC practitioners such as school counselors, social workers, and psychologists, but also by teachers and parents. It provides many suggestions for how to support children mentally in times of crisis and disaster."

Yuto Kitamura, *PhD, Professor, Graduate School of Education, The University of Tokyo*

"This book describes the pivotal role schools and families can play in reducing the destructive effects of disaster and crisis on children, families, and schools. Written by experts in the field in an easy-to-use manner, this book contextualizes disasters ranging from Covid 19 global pandemic to the refugee crisis that is a result of Russia-Ukraine war. Fourteen of the chapter authors were actively involved in providing psychological services in different countries to children, families, and schools affected by both disasters. School-based family counseling (SBFC) is described as an interdisciplinary mental health meta-model that can be used to strengthen children, families, and school personnel in times of crisis and disaster. Counselors, social workers, mental health professionals, as well as parents, will value this book's evidence-based practices for K-12."

Huda Ayyash-Abdo, *PhD, Associate Professor of Psychology, Department of Social Sciences, Lebanese American University, Beirut, Lebanon*

School-Based Family Counseling for Crisis and Disaster

School-Based Family Counseling for Crisis and Disaster is a practical handbook with a school-based family counseling and interdisciplinary mental health practitioner focus that can be used to mitigate crises and disasters that affect school children.

Anchored in the school-based family counseling (SBFC) tradition of integrating family and school mental health interventions, this book introduces interventions according to the five core SBFC metamodel areas: school intervention, school prevention, family intervention, family prevention, and community intervention. The book has an explicit "how to" approach and covers prevention strategies that build student, school, and family resilience for handling stress and interventions that can be provided during and immediately after a disaster or crisis has occurred. The chapter authors of this edited volume are all experienced professors and/or practitioners in counseling, psychology, social work, marriage and family therapy, teaching, and educational administration.

All mental health professionals, especially school-based professionals, will find this book an indispensable resource for crisis planning and developing a trauma-sensitive school.

Brian A. Gerrard, PhD, is a Chief Academic Officer of the Western Institute for Social Research, Berkeley, California, and the Chair of the Institute for School-Based Family Counseling.

Emily J. Hernandez, EdD, LMFT, is an Associate Professor and the Program Coordinator of the School-Based Family Counseling Program at California State University, Los Angeles.

Prof. Sibnath Deb, PhD, DSc, is the Director of the Rajiv Gandhi National Institute of Youth Development, Government of India. Currently, he is also an Adjunct Professor of the School of Justice, Queensland University of Technology (QUT), Australia.

School-Based Family Counseling for Crisis and Disaster

Global Perspectives

**Edited by
Brian A. Gerrard,
Emily J. Hernandez,
and Sibnath Deb**

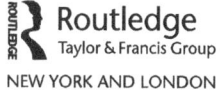

Routledge
Taylor & Francis Group

NEW YORK AND LONDON

Designed cover image: © Getty Images

First published 2023
by Routledge
605 Third Avenue, New York, NY 10158

and by Routledge
4 Park Square, Milton Park, Abingdon, Oxon, OX14 4RN

Routledge is an imprint of the Taylor & Francis Group, an informa business

© 2023 selection and editorial matter, Brian A. Gerrard,
Emily J. Hernandez, and Sibnath Deb; individual chapters, the
contributors

The right of Brian A. Gerrard, Emily J. Hernandez, and Sibnath
Deb to be identified as the authors of the editorial material, and
of the authors for their individual chapters, has been asserted in
accordance with sections 77 and 78 of the Copyright, Designs
and Patents Act 1988.

All rights reserved. No part of this book may be reprinted
or reproduced or utilised in any form or by any electronic,
mechanical, or other means, now known or hereafter invented,
including photocopying and recording, or in any information
storage or retrieval system, without permission in writing from
the publishers.

Trademark notice: Product or corporate names may be trademarks
or registered trademarks, and are used only for identification and
explanation without intent to infringe.

Library of Congress Cataloging-in-Publication Data
Names: Gerrard, Brian A., editor. | Hernandez, Emily J., editor. |
Deb, Sibnath, editor.
Title: School-based family counseling for crisis and disaster : global
perspectives / edited by Brian A. Gerrard, Emily J. Hernandez,
Sibnath Deb.
Description: New York, NY : Routledge, 2023. | Includes
bibliographical references and index.
Identifiers: LCCN 2022049507 (print) | LCCN 2022049508 (ebook) |
ISBN 9781032063720 (hardback) | ISBN 9781032063713 (paperback) |
ISBN 9781003201977 (ebook)
Subjects: LCSH: Family psychotherapy. | Educational counseling. |
Students—Mental health. | Parent-student counselor relationships. |
Home and school. | School crisis management.
Classification: LCC RC489.F33 .S358 2023 (print) | LCC
RC489.F33 (ebook) | DDC 616.89/156—dc23/eng/20230202
LC record available at https://lccn.loc.gov/2022049507
LC ebook record available at https://lccn.loc.gov/2022049508

ISBN: 978-1-032-06372-0 (hbk)
ISBN: 978-1-032-06371-3 (pbk)
ISBN: 978-1-003-20197-7 (ebk)

DOI: 10.4324/9781003201977

Typeset in Baskerville
by codeMantra

Contents

Figures

Boxes

Tables

Tables

About the editors

Brian A. Gerrard has a PhD in Sociology, from the University of New South Wales, Sydney, Australia and a PhD in Counseling Psychology, from the University of Toronto. He has extensive experience teaching a wide variety of Master's and Doctoral level courses in Counseling Psychology and holds teaching awards from two universities. Brian is an Emeritus Faculty Member of the University of San Francisco where he developed the Master's MFT Program and for 14 years served as the MFT Coordinator. His orientation emphasizes an integration of family systems and problem-solving approaches. He is an experienced administrator and has been the Chair of the USF Counseling Psychology Department three times. Currently, Brian is the Chief Academic Officer, and a core faculty member, for the Western Institute for Social Research (WISR) in Berkeley, California. He is a member of the Board, Center for Child and Family Development, at WISR. The Center, co-founded by Brian, has for years managed the largest and longest-running School-Based Family Counseling Program of its type in the USA. Its Mission Possible Program has served more than 20,000 children and families in over 70 Bay area schools. Brian is also the Chair of the Institute for School-Based Family Counseling and the Symposium Director for the Oxford Symposium in School-Based Family Counseling. He is the senior author of several books on School-Based Family Counseling. During the 2020 pandemic, he was actively involved in co-leading the Disastershock Global Volunteer Team which developed 26 different language translations of the book *Disastershock: How to Cope with the Emotional Stress of a Major Disaster* which are available free on disastershock.com. Brian lives in Stuart, Florida with his wife Olive Powell.

Emily J. Hernandez is an Associate Professor and Program Coordinator of the School-Based Family Counseling Program at Cal State University, Los Angeles. She brings over 20 years of experience working in public education and mental health. Her professional background includes working directly with schools, families, and communities, including child welfare and attendance, counseling, K-12, administration, clinical mental health, employee assistance services in education, and counselor preparation/education. She is a Licensed Marriage and Family Therapist with areas of expertise in working with children, couples and families, educators, victims of violence, trauma, and crisis counseling. As a leader in the field, she has presented locally, regionally, nationally, and internationally and has authored a variety of scholarly work. She has participated in leadership organizational decision making through board and advisory memberships and has served by advocating for the need for mental health services in education in various capacities. She brings a unique lens to working with educators and school systems understanding the importance of bridging the gap toward more access to mental health in prevention and intervention in education. She holds a bachelor's degree in Psychology and a master's degree in Counseling and Marriage and Family Therapy and School Counseling from Cal State University, Los Angeles, and a doctoral degree in Educational Leadership focusing on educational psychology from the University of Southern California (USC).

Prof. Sibnath Deb, PhD, DSc, is the Director of the Rajiv Gandhi National Institute of Youth Development – an institute of national importance, Government of India. Prior to joining the RGNIYD, he was teaching in the Department of Applied Psychology, Pondicherry University (A Central University) and University of Calcutta. Currently, he is also attached to the School of Justice, Queensland University of Technology (QUT), as an Adjunct Professor. From 2004 to 2008, he served the International Society for Prevention of Child Abuse and Neglect (ISPCAN) as a Council Member. In brief, Prof. Deb has 31 years of teaching, research, and administrative experience and has published a large number of research articles and 20 books. Some of his latest books include *Child Safety, Welfare and Well-being, Second Edition* (Springer, 2022), *Health and Well-being: Challenges, Strategies and Future Trends* (Springer, 2022), *Youth Development in India: Future Generations in a Changing World* (Routledge, 2022), *Community Psychology: Theories and Applications* (Sage, 2020), *Disadvantaged Children in India: Empirical Evidence, Policies and Actions* (Springer, 2020), *Social Psychology in Everyday Life* (Sage, 2019), *Childhood to Adolescence: Issues and Concerns* (Pearson, 2019) and so on. His research interests include child safety, students' mental health, youth development, adolescent reproductive health, family relationships and child protection. In recognition of his academic and research contribution, Prof. Deb has received a number of national and international awards, including an Award from the Asiatic Society, Kolkata (an institute of national importance under the Ministry of Culture, Government of India) in 2018 and the "Visitor's Award 2019" from the Hon'ble President of India Shri Ram Nath Kovind.

Contributors

Nyna Amin, DEd, University of KwaZulu-Natal, Durban, KwaZulu-Natal, South Africa

Karen S. Buchanan, EdD, George Fox University, Newberg, Oregon, USA

Thomas D. Buchanan, EdD, George Fox University, Newberg, Oregon, USA

Carol E. Buchholz Holland, PhD, North Dakota State University, Fargo, North Dakota, USA

Michael J. Carter, PhD, California State University, Los Angeles, Los Angeles, California, USA

Jeff Chang, PhD, Athabasca University, Calgary, Alberta, Canada

Ralph S. Cohen, PhD, Central Connecticut State University, New Britain, Connecticut, USA

Shayana Deb, MSc Behavioral Science graduate of Department of Psychology, CHRIST (Deemed to be) University, Bengaluru, India

Sibnath Deb, PhD, DSc, Rajiv Gandhi National Institute of Youth Development (RGNIYD), Ministry of Youth Affairs and Sports, Govt. of India, Pennalur, Sriperumbudur, Tamil Nadu, India

Nidup Dorji, PhD, Khesar Gyalpo University of Medical Sciences of Bhutan, Thimphu, Bhutan

Alia R. Elasmar, MS, California State University, Los Angeles, Los Angeles, California, USA

Maya Sophia Fujimura, PhD, University of California, Los Angeles, California, USA

Brian A. Gerrard, PhD, Western Institute for Social Research, Berkeley, California, USA

Judith E. Giampaoli, MA, Center for Child & Family Development, Western Institute for Social Research, Berkeley, California, USA

Anjali Gireesan, PhD, Defense Research and Development Organisation, Government of India, Kapurthala, Punjab, India

Kezia Gopaul-Knights, PhD, California State University, Los Angeles, California, USA

Belinda Hernández-Arriaga, PhD, Counseling Psychology Department, University of San Francisco, San Francisco, California, USA

Emily J. Hernandez, EdD, California State University, Los Angeles, Los Angeles, California, USA

Masamine Jimba, PhD, The University of Tokyo, Bunkyo-ku, Tokyo, Japan

Celina Korzeniowski, PhD, Human, Social and Environmental Science Institute of the National Scientific and Technical Research Council (CONICET), Mendoza, Argentina

Robyne Le Brocque, PhD, University of Queensland, Brisbane, Queensland, Australia

Bishakha Majumdar, Indian Institute of Management, Visakhapatnam, India

Juan Carlos Ruiz Malagon, MA, MS, Department of Pediatrics, Stanford University, Stanford, California, USA

Maria C. Marchetti-Mercer, PhD, University of the Witwatersrand, Johannesburg, South Africa

Reshelle Marino, PhD, Southeastern Louisiana University, Hammond, Louisiana, USA

Helen Nelson, PhD, Carey Community Resources, Harrisdale, Western Australia, Australia

Toni Nemia, MS, Center for Child and Family Development (WISR), San Francisco, California, USA

Sudia Paloma McCaleb, EdD Western Institute for Social Research, Berkeley, California, USA

Wendy D. Rock, PhD, LCP-S, NCC, NCSC, Southeastern Louisiana University, Hammond, Louisiana, USA

Elina Saeki, PhD, California State University, Los Angeles, Los Angeles, California, USA

Zipora Shechtman, PhD, Emerita professor, Haifa University, Haifa, Israel

Akira Shibanuma, PhD, The University of Tokyo, Bunkyo-ku, Tokyo, Japan

Phillip T. Slee, PhD, Flinders University, Adelaide, South Australia, Australia

Nurit Kaplan Toren, PhD, Oranim Academic College of Education, Kiryat Tiv'on, University of Haifa, Haifa, Israel

Nikki Triggell, MEdSt, Queensland Department of Education, Queensland, Australia

Jaffa Weiss, MEd, Former Hugim High School principal, Haifa, Israel

We are in this together

Foreword to School-based family counseling for crisis and disaster: Global perspectives

At this moment, in the aftermath of a health-triggered pandemic and the advent of disruptive geopolitical war and conflict, we are in the harsh grip of global challenge. Global challenge is of course not new. It has been going on since the dawn of time. Its impact is evident in world-wide movements to sustain development through joint agendas and strategies. World-wide challenges require complex, global thinking such as Sustainable Development Goals (The World Bank, 2020).

Sustainability science (Wiek et al., 2014) advocates that, in the face of world-wide challenges, global thinking and local action are complementary. Global challenge impacts on the individual level, in homes, in schools and in neighborhoods. Extreme adversity means that, in their everyday lives, children, parents, teachers and school-leaders alike may all feel uncertain, anxious, helpless and without hope. They may have no examples from comparable previous life experiences to support one another on how to act to protect themselves and others from impending catastrophe. From a resilience perspective (Ungar, 2018), extreme crises – if unchecked – can lead to disastrous outcomes. Crises and disaster indicate an urgency to access trustworthy sources on what to do to support quality of life.

In this timely and much-needed collection of evidence-based practices, authors flocked together to share their joint knowledge as a resource to support the collective well-being of children, families and schools in distress. Flocking (Ebersöhn, 2019) is an alternative, Afrocentric response to collective distress. Other than familiar fight, flight, faint, freeze and swarm responses in resilience literature, flocking aims at collective well-being – rather than individual-level well-being. Flocking implies mobilizing existing social resources to provide social support in order to buffer against adversity and promote better-than-expected outcomes.

The content of the volume similarly reflects flocking responses to crises and disaster. In meaningful chapter-clusters, editors present quality insights from authors that demonstrate how school-based family counseling constitutes flocking. The School-Based Family Counseling (SBFC) metamodel shows how students, parents, families, teachers, mental health professionals counselors and school leadership flock. Flocking, according to SBFC, on the one hand, buffers against a range of systemic crises (the uncertainty of a pandemic; school and societal violence; border-migrant circumstances; high-conflict couples; suicidal ideation; death, grief and loss; self-harm; stress and coping). Flocking in SBFC scenario creates a caring supportive education environment that, on the other hand, promotes unpredicted positive well-being and learning outcomes for students and their families – despite the presence of a challenge.

The volume shows how student-family care and support may be grafted onto the "business-as-usual" practices of schools in low-threshold ways which are as much pragmatic as they are innovative. The portrayals are varied enough to provide the reader with transferability options in order to craft interventions relevant to different contextual and cultural perspectives.

In a closing of this brief contribution, it is significant to recognize how meaningfully *SBFC for Crisis and Disaster: Global Perspectives* contributes to distilling hands-on and quality evidence for use by mental health professionals, teachers, school-leaders and education officials desperate for reliable and relevant guidelines on "what to do." The value of this intellectual contribution is to expand the base of go-to-resources of those who need to support others when coping with crises' severe adversity.

Liesel Ebersöhn, PhD, Director of the Centre for the Study of Resilience; Professor: Department of Educational Psychology, Faculty of Education, University of Pretoria, South Africa; President-Elect: World Education Research Association (WERA)

References

Ebersöhn, L. (2019). *Flocking Together: An Indigenous Psychology Theory of Resilience in Southern Africa*. Cham, Switzerland: Springer Nature. doi.org/10.1007/978-3-030-16435-5

The World Bank. (2020). Sustainable Development Goals and Targets. https://datatopics.worldbank.org/sdgatlas/targets/

Ungar, M. (2018). Systemic Resilience: Principles and Processes for a Science of Change in Contexts of Adversity. *Ecology and Society, 23* (4), 34–52. https://doi.org/10.5751/ES-10385-230434

Wiek, A., Harlow, J., Melnick, R., van der Leeuw, S., Fukushi, K., Takeuchi, K., Farioli, F., Yamba, F., Blake, A., Geiger, C., & Kutter, R. (2014). Sustainability Science in Action: A Review of the State of the Field through Case Studies on Disaster Recovery, Bioenergy, and Precautionary Purchasing. *Sustainability Science Online First*. https://doi.org/10.1007/s11625-014-0261-9

Part I

Overview

1 The school-based family counseling approach to strengthening families and schools in crisis and disaster

Brian A. Gerrard, Emily J. Hernandez, and Sibnath Deb

Overview

This chapter describes the unique role schools can play in mitigating the destructive effects of disaster and crisis on children, families, and schools. School-based family counseling (SBFC) is described as an interdisciplinary mental health metamodel that can be used to strengthen children, families, and school personnel in times of crisis and disaster. Research is presented that supports schools taking an active role in intervening in disasters and crises. Evidence-based support for SBFC is also presented.

Introduction

This is a practical "how to" book on ways school personnel can prepare school communities (students, families, and school personnel) on how to cope with the stress of major crises and disasters. Common school crises are school shootings, death of a teacher or student, acts of violence between students or students and school personnel, suicide or suicide attempts of students or school personnel. Common disasters are natural: pandemics, earthquakes, floods, fires, tsunamis, hurricanes, and human-caused: war, terrorist attacks, chemical spills, crime.

These crises and disasters have a strong negative effect on the mental health of children and adolescents (Becker-Blease et al., 2010; Catani et al., 2008; Gkatsa, 2020; Kar, 2009; Leeb et al., 2020; Marques de Miranda et al., 2020; Senft et al., 2022).

However, there is research demonstrating that schools can play an important role in helping children cope with disaster and crisis-related stress (see Box 1.1). This is important because – particularly in disasters – community mental health resources quickly become overwhelmed. The population of an entire city or country may be affected by severe stress and large numbers of children and families may lack mental health resources for coping with disaster-related stress (Edmeade & Buzinde, 2021). In these situations, schools that are "trauma sensitive" can be safe havens during times of crisis and disaster because the school personnel are trained in ways that relate to students that promote student resilience.

DOI: 10.4324/9781003201977-2

Box 1.1 Studies on the calming role school personnel have on children coping with disasters and trauma

Alisic, E. (2012). Teachers' perspectives on providing support to children after trauma: A qualitative study. *School Psychology Quarterly*, *27*(1), 51–59. https://doi.org/10.1037/a0028590

Alisic, E., Bus, M., Dulack, W., Pennings, L., & Splinter, J. (2012). Teachers' experiences supporting children after traumatic exposure. *Journal of Traumatic Stress*, *25*(1), 98–101. https://doi.org/10.1002/jts.20709

Berger, R., & Gelkopf, M. (2009). School-based intervention for the treatment of tsunami-related distress in children: A quasi-randomized controlled trial. *Psychotherapy and Psychosomatics*, *78*(6), 364–371. https://doi.org/10.1159/000235976

Cole, S. F., Eisner, A., Gregory, M., & Ristuccia, J. (2013). *Helping traumatized children learn: Creating and advocating for trauma-sensitive schools*. Trauma and Learning Policy Initiative, Massachusetts Advocates for Children, & Harvard Law School.

Edmeade, J. N., & Buzinde, C. N. (2021). The role of educators in community resilience in natural disaster-prone communities. *Community Development Journal*. https://doi.org/10.1093/cdj/bsab010

Jaycox, L. H, Morse, L. K., Tanielian, T. & Stein, B. D. (2006). *How schools can help students recover from traumatic experiences: A tool kit for supporting long-term recovery*. RAND Corporation Retrieved from https://www.rand.org/pubs/technical_reports/TR413.html

Johnson, V. A., & Ronan, K. R. (2014). Classroom responses of New Zealand school teachers following the 2011 Christchurch earthquake. *Natural Hazards*, *72*(2), 1075–1092. https://doi.org/10.1007/s11069-014-1053-3

Le Brocque, R., De Young, A., Montague, G., Pocock, S., March, S., Triggell, N., Rabaa, C., & Kenardy, J. (2016). Schools and natural disaster recovery: The unique and vital role that teachers and education professionals play in ensuring the mental health of students following natural disasters. *Journal of Psychologists and Counsellors in Schools*, *27*(1), 1–23. https://doi.org/10.1017/jgc.2016.17

Liu, Z., Zhu, Z., Kao, H. S., Zong, Y., Tang, S., Xu, M., Liu, I. C., Lam, S. P., & Wang, R. (2014). Effect of calligraphy training on hyperarousal symptoms for childhood survivors of the 2008 China earthquakes. *Neuropsychiatric Disease and Treatment*, 977. https://doi.org/10.2147/ndt.s55016

Minahan, J. (2019). Trauma-informed teaching strategies. *Educational Leadership*, *77*(2), 30–35.

Ophir, Y., Rosenberg, H., Asterhan, C. S., & Schwarz, B. B. (2015). In times of war, adolescents do not fall silent: Teacher–student social network communication in wartime. *Journal of Adolescence*, *46*(1), 98–106. https://doi.org/10.1016/j.adolescence.2015.11.005

Plumb, J., Bush, K., & Kersevich, S. (2016). Trauma-sensitive schools: An evidence-based approach. *School Social Work Journal*, *40*(2), 37–60.

Stevens, J. E. (2012, June 26). Trauma-sensitive schools are better schools. *Huffington Post*. Retrieved from https://www.huffingtonpost.com/jkane-ellen-stevens/trauma-sensitive-schools b 1625924.html

Teaching Tolerance Staff (2020). A trauma-informed approach to teaching through coronavirus. Retrieved from https://www.tolerance.org/magazine/a-trauma-informed-approach-to-teaching-through-coronavirus

Toros, K. (2013). School-based intervention in the context of armed conflict: Strengthening teacher capacity to facilitate psychosocial support and well-being of children. *International Journal of Humanities and Social Science*, *3*(7), 228–237.

Wisconsin Department of Public Instruction (2013). Mental health: Creating trauma-sensitive schools to improve learning: A response to intervention (RTI) model. Retrieved from http://sspw.dpi.wi.gov.sspw_mhtrauma

Wolmer, L., Hamiel, D., & Laor, N. (2011). Preventing children's post-traumatic stress after disaster with teacher-based intervention: A controlled study. *Journal of the American Academy of Child & Adolescent Psychiatry*, *50*(4), 340–348.e2. https://doi.org/10.1016/j.jaac.2011.01.002

School-based family counseling

School-based family counseling (SBFC) is an integrated systems approach to helping children succeed academically and personally through linking home, school, and community interventions. SBFC has nine strengths:

- School and Family Focus
- Systems Orientation
- Educational Focus
- Parent Partnership
- Multicultural Sensitivity
- Child Advocacy
- Promotion of School Transformation
- Interdisciplinary Focus
- Evidence-Based Support

School and family focus

The two most influential microsystems affecting children are the family and the school. Children spend most of their time either in families or in schools. Both have a powerful socializing influence on child development. SBFC practitioners collaborate with families and schools in order to better mobilize constructive resources that can help a child to overcome personal problems.

Systems orientation

SBFC draws heavily on systems theory to conceptualize the multiple school, family, and community relationships that affect children. The strength of the family systems approach is that it helps the SBFC practitioner to look beyond the "identified patient" (e.g. the child) to the family and school relationships that may be negatively affecting a child's behavior. On the rare occasions when an SBFC practitioner works only with an individual (such as a child, a parent, or a teacher), the SBFC practitioner always conceptualizes the "case" from a systems perspective.

Educational focus

SBFC has an explicit focus on working with families and teachers to help children overcome personal problems and succeed academically. This approach appeals to parents and guardians because it avoids a "therapy" emphasis that many families find stigmatizing.

Parent partnership

SBFC emphasizes using a collaborative approach with parents and guardians who are viewed as valuable persons for helping children to become more resilient.

Multicultural sensitivity

SBFC is a multiculturally sensitive approach. It avoids the Eurocentric focus on individuals and instead places an emphasis on family. In addition, SBFC avoids the stigmatizing labeling that therapy may have for many minority families by placing an emphasis on SBFC practitioners and parents/guardians collaborating to promote child success at school.

Child advocacy

Although the SBFC practitioner views the child, family, and school as an integral part of the "client system", the SBFC practitioner is first and foremost a child advocate. Children are more vulnerable than parents/guardians or teachers and therefore need more protection from adverse relationships, whether at school or at home.

Promotion of school transformation

SBFC emphasizes that just as families may need to change in order to help children, so to must schools. Families need to change when child abuse, marital discord, divorce, sibling rivalry, and other family problems negatively affect a child. Similarly, schools need to change when bullying, racial discrimination, authoritarian teaching, and other problems at school negatively affect a child.

Interdisciplinary focus

Just as family therapy as a discipline developed separately from the other mental health approaches and later was incorporated into all of them, SBFC is an approach that can be used by any of the other mental health approaches. Many SBFC functions, especially involving school prevention, can be performed by teachers. SBFC is not intended to replace other mental health professions, e.g. Counseling, Social Work, Psychology, and Psychiatry. Rather, it is an adjunct approach that can be value-added for any mental health approach. Many SBFC functions, especially involving school prevention and school intervention, can be performed by teachers.

Evidence-based support

Moderate evidence-based support for the effectiveness of SBFC is demonstrated in a number of randomized control group studies that compared school-only, or family-only, intervention with combined school and family intervention. These studies found the combined intervention superior (see Box 1.2).

Box 1.2 Evidence-based support for SBFC

Apisitwasana, N., Perngparn, U., & Cottler, L. (2018). Effectiveness of school and family-based interventions to prevent gaming addiction among grades 4–5 students in Bangkok, Thailand. *Psychology Research and Behavior Management*, *11*, 103–115. https://doi.org/10.2147/PRBM.S145868

Conduct Problems Prevention Research Group. (2007). Fast track randomized controlled trial to prevent externalizing psychiatric disorders: Findings from grades 3 to 9. *Journal of the American Academy of Child and Adolescent Psychiatry*, *46*(10), 1250–1262. https://doi.org/10.1097/chi.0b013e31813e5d39

Crozier, M., Rokutani, L., Russett, J., Godwin, E., & Banks G. (2010). A multisite program evaluation of families and schools together (FAST): Continued evidence of a successful multifamily community-based prevention program. *The School Community Journal, 20*(1), 187–207. ERIC: EJ891838.

Eddy, J. M., Reid, J. B., & Fetrow, R. A. (2000). An elementary school-based prevention program targeting modifiable antecedents of youth delinquency and violence. *Journal of Emotional and Behavioral Disorders, 8*(3), 165–176. https://doi.org/10.1177/106342660000800304

Flay, B., Graumlich S., Segawa, E., Burns, J., Amuwo, S., Bell, C., Campbell, R., Cowell, J., Cooksey, J., Dancy, B., Hedeker, D., Jagers, R., Levy, S., Paikoff, R., Punwani, I., & Weisberg, R. (2004).Effects of 2 prevention programs on high-risk behaviors among African American youth: A randomized trial. *Archives of Pediatrics and Adolescent Medicine, 158*(4), 377–384. https://doi.org/10.1001/archpedi.158.4.377

Kratochwill, T., McDonald, L., Levin, J., Scalia, P., & Coover, G. (2009). Families and schools together: An experimental study of multi-family support groups for children at risk. *Journal of School Psychology, 47,* 245–265. https://doi.org/10.1016/j.jsp.2009.03.001

Kratochwill, T.R., McDonald, L., Levin, J.R., YoungBear-Tibbetts, H., & Demaray, M. K. (2004). Families and schools together: An experimental analysis of a parent-mediated multi-family group program for American Indian children. *Journal of School Psychology, 42*(5), 359–383. https://doi.org/10.1016/j.jsp.2004.08.001

Lochman, J. E., & Wells, K. C. (2004). The coping power program for preadolescent aggressive boys and their parents: Outcome effects at the 1-Year follow-up. *Journal of Consulting and Clinical Psychology, 72*(4), 571–578. https://doi.org/10.1037/0022-006x.72.4.571

The SBFC metamodel

The SBFC metamodel may be used to illustrate the SBFC approach to crisis (Gerrard et al., 2019). It is a diagram that identifies the different systems in which the SBFC practitioner does prevention or intervention work (see Figure 1.1).

The heart of the diagram consists of two axes: Family-School and Intervention-Prevention which create a square with four quadrants: School Prevention, School Intervention, Family Prevention, and Family Intervention. The School Prevention quadrant is where strategies to prevent problems from occurring are used. These include classroom meetings, guidance groups, psychoeducation presentations on dealing with stress and bullying, socio-emotional learning topics, and classroom management for educators. The School Intervention quadrant refers to mental health interventions intended to remediate existing student challenges such as school refusal, school failure, depression, anxiety, peer-related problems, and classroom

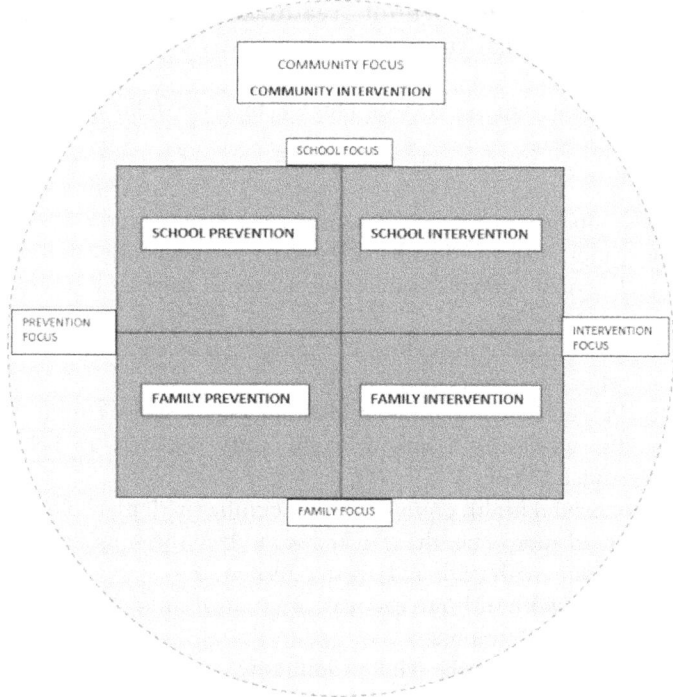

Figure 1.1 The SBFC metamodel.

behavior. The Family Prevention quadrant deals with psychoeducational strategies such as parenting skills workshops, seminars on dealing with bullying or mental health topics, and parent support groups. The Family Intervention quadrant deals with traditional family counseling interventions such as parent consultation, conjoint family therapy, and couples therapy. The Community Intervention level refers to situations in which (a) resources from the community are needed to be mobilized to help students, teachers or families; and (b) situations in which the SBFC practitioner should intervene to reduce a negative community behavior (e.g. discrimination by an employer that affects an immigrant family).

The SBFC approach to crisis and disaster

The SBFC approach to crisis and disaster emphasizes prevention at the school and family levels. Assessing the school community for its readiness to provide psychological support should a crisis or disaster occur is a critical first step. Box 1.3 shows some common indicators that a school community is prepared for providing psychological support during and following a disaster.

Box 1.3 Indicators of school readiness for providing psychological support during crisis and disaster

Instructions: Please indicate Yes or No whether the following are present in your school.

Yes/No

____1 The school has a Crisis and Disaster Safety Plan

____2 The school Crisis and Disaster safety plan is comprehensive. It has:

   ____a Detailed safety procedures for handling different kinds of crisis and disaster.

   ____b Resources for providing psychological first aid to students, school personnel, and families.

   ____c Procedures for sharing information with students' families.

   ____d Procedures for involving community resources to help students cope.

____3 School mental health professionals are familiar with psychological first aid approaches that can be used to help the school community cope with crisis and disaster-related stress.

____4 School mental health professionals are trained in best practices for dealing with trauma.

____5 The relationships in the school community are supportive.

   ____a the students relate to each other in a supportive way.

   ____b the teachers and students have a supportive relationship.

   ____c the school administration relates in a supportive way to students.

   ____d the teachers and school administration relate is a supportive way to students' families.

____6 The school administration has identified community resources that can be utilized in a crisis or disaster.

If the school has:

1 an existing Crisis and Disaster Plan that is comprehensive in providing psychological support resources for teachers, students, and their families;

2 the school mental health professionals that can provide psychological first aid to the school community and effectively deal with psychological trauma; and

3 a positive social climate characterized by supportive relationships, then the school is likely prepared for dealing with crisis and disaster.

Of these three attributes, a positive school climate is likely the most important. Schools that are cohesive and have strong supportive relationships between members of the school community are more likely to be resilient in the face of disaster-related stress. However, research on social climate in schools suggests that there are many schools that fall short of the social climate necessary for student school engagement:

> An analysis of students' engagement and literacy results in 43 countries, based on large and nationally-representative samples of 15-year-old students from PISA 2000 (Organisation for Economic Co-operation and Development [OECD] 2003), concluded that there is a high prevalence of students who are disaffected from school, that the prevalence varies significantly among schools, and that it is influenced by school policies and local practices. Schools have higher levels of students' engagement when there is a positive climate, good relations between teachers and students, and high expectations for students' success. Teachers and principals can play a strong role in creating a positive culture at school. The importance of engagement is discussed for its association with other positive outcomes, such as well-being and quality of school life. Schools with high levels of engagement among the students did not achieve it at the expense of literacy skills: high student engagement was associated on average with higher literacy skills.
>
> (Allodi, 2010, p. 92)

How to use this book

Step one in the SBFC approach to helping schools deal with crisis and disaster is to ensure that the school has a positive social climate with strong student engagement. When an earthquake has already occurred, building a strong school climate is too late because the school may be destroyed. The old saying "an ounce of prevention is worth a pound of cure" applies here. In this book, the reader will find several chapters on how to create a positive climate in schools through promoting children's well-being and resilience, reducing bullying, promoting student engagement, and developing trauma-sensitive schools. Because students are part of families, family prevention is also central to promoting student resilience. This book contains chapters on how to build family resilience using the Internal Family Systems and Intimate Parenting approach, strengthen teacher-parent engagement, and empower immigrant families.

Step two in the SBFC approach to helping schools deal with crisis and disaster involves effective interventions to use when a crisis or disaster has already occurred. Chapters on school intervention describe psychological approaches and teaching approaches that school personnel can use to help students cope, crisis intervention with school personnel, and solution-focused therapy and grief therapy strategies for dealing with student trauma. In addition, there are chapters describing community intervention strategies for strengthening schools dealing with crisis and disaster.

This book was written during the COVID-19 global pandemic and the refugee crisis during the war on Ukraine. Fourteen of the chapter authors were actively involved in providing psychological first aid globally to children, families, and schools affected by both disasters. The final chapter in this book describes our SBFC approach as we actively carried it out.

Resources

Gerrard, B., Carter, M., & Ribera, D. (Eds.) (2019). *School-based family counseling: An interdisciplinary practitioner's guide.* Routledge.
This is a comprehensive text describing how to implement SBFC for school intervention, school prevention, family intervention, family prevention, and community intervention.
Gerrard, B., Selimos, E., & Morrison, S. (Eds.) (2022). *School-based family counseling with refugees and immigrants.* Routledge.
This book describes how to use a collaborative SBFC approach to empower refugees and immigrant children and families.
Gerrard, B., & Soriano, M. (Eds.) (2013). *School-based family counseling: Transforming family-school relationships.* Createspace.
This book was the precursor to the 2019 SBFC book and gives a thorough overview of the SBFC approach.

References

Allodi, M. W. (2010). The meaning of social climate of learning environments: Some reasons why we do not care enough about it. *Learning Environments Research, 13*(2), 89–104. https://doi.org/10.1007/s10984-010-9072-9
Becker-Blease, K. A., Turner, H. A., & Finkelhor, D. (2010). Disasters, victimization, and children's mental health. *Child Development, 81*(4), 1040–1052. https://doi.org/10.1111/j.1467-8624.2010.01453.x
Catani, C., Jacob, N., Schauer, E., Kohila, M., & Neuner, F. (2008). Family violence, war, and natural disasters: A study of the effect of extreme stress on children's mental health in Sri Lanka. *BMC Psychiatry, 8*(1). https://doi.org/10.1186/1471-244x-8-33
Edmeade, J. N., & Buzinde, C. N. (2021). The role of educators in community resilience in natural disaster-prone communities. *Community Development Journal.* https://doi.org/10.1093/cdj/bsab010
Gerrard, B. A., Carter, M. J., & Ribera, D. (Eds.) (2019). *School-based family counseling: An interdisciplinary practitioner's guide.* Routledge.
Gkatsa, T. (Sep 2021). Mental health and behavior difficulties for children and adolescents, during the COVID-19 pandemic lockdown. *International Journal of Scientific Advances, (2).* https://doi.org/10.51542/ijscia.spi2.02Kar, N. (2009). Psychological impact of disasters on children: Review of assessment and interventions. *World Journal of Pediatrics, 5*(1), 5–11. https://doi.org/10.1007/s12519-009-0001-x
Leeb, R. T., Bitsko, R. H., Radhakrishnan, L., Martinez, P., Njai, R., & Holland, K. M. (2020). Mental health–related emergency department visits among children aged <18 Years during the COVID-19 pandemic — United

States, January 1–October 17, 2020. *Morbidity and Mortality Weekly Report, 69*, 1675–1680. http://dx.doi.org/10.15585/mmwr.mm6945a3

Marques de Miranda, D., da Silva Athanasio, B., Sena Oliveira, A. C., & Simoes-E-Silva, A. C. (2020). How is COVID-19 pandemic impacting mental health of children and adolescents? *International Journal of Disaster Risk Reduction, 51*, 101845. https://doi.org/10.1016/j.ijdrr.2020.101845

Senft, B., Liebhauser, A., Tremschnig, I., Ferijanz, E., & Wladika, W. (2022). Effects of the COVID-19 pandemic on children and adolescents from the perspective of teachers. *Frontiers in Education, 7.* https://doi.org/10.3389/feduc.2022.808015

2 Chronic disaster

A South African perspective

Nyna Amin

Overview

Disaster, in this book, is premised on the idea that it is a significant event that leads to wide-reaching death, destruction and devastation. Thus, the focus is on the emotional and psychological effects on survivors and the successful use of the SBFC model in educational settings for restorative intervention. In this chapter, however, I argue that the accepted definitions of disaster as natural or human-generated phenomena do not apply to situations where individuals are affected by a series of calamitous events over a very long period. In other words, disaster is chronic. Chronic disaster, as a notion, captures the persistent trauma of individuals whose childhoods, present existences and futures are ravaged by poverty and disadvantage. It is characterized by physical, socioeconomic, psychological and emotional trauma in disconcerting family structures – orphans living without adults, physical abuse, lack of safety, security, shelter and nutrition. The schools they attend provide minimal support – inadequate to ameliorate the material conditions of their lives. The chronically affected require intensive, extensive and prolonged intervention. In resource-constrained schools, however, the teachers are unqualified and ill-prepared to support adequately those suffering from the psychological effects of chronic disasters. Given these circumstances, an adapted SBFC approach is recommended.

Background: Conceptions of disasters

Disasters are characterized by sudden, unexpected natural events like avalanches, cyclones, droughts, earthquakes, floods, forest fires, hurricanes, mudslides and tsunamis. From a human perspective, these are cataclysmic events characteristic of the forces of nature. Disasters can also be human-generated, as exemplified by wars, civil conflicts and genocide. Both conceptions, natural and human, are conflated as "cultural" events (Dombrowsky, 1995). The conflation is understandable, seeing that it affects human (and animal and vegetal) existence in significant ways: damaging homes, interrupting services, ruining infrastructure and causing death, destruction, disruption and disturbance. Furthermore, they affect a community or many communities at the same time, and the destruction caused cannot be resolved or rebuilt by an individual.

DOI: 10.4324/9781003201977-3

However, there is a distinction from the abovementioned forms of disaster and that experienced by an individual who, for example, may have been injured in an automobile accident or diagnosed with a life-threatening condition. Nevertheless, long-term psychological trauma and psychic pain can occur, whether the disaster is natural, human or individual in essence. Disasters result in loss and grief, and therapeutic intervention is vital to rebuild affected individuals' shattered spirits. Educational institutions, which are important social hubs (Azada-Palacios, 2021), can be significant spaces where school-going survivors can share their experiences and receive psychological support.

Under the abovementioned conditions, the SBFC metamodel is an ideal intervention to assist students to cope with and improve their mental well-being. It is an invaluable multimodal attempt to buttress students' mental health and negate their fears and anxieties. Trained and experienced SBFC can quickly identify the causes of distress and work with school and family members to aid the recovery of those affected by disasters. However, the SBFC approach may need to be modified for some contexts, especially when the disaster is not an event but a chronic feature of life.

Chronic disaster: The case of South Africa

In 1994, democracy replaced apartheid as a political system in South Africa. One of apartheid's sociopolitical designs and consequences was the creation of two distinct societies: a wealthy, privileged class and a poor, underprivileged class. Since the inception of a democratic dispensation, the State has attempted to undo and eradicate the harmful policies based on race profiles, language spoken and skin color, albeit with limited success to date (Hino et al., 2018). Studies show that inequalities have widened in the post-apartheid era and become more deeply entrenched (Phaswana, 2021; Hiroyuki et al., 2018), as has psychological stress, which has not only proliferated but also become racialized (Harriman et al., 2021).

Materially, much has been accomplished in providing universal access to education, although quality education for all students is yet to be achieved (Kubow, 2018; Strassburg et al., 2010). There are two parallel public education systems in the country (Spaull, 2013): one system serves a prosperous group and the other serves a group of people living in poverty (Kubow, 2018; Spaull, 2013), mirroring the social stratifications which existed during apartheid.

Though not sanctioned by law, it is an unfortunate consequence of the State's inability to improve the conditions of impoverished schools. The South African bimodal education system means that there are doubly disadvantaged students: a combination of the policies of the past and their marginalization at present. Similarly, some schools are disadvantaged due to a lack of resources, large teacher-student ratios and poor educational leadership (Amnesty International, 2020).

The inequalities and inequities in education affect poor, unemployed families to a greater degree than middle- and upper-class families (Stats SA, 2020).

The Stats SA (2020) report reveals that most children in the country (70%) live with one parent only. Fathers are present in the lives of only 31.7% of children. An earlier study by Meintjes et al. (2009) identified 122,000 children living without adults (child-headed households). Furthermore, studies indicate that parent involvement in school is erratic, with a low response by parents summoned by school personnel (Segoe & Bisschoff, 2019; Michael et al., 2012). Some factors that explain the lack of parent participation include employment complications (Harris & Goodall, 2008), student underachievement (Ingram et al., 2007), feeling unwanted (Crozier, 1999) and unconventional family configurations (Amin, 2020).

Complicating matters further, teachers, employed in schools most affected by inequities and inequalities, are more likely to be underqualified and inadequately knowledgeable about curriculum content and pedagogical approaches (De Wet, 2016). They also work in overcrowded rooms with many students and a dearth of teaching and human resources (Amnesty International, 2020). In practice, it means that in their classrooms, teachers have a large cohort of students who are "multidimensionally poor" (Stats SA, 2020).

The multidimensionally poor are malnourished, victims of physical and emotional abuse, living in unsafe environments without adult support or supervision, drug and substance abusers, engaging in petty criminal behavior, and lack clean water, electricity and ablution facilities. In these circumstances, overworked teachers employed in under-resourced schools experience work intensification brought on by multiple curriculum changes, large class sizes and emotional work due to the extent and intensity of trauma endured by students (Williamson & Myhill, 2008). Expecting teachers to provide emotional and psychological support creates an additional layer of burden that could lead to burnout (Bodenheimer & Shuster, 2020). In that respect, the SBFC model seems to offer a viable and relevant intervention for improving the mental health of both students and teachers. Several SBFC presuppositions need to be unpacked to understand the approach.

The first is that a family, however configured, is willing to cooperate with the school and the SBF counselor. The SBFC-involved parents want to improve their children's well-being and harmonize and strengthen the bonds between school and family. The family, school and SBFC are equal and willing partners, working in students' interests.

Second, teachers are willing and active partners in efforts to provide stability and psychosocial safety for students who are traumatized and have experienced a disaster.

Third, SBFC uses successful strategies for countering both the immediate and the long-term effects of a disaster, especially since time plays a vital role in reducing or eradicating emotional trauma. The longer the passage of time after the event, the more likely it is that the students' trauma will subside, and they will continue with their activities, roles and functions as the memory of the stressful event fades and support received is available when needed (Le Brocque et al., 2017).

However, when providing psychological support, deeper introspection is necessary in the following situations: families and teachers are unwilling or unable to engage in joint counseling ventures with schools; there are no SBFC counselors; most children in a school or classroom are experiencing trauma and where human resources (counselors) are non-existent.

Given the many complications and complexities outlined in this section, rethinking the notion of disaster and modifying the SBFC approach are vital.

Chronic disaster

The established conceptions of disaster cannot account for all situations. For instance, in South Africa, for some children, disaster is not an event; it is a series of events or a prolonged event accompanied by hardship and trauma. Imagine situations like:

A   *A child is born to an unmarried couple. The mother is abandoned by the father and the baby has to be brought up by a young, single, unemployed individual living in an informal settlement (a makeshift home that is vulnerable to damage and danger). Without a regular income, they survive on an inadequate grant from the State. The baby faces an uncertain future as a child and adult due to deprivation, disadvantage, hunger and inadequate shelter (amongst other deprivations and desires). Due to her dire situation, the mother is unable to pay attention to the child's education needs. Every day is a struggle for survival.*

B   *Annie is a young girl who has been living in a family structure headed by a matriarch, her grandmother, who makes all the decisions in the household. The matriarch supports and actively encourages the use of violence on Annie, the siblings and mother. Annie does not share her home experiences with her teachers. She survives the regular physical assaults, and when an adult, Annie gets involved with a violent, toxic male and violence is again a prominent feature of her life.*

C   *Kanye is 14 years old. His parents are deceased. He lives in a makeshift home with his eight-year-old brother and six-year-old sister. There is no income and they survive on food they receive at school and from neighbors. The future is bleak. He drops out of school to take on menial work and begs on street corners to support his siblings. Mafia-type gangs run the streets and a portion of the begged earnings, sometimes all, are given to the gangs as payment for "protection".*

D   *Dolly is 16 years old and is regularly beaten and coerced to find work. During weekends and some weeknights, she works as a prostitute, which is the only employment available. Her mother collects and controls the money earned from the sex work she is forced to engage in. Her work results in three pregnancies by the time she is 20 years old and she turns to drug use to deal with the situation. To keep the family alive, she continues with sex work and endures the imminent dangers. As they grow, the children are neglected, exposed to danger and attend school intermittently.*

In each case, life is complicated and tough and the material conditions are severe. There seems to be no escape from hardship and trauma. Staying alive means having to negotiate one's life using risky survival strategies.

Since the lives of chronic disaster victims are unsafe, unhealthy and unusual, they are reluctant to share their home experiences with others, particularly teachers (see, e.g., Amin & Vithal, 2015). The intensity of the psychological damage of chronic disaster may surpass that experienced by communities of a natural or human disaster. For instance, after the occurrence of a natural or human disaster, there is a period of recovery and reconstruction. Even though the effects may be long-term, the damage is visible and known to others, and there are opportunities for collective grieving. The State also gets involved in reconstruction efforts. In the case of chronic disaster, there may be signs of suffering, but few persons, especially teachers, may know the actual circumstances of the affected persons' lives. There is no time for recovery and reconstruction due to the repetitive nature of the chronic disaster. However, there could be long-term pain, shame, embarrassment, psychological scarring, social isolation and more, which, probably, are borne alone by the victim. Teachers may be unaware of the chronic character of disaster that stalks students' lives in their classes as there is no visible or witnessed event (like a natural or human-caused disaster). As each chronic disaster case is different, they may not even be aware of such a situation if the symptoms and signs of suffering are hidden. More likely, because of large numbers of chronic disaster cases in a school, prioritizing teaching offers teachers a way to cope in "untenable situations and contexts where social, economic and emotional traumas are so intricately bound together" (Amin & Vithal, 2015, p. 6). As a result, even though poor, under-resourced schools may want to help, they face resource constraints and the absence of parental involvement.

A way to understand the notion of disaster as a chronic condition is to draw parallels to a water organism: the hydra, a small sea creature studied for centuries because of its unique ability to resist aging (Chapman et al., 2010). Made up of a head, column and foot, its most fascinating and vital characteristic is its ability to regenerate the head and foot and survive for many years (Bode, 2003).

In some ways, chronic disasters are like a hydra: they continue to torment individuals long after reaching adulthood, regenerating at each stage of life, compounded by poverty, insufficiency, underprivilege and marginalization. For many students, life is a disaster, activated by the geography of birth in the ecology of poverty, which resists dissipation over time. Trapped in a circuit of poverty without redemptive measures, chronic disaster and its consequences become an endemic feature of their lives.

Chronic disaster challenges and solutions for the SBFC approach

The four life situations described above reveal the challenges of deploying the SBFC strategy. The SBFC approach depends on a partnership comprising SBFC counselors, schools and families.

The first challenge is the absence of an SBFC system. Over the past two decades, the South African government's priority has been to ensure that every child receives quality education with district-based support for schools to implement inclusive education and eradicate learning barriers (Department of Basic Education, 2010). However, district-based support is insufficient and inefficient due to inadequate human resources (Engelbrecht et al., 2016; Makhalemele & Nel, 2016). The district structures are unlikely to provide sustained psychological assistance to schools, teachers, parents and students.

A second challenge is erratic or non-involvement in school activities by parents. Chronic disaster victims' school attendance is irregular and parents are absent or uncooperative. It implies that one sector of the school-parent-child triad is missing which can compromise the success of SBFC.

The third challenge is school involvement in an SBFC approach, as teachers are overwhelmed by work demands. Furthermore, the issues connected to chronic disaster are psychological and emotional distress combined with economic and financial hardships beyond the support capacities of impoverished schools. Chronic disaster cases may require prolonged intervention that will need to continue beyond the years of schooling.

It seems that in the abovementioned situations, state intervention is necessary, comprising primary health care, welfare/child grants, removal from families and placement of children in other families. Long-term psychological counseling may be necessary. Schools with many chronic disaster victims need more human and material resources than is available at present. If the traditional SBFC approach is applied to chronic disaster victims currently, it would encounter limitations (information, time, resources, cooperation) for successful implementation. So, what can be done, knowing that known solutions at present are impractical? Rethinking family and modifying the SBFC approach may offer viable solutions.

Supporting chronic disaster victims – strategic modifications

Some modifications are necessary for addressing the challenges an SBFC approach may encounter to support chronic disaster victims. The first is to acknowledge that though teachers may be untrained as SBFC practitioners, they can, nevertheless, offer SBFC support (see e.g. Chapter 7 in this book: How to Lower Stress and Strengthen Student Executive Functions During Crisis and Disasters by Korzeniowski). Teachers are vital components of school-based intervention strategies. The second is to imagine the classroom as a family unit so that victims who live without adults or whose family situations are toxic can experience a sense of belonging. It is a crucial step as many chronic disaster cases have complex and unusual family arrangements. They may not even have experienced a positive family life or experienced positive interactions with family members. The classroom family, in this instance, is not about blood connections. Instead, it is a social connection in which an entire classroom of students is treated as if they belong together as a unit with shared values, needs and strengths. It may require additional organization for the class teacher to create a conducive environment where each child is connected to others, with the teacher enacting a parent role.

Each day, even for ten minutes, time could be spent greeting each other, wishing each other a good day and singing a song of joy/resilience/survival together. To counteract alienation and sadness, the daily ritual, over time, creates a sense of belonging and attachment (Joerdens, 2014; Levine, 2011). It means that teachers do not have to identify each child's trauma or attempt counseling when they are not trained. Treating the entire class of students as a family makes it a doable, time-saving intervention.

The third is to share folk tales and stories at the school assembly weekly. The stories should be culturally relevant, inspirational and interesting to the children. Stories are essential therapeutic tools, but as they are time-consuming (Tin et al., 2013), short stories are recommended. Telling stories to a large group of students with teachers taking turns to narrate them makes it less labor-intensive and, more importantly, does not come across as therapy. Community leaders can also be invited regularly to share stories. Research shows that constant interaction with community members can improve awareness of issues that victims of chronic disasters face and ways to resolve them (West-Olatunji et al., 2011).

In situations of chronic disaster, the options are limited and group intervention, which has limited success, may be the only way for both teachers and victims to navigate lives of hardship, psychological trauma, emotional pain and deprivation.

Conclusion

Whether disaster is natural, human or chronic, the victims suffer trauma that will require therapeutic intervention, support and empathy. In schools, parents', teachers' and professionals' involvement is vital, and in ideal contexts, SBFC approaches are effective and successful.

In contrast, in some school contexts in South Africa, chronic disaster is an unfortunate circumstance that some individuals have to negotiate and live through. It is characterized by poverty, trauma, hardship, alienation and marginalization. It is a situation that no individual should face but it is a reality for many young victims. Some schools are severely constrained by a short supply of professionally trained personnel to assist the victims of on-going physical, psychological and emotional trauma. Alternative, group-based interventions are the only possibilities available in these circumstances. Though group-based effectiveness is limited for chronic disaster cases, they are better than no intervention.

Resources

10 most inspirational short stories I've heard. Available at https://wealthygorilla. com/10-most-inspirational-short-stories/
These are very short stories that can be read at the school assembly. Each has a moral message that inspires creative thinking, resilience, insight about life's challenges and also when being helpful has the opposite effect.

The hugging tree: A story about resilience by Jill Neimark and illustrated by Nicole Wong.

A beautifully illustrated tale of a tree that survives challenges and thrives until it can provide shelter for others. Appropriate skills to cope with life's challenges are embedded in the story. Suitable for preschoolers and early grades students.

Theron, L., Cockcroft, K., & Wood, L. (2017). The resilience-enabling value of African folktales: The read-me-to-resilience intervention. *School Psychology International, 38*(5), 491–506. Available at https://doi.org/10.1177/0143034317719941

This article provides insights about the value of African stories that enable resilience.

Songs of joy

Happy by Pharrell Williams

Jerusalema By master KG - Https://www.youtube.com/watch?v=fCZVL_8D048Mawujabulile (If you happy and you know it) in isiZulu Https://www.youtube.com/watch?v=s153a85F3Xo

References

Amin, N. (2020). Teachers' perspectives of the parent involvement hexis in under-resourced urban schools. In G. van Schalkwyk & N. Toren (Eds.). *Parental involvement: Practices, improvement strategies and challenges* (pp. 143–170). Nova Science Publishers.

Amin, N. & Vithal, R. (2015). Teacher knowing or not knowing about students. *South African Journal of Education, 35*(3), 1–9. Doi.10.15700/saje.v35n3a1078

Amnesty International. (2020). *Broken and unequal: The state of education in South Africa*. Amnesty International Inc.

Azada-Palacios, R. (2021). Schools as social spaces: Towards an Arendtian consideration of multicultural education. *Journal of Philosophy of Education, 55*(4–5), 564–576.

Bode, H.R. (2003). Head generation in hydra. *Developmental Dynamics, 226*(2), 225–236. Doi.10.1002/dvdy.10225

Bodenheimer, G., & Shuster, S.M. (2020). Emotional labour, teaching and burnout: Investigating complex relationships. *Educational Research, 62*(1), 63–76. Doi: 10.1080/00131881.2019.1705868

Chapman, J., Kirkness, E., Simakov, O., Hampson, S.E., Mitros, T., Weinmaier, T., Rattei, T., Balasubramanian, P.G., Borman, J., Busam, D., & Disbennett, K. (2010). The dynamic genome of hydra. *Nature, 464*(7288), 592–596. Doi.10.1038/nature08830

Crozier, G. (1999). Is it a case of 'We know when we're not wanted'? The parents' perspective on parent-teacher roles and relationships. *Educational Research, 41*(3), 315–328.

De Wet, C. (2016). The status of teaching as a profession in South Africa. *Proceedings of the Bulgarian Comparative Education Society, 14*(1), 143–149. Paper presented at the Annual International Conference of the Bulgarian Comparative Education Society (June 14–17, 2016).

Department of Basic Education. (2010). *Guidelines for full service/inclusive schools*. Government Printer.

Dombrowsky, W.R. (1995). Again and again: Is a disaster what we call a 'disaster'? *International Journal of Mass Emergencies and Disasters, 13*(3), 241–254.

Engelbrecht, P., Nel, M., Smit, S., & van Deventer, M. (2016). The idealism of education policies and the realities in schools: The implementation of inclusive education in South Africa. *International Journal of Inclusive Education, 20*(5), 520–535. Doi:10.1080/13603116.2015.1095250

Harriman, N.W., Williams, D.R., Morgan, J.W., Sewpaul, R., Manyaapelo, T., Sifunda, S., Mabaso, M., Mbewu, A.D., & Reddy, S.P. (2021). Racial disparities in psychological distress in post-apartheid South Africa: Results from the SANHANES-1 survey. *Social Psychiatry and Psychiatric Epidemiology*, 1–15. Doi.10.1007/s00127-021-02175-w

Harris, A., & Goodall, J. (2008). Do parents know they matter? Engaging all parents in learning. *Educational Research, 50*(3), 277–289. Doi: 10.1080/00131880802309424

Hiroyuki, H., Leibbrandt, M., Machema, R., Shifa, M., & Soudien, C. (2018). *Identity, inequality and social contestation in the post-apartheid South Africa* [Working Paper 23]. Southern African Labour and Development Unit, Open SALDRU Publications Repository. http://www.opensaldru.uct.ac.za/handle/11090/946

Ingram, M., Wolfe, R.B., & Lieberman, J.M. (2007). The role of parents in high-achieving schools serving low-income, at-risk populations. *Education and Urban Society, 39*(4), 479–497.

Joerdens, S. H. (2014). 'Belonging means you can go in': Children's perspectives and experiences of membership of kindergarten. *Australasian Journal of Early Childhood, 39*(1), 12–21.

Kubow, P.K. (2018). Schooling inequality in South Africa: Productive capacities and the epistemological divide. In A.W. Wiseman (ed.). *Annual review of comparative and international education 2017. (International Perspectives on Education and Society, volume 34)* (pp. 161–185). Emerald Publishing Limited. Doi.10.1108/S1479-367920180000034016

Le Brocque, R., De Young, A., Montague, G., Pocock, S., March, S., Triggell, N., Rabaa, C., & Kenardy, J. (2017). Schools and natural disaster recovery: The unique and vital role that teachers and education professionals play in ensuring mental health of students following natural disasters. *Journal of Psychologists and Counsellors in Schools, 27*(1), 1–23. Doi:10.1017/jgc.2016.17

Levine, D. (2011). *Building classroom communities: Strategies for developing a culture of caring*. Solution Tree Press.

Makhalemele, T., & Nel, M. (2016). Challenges experienced by district-based support teams in the execution of their functions in a specific South African province. *International Journal of Inclusive Education, 20*(2), 168–184. Doi:10.1080/13603116.2015.1079270

Meintjes, H., Hall, K., Marera, D., & Boulle, A. (2009). *Child-headed households in South Africa: A statistical brief.* Children's Institute, University of Cape Town.

Michael, S., Wolhuter, C.C., & van Wyk, N. (2012). The management of parental involvement in multicultural schools in South Africa: A case study. *CEPS Journal, 2*(1), 57–82.

Phaswana E.D. (2021). Women, gender, and race in post-apartheid South Africa. In O. Yacob-Haliso & T. Falola (Eds.). *The Palgrave handbook of African women's studies* (pp. 197–215). Palgrave Macmillan, Cham. Doi. 10.1007/978-3-030-28099-4_141

Segoe, B.A., & Bisschoff, T. (2019). Parental involvement as part of curriculum reform in South African schools: Does it contribute to quality education? *Africa Education Review, 16*(6), 165–182.

Spaull, N. (2013). Poverty & privilege: Primary school inequality in South Africa. *International Journal of Educational Development, 33*(5), 436–447.

Strassburg, S., Meny-Gibert, S., & Russell, B. (2010). More than getting through the school gates: Barriers to participation in schooling, (Vol. 3). *Johannesburg: South Africa: Social Surveys Africa.*

Stats SA. (2020). *Education Series. Vol. 8: Children's well-being and education in South Africa.* 2018. Statistics South Africa.

Tin, H.W., Nonis, K.P., Lim, S.E.A., & Honig, A.S. (2013). Teachers' perceptions of the importance of stories in the lives of children in Myanmar. *Early Child Development and Care, 183*(10), 1449–1467.

West-Olatunji, C., Goodman, R.D., Mehta, S., & Templeton, S. (2011). Creating cultural competence: An outreach immersion experience in Southern Africa. *International Journal for the Advancement of Counselling, 33*(4), 335–346. Doi.10.1007/s10447-011-9138-0

Williamson, J., & Myhill, M. (2008). Under 'constant bombardment': Work intensification and the teachers' role. In D. Johnson & R. Maclean (Eds.). *Teaching: Professionalization, development and leadership.* Springer. Doi.10.1007/978-1-4020-8186-6_3

3 A positive deviance approach for overcoming crisis and disaster

Masamine Jimba, Maya Sophia Fujimura,
and Akira Shibanuma

Overview

Looking for outliers who succeed against all odds. This is the basic concept of positive deviance. Rather than focusing on the glass being half-empty, it makes the best use of the glass half-full in a person or a community. Successful cases of using positive deviance approach have been reported in the Netherlands, Singapore, and other countries within the schools. However, it is equally important to describe how it works in community settings during crisis and disaster, as school students are obliged to stay at shelters, camps, or more broadly in the communities. This chapter describes the steps to be taken for conducting a positive deviance approach by focusing on Community Intervention of the SBFC metamodel, by mobilizing children's positive deviant practices and available community resources. Two case studies from Israel and Uganda illustrate how suffering children are creative in solving their own problems, not as beneficiaries, but as real actors. The role of school teachers and parents in the community is to find positive deviance actors during crisis and disaster and share their practices within the community and beyond.

Background

Some schools succeed more than others though they face similar hardships. Some school-aged children perform better than their peers even if they live in limited-resource settings. These schools and children can be called positive deviants. These positive deviants can be found

> based on the observation that in every community there are certain individuals or groups whose uncommon behaviors and strategies enable them to find better solutions to problems than their peers, while having access to the same resources and facing similar or worse challenges.
>
> (https://positivedeviance.org/)

Schools have been a good place for using a positive deviance approach in many countries. In the Netherlands, for example, a unique case study was conducted among students aged 12–16 who attend VMBO schools (preparatory

DOI: 10.4324/9781003201977-4

vocational training schools). About 22% of roughly 1 million students attend VMBO schools and most of them are migrants and/or have a lower socio-economic background. The research team used a positive deviance approach among VMBO schools in Rotterdam and the Strengths and Difficulties Questionnaire (SDQ) score was used to identify three positive deviant schools and ten positive deviant behaviors in these schools. For example, the schools contacted parents by telephone when the students achieved positive results and grades. The school administration also sent out personalized birthday cards and celebratory cards to all students via post to congratulate them (Bouman et al., 2014).

In Singapore, another positive deviance approach was taken to understand the reason "why some children from poor families do well." They identified ten positive deviant children aged 10–13 from low-income families, whose overall academic performance was at the 70th percentile or greater. As a result, they found that the "children's awareness of their family circumstances motivated them to work hard and enabled them to devise creative ways to manage their limited financial resources" (Cheang & Goh, 2019). At a global level, UNICEF's "Data Must Speak" project has investigated how the positive deviance approach could be applied in lower performing schools in fourteen countries in Asia, Africa and South America. These school-based activities can fit into the School Prevention quadrant in the SBFC metamodel (Gerrard et al., 2020, pp. 9–12). However, in crisis and disaster, schools are often closed as it was in the case for COVID-19, and school-aged children are obliged to stay at home, shelters, and refugee or internally displaced people (IDP)'s camps. Even under such circumstances, a positive deviant approach can be taken. This chapter focuses on Community Intervention of the SBFC meta-model, which refers to interventions aimed at bringing solutions that advocate particularly for school-aged children through the mobilization of children's positive deviant behaviors and available community resources.

Procedure

Prerequisite for the positive deviance approach

During the Great East Japan Earthquake in 2011, a positive deviant approach was taken in Kesennuma, Miyagi prefecture. Due to the earthquake and tsunami, school children and their families had to remain in an evacuation shelter for more than three months. One week after the disaster, seven-year-old Lisa Yoshida issued an original newspaper on the bulletin board at the shelter, called *FIGHT Shimbun newspaper*. She was only in the second grade at a local primary school but Lisa found that the adults were discouraged and she was motivated to cheer everybody up at the shelter. Satoko and her 11 friends reported only positive news each day, resulting in nearly 50 editions of *FIGHT Shimbun newspaper* over three months. Satoko said adults were "now living in unfavorable circumstances but let's fight for future! We will do our best" (Fight Shimbun Sha, 2011). Although she and her team were not familiar with the concept of positive deviance, they demonstrated being the epitome of positive deviants during crisis.

Despite their admirable action, the whole process as a positive deviance approach had not been well documented. Therefore, in this chapter, two well-documented cases are provided to illustrate the process of this approach in crisis and disaster. The general process of taking a positive deviance approach is similar to that in non-crisis and non-disaster situations. The task is to find uncommon and successful practices that have already been exercised among people in a community and can be adopted at a low cost.

In a community, whether it may be at an evacuation shelter or an IDP camp, it is the school-aged children, their family members, and teachers who play a central role in conducting the positive deviance approach. Positive deviants are not necessarily people who are known to be skillful, knowledgeable, economically successful, or politically influential in the community. Rather, they can be found at the periphery of the community.

Steps in the positive deviance approach

Various steps have been proposed for this approach. Most commonly, the following steps are taken: (1) identify a problem and outcome, (2) conduct positive deviance inquiry, and (3) develop and disseminate solutions. This section introduces tasks required at each step. However, the steps are not a fixed template applied to every problem but rather steps which can be modified flexibly and at an ad hoc basis to reflect participants' intentions (Table 3.1).

The general description of the three steps is as follows:

Step 1: Identify a problem and outcome

Step 1 analyzes the problems in the community. In this step, the team discusses what problems they must address and what are the desired outcomes that are expected to solve this. In this approach, experts and community leaders are often the ones to recognize the problem in the community, while people of

Table 3.1 Steps in the positive deviance approach

Steps	Tasks[a]
Step 1: Identify a problem and outcome	1. Define the problem and desired outcome
	2. Determine common practices
Step 2: Conduct positive deviance inquiry	3. Discover uncommon but successful behaviors and strategies through inquiry and observation
Step 3: Developing and disseminating solutions	4. Design an action learning initiative based on findings
	5. Monitor and evaluate

[a]Pascale et al. (2010, p. 202). Monitor and evaluate was later added on the website.

the community are the ones to discuss ways to identify the root causes. It is essential during this step for the team to reach an agreement on the potential of the positive deviance approach to solve the problems which are identified.

When in-depth data are available to the team, it is recommended to examine whether the data contains sufficient information to analyze the problems and desired outcomes. Specifically, data should be used to identify who lives under difficult circumstances, suffers from the problem, and exhibits favorable outcomes despite the obstacles.

Step 2: Positive deviance inquiry

Step 2 involves the team screening residents who demonstrate the desired outcome despite the common problems faced in the community. Community members should be a part of the research team because it provides an advantage to help navigate the whereabouts of the target population. The team will then visit these selected groups of people, communicate their objectives, and observe their daily lives.

Step 3: Solution building and dissemination

The team discusses the identified successful practices and ways to design them as a sustainable solution for the rest of the community to implement. As the practices may not be immediately adopted by others, Step 3 calls for the team to design solutions and consider ways which non-positive deviants can easily exercise and adopt the behaviors. The positive deviants themselves can contribute to building solutions and disseminating the knowledge. They become key persons to spreading insight on how they adapted the behaviors and it leads to achieving successful outcomes for the rest of their community.

Two cases of the positive deviance approach

In this section, two positive deviant cases are shown: one in Israel, another in Uganda.

Case 1: Childhood injury prevention in Israel

The first case of positive deviance is childhood injury prevention in Israel. It targeted the Arab Bedouin population living in Negav, the Southern District of Israel. The Arab Bedouin population is among IDPs in Israel (Boqa'i, 2008). Under the Israeli government, they abandoned their traditional nomadic lifestyles. In the 1950s, approximately 110,000 Bedouins had to settle in the designated zones in Nagav (Boqa'i, 2008). According to the Israel government's report in 2013, about 120,000 people were settled in the regulated, planned settlements, while 90,000 people lived in unrecognized zones (Israeli Mission Around the World. The Bedouin in Israel). Particularly, in unregulated zones, land ownership is restricted and housing without the government's regulation is prevalent. Reflecting unstable living conditions, the Arab Bedouin population lived in low levels of socioeconomic conditions, housing, and community infrastructure (Gesser-Edelsburg et al., 2021).

Box 3.1 Childhood injury prevention in Israel (Gesser-Edelsburg et al., 2021)

Step 1: Identify a problem and outcome

Theater-based performing arts were used to present stories about unintended accidents to participants, both adults and children in the Arab Bedouin community. Through the arts, they could learn vicariously about unintended child injuries and understand the ways of preventing these injuries. Participants not only listened to stories about injuries but they had also reenacted the scenarios themselves.

Step 2: Positive deviance inquiry

In this step, the participants proposed the following practices: socially involving community members, suggesting reminders for parents by using checklists and cell phones, establishing visual boundaries for play areas, and providing tips to prevent children from being run over by vehicles and being left unattended inside cars. For children, performing arts were used instead of observing practices of the positive deviants. After experiencing child injury cases through acting in a scene, participants were asked to modify the scenarios to prevent similar injuries. Children were also asked to draw pictures regarding safe and secure places to play. Through eliciting this positive deviance practice, some children drew pictures of mosques as a place where they considered safe and secure. This surprised the adults as mosques were only used for the place of worship and events for men, not typically a place for children to visit.

Step 3: Solution building and dissemination

Finally, a social-network map was drawn to visualize the connections among people in the community, including positive and non-positive deviants. This map was used to disseminate positive deviant practices. A video was then created in which children explained how they lacked a safe place to play and requested the leaders to arrange an environment for them. It was widely disseminated to people in the community. After recognizing that some children felt mosques were a safe place, the team worked with religious leaders to set up a playroom inside the building. This initial idea brought forth by children was adapted into a viable solution.

Unintentional injuries refer to motor vehicle accidents, accidental falls, accidental poisoning and drowning, and suffocation. Almost all of them are preventable but were prevalent among children and adolescents of this population. Among Arab Bedouin parents with low socioeconomic status, home injuries tended to be believed as a matter of fate and not preventable (Gesser-Edelsburg et al., 2021). To overcome this situation, Beterem Safe Kids Israel, an organization involved in child safety issues, implemented a unique community-based program in Negav. They combined the positive deviance approach with community-based participatory research and entertainment education. Beyond school prevention activities, parents and children from the Arab Bedouin community participated in this Community Intervention program together with the local figures and religious leaders.

Case 2: Former girl soldiers in Uganda

The second positive deviance case is about former girl soldiers living in Northern Uganda. In Uganda, many girls and boys had been abducted by the Lord's Resistance Army (LRA) during the late 1980s. It is estimated that LRA abducted 54,000–75,000 people between 1986 and 2006, including 25,000–38,000 children (Pham et al., 2008). Girls tended to be abducted for a longer period compared to boys and girls were forced to be sexual partners and domestic workers for LRA commanders during their abduction.

According to a survey conducted among former girl soldiers, 90% had experienced being tortured, 56% were sexually abused, and 41% committed crimes such as killing (Vindevogel et al., 2011). They were often forced to attack the community where they were raised, including their own family members. Therefore, even after escaping from LRA, girls were not always welcomed back by family members and people of their community (Allen et al., 2020). In the IDP camps, girls were often isolated and experienced difficulty sustaining their livelihood, especially ones who were raising small children.

In 2007 and 2008, Save the Children and the Ork Foundation in Geneva started a pilot project for empowering former girl soldiers. Save the Children supported those who returned to an IDP camp in Pader District of Northern Uganda to integrate back into their original community.

Box 3.2 Former girls soldiers in Uganda (Singhal & Dura, 2009, Pascale et al., 2010)

Step 1: Identify a problem and outcome

Approximately 1,000 child mothers and 7,500 vulnerable girls were potential project participants in the target area. In this positive deviance project, 500 young mothers, vulnerable girls survivors, and 50 adult mentors were targeted. Of 500 girls, 40% were formerly abducted child mothers, 50% were vulnerable mothers having one or more early pregnancies, and 10% were heads of households. Discussions were conducted among a group of former girl soldiers, together with other family members and camp officials. It was revealed that unwanted pregnancies were one of the true obstacles which prevented them from being integrated back into the community.

Step 2: Positive deviance inquiry

A team of peer educators, mentors, sub-county representatives, and NGO staff facilitated a community process to identify positive deviant girls (called PD girls). They identified the following three PD practices among PD girls: (1) work harder, smarter, and together; (2) respect oneself and others; (3) display business acumen, save, invest, and learn. For example, a 16-year-old old PD girl said:

> With the small money I received from Save the Children, I hired a sewing machine. Now I'm reparing and selling second-hand clothes. I have made some sales and I have the money in my pocket. I have three sacks of maize saved from my garden, and I also have another garden in which I grow eggplant and other vegetables. I have hired a boy who helps sell in the market when I'm not there.
> (Singhal & Dura et al., 2008, p. 2)

Step 3: Solution building and dissemination

After identifying the positive deviants, the team implemented a training program for peer educators among PD girls. They worked as mentors to educate and empower other girls who also experienced isolation. The training strengthened coping mechanisms to reduce transactional sex and enhance the reintegration of girls into the community. The team also implemented a business skill training for girls, including how to conduct income generation activities as a group. The solutions were designed to involve people in the community and focus on the girls' coping skills, not simply by addressing the reduction of unwanted pregnancies and the improvement in girls' livelihood.

The positive deviance approach highlighted issues beyond the capacity of the former girl soldiers to solve on their own. In other words, targeting an intervention only for girls to improve their livelihood might not solve the structural issue behind unwanted pregnancies. The team agreed that the new desired outcome could be achieved by behavior changes, not only among former girl soldiers but also among the other people in the community. This approach was therefore used as a means of involving people, stimulating conversations, and motivating them for behavior changes.

Multicultural considerations

As of April 2022, the positive deviance approach has a history of more than 30 years, is widespread across 65 countries, and has impacted more than 30 million people. The process of identifying positive deviant practices has been well described but a special cultural consideration is necessary when it comes to expansion.

In anthropology, the term "scaling across" is preferred rather than "scaling up," which is relevant to the positive deviance approach. Scaling up means exporting something like a vaccine from one place to another as it is, despite the differences in culture between the two places. It is acceptable for vaccines but not always true for some human behaviors and practices.

> Scaling across puts an emphasis on a constantly moving set of targets and circumstances that requires sustained adaptability. The success here is in adaptability and flexibility for expansion, rather than fidelity to a normative structure (where it is with global policies or RCT designs).
>
> (Adams et al., 2015)

Positive deviance experts Jerry and Monique Sternin also have one view about scalability.

> PD may be less effective on scale if we talk about geographic scaling (from a village community, to a district, to a region), but scaling may also mean influencing policy, or promoting the emergence of new leadership, unleashing new social networks, or building community capacity...So, PD approach...is scalable in a different way than geographical scaling.
>
> (Singhal & Dura, 2009, p. 74)

That is why an "approach" is used for positive deviance instead of a "model." In the first positive deviance approach case in Vietnam, the process of self-discovery was replicated in new villages at the time of expansion after identifying three common practices for improving undernutrition of children, not modeling of three practices identified in the first villages. This process was later called "Living University." Cultural appropriateness is highly valued in this approach, as it was also shown in the case of Israel and Uganda.

Challenges and solutions

Although the positive deviance approach can make a difference in schools and communities, it faces several challenges. First, it may not be suitable for a problem that can be solved by advanced science and technology input, such as a highly efficacious immunization program at the population level for an infectious disease. The positive deviance approach is expected to work where the problem is intertwined in a complex social system, and where behavior and social changes are required to solve the problem.

Second, the positive deviance approach is often time-consuming and labor-intensive because it needs in-depth observations and direct interactions with people in the community. Once the positive deviants are identified, it relies on the community to scale across their practices. Because of this, positive deviance studies are often conducted on small scales, limiting the generalizability of the identified positive deviant practices (Marsh et al., 2004).

Although Jerry and Monique Sternin have shown insightful views about scalability as mentioned above, a larger-scale approach, such as "big data-based positive deviance," has been proposed. It is defined as "a problem-solving asset-based approach that uses big data sources to identify objects (positive deviants) performing unexpectedly well in a specific outcome measure that is digitally recorded, mediated or observed" (Albanna & Heeks, 2019). In the big data-based positive deviance approach, the positive deviants are considered as "individuals, communities, entities, areas, or countries whose uncommon behaviors and strategies, in a specific context, can be translated into a performance measure that is digitally recorded, mediated or observed" (Albanna & Heeks, 2019). Although a big data-based approach cannot solve all the challenges of a positive deviance approach, it can reduce time, labor, and cost. It enables the positive deviance approach to be utilized in fields other than public health, such as agriculture, education, and urban planning (Albanna & Heeks, 2019).

Finally, obstacles usually do not come from the community members but from the outside experts trying to help solve the problem (Pascale et al., 2010). In Uganda's case, experts of NGOs initially identified a problem (former girl soldiers and their lack of reintegration), their expected outcome from their own perspectives (developing life skills for livelihood), and defined the positive deviants (those who were successful with reintegration through work). However, these practices imposed by the experts were not adopted by other former girl soldiers. Those who are experts in their own specific field are supposed to know what to do or know what are the problems. However, it does not always mean that they also know "how to do" and can solve the problems in different contexts in a sustainable way. The people in the community rather know "how to do" much better.

Conclusion

Paska Aber, the project coordinator of the Uganda's positive deviance project, once mentioned about her experience:

> PD questions the assumption that beneficiaries are helpless...that they know nothing and can do nothing without outside help. My experience in northen Uganda tells me that the beneficiaries are the real actors. They drive the PD wagon. At best, Save the Children staff members help them to access some fuel.
>
> (Singhal & Dura, 2009, p. 62)

During crisis and disaster, the beneficiaries often cannot know when and where they will receive "the support." It is the empowered community people who can take action first. It can be a seven-year-old school child in times of when the adults are in distress as it was shown in Japan. The role of school teachers and parents in the community can be to find such positive deviants in children or they themselves behave as positive deviants who have "glass-half-full energy, even under such critical situations." Nevertheless, this will "help them (and themselves) to access some fuel" and scale across the positive deviant practices within the community and beyond.

Resources

Bedouin Society in the Negev PD Project https://positivedeviance.org/case-studies-all/2021/1/25/bedouin-society-in-the-negev-pd-project
This site shows a video with activities of the "Bedouin Society in the Negev PD Project."
Pascale R., Sternin, J., & Sternin, M. (2010). The power of positive deviance: *how unlikely innovators solve the world's toughest problems.* Harvard Business Review Press.
This is the Bible of the positive deviance approach. A book review is available in the following site. https://positivedeviance.org/the-power-of-positive-deviance
Positive deviance collaborative https://positivedeviance.org/
This is the headquarter website of the positive deviance approach. Starting with a 3-minute video "what is positive deviance," there are many positive deviance resources.
UNICEF: Data Must Speak https://www.unicef-irc.org/research/data-must-speak/
This website introduces UNICEF's positive deviance project in schools in 14 countries. A short video and 5 stage model are shown on this website.

References

Adams, V., Craig, S.R., & Samen, A. (2016). Alternative accounting in maternal and infant global health. *Global Public Health*, 11(3), 276–294.

Albanna, B., & Heeks, R. (2019). Positive deviance, big data, and development: A systematic literature review. *Electronic Journal of Information Systems in Developing Countries*, 85(1), 1–22.

Allen, T., Atingo, J., Atim, D., Ocitti, J., Brown, C., Torre, C., Fergus, C.A., & Parke, r M. (2020) What happened to children who returned from the Lord's Resistance Army in Uganda? *Journal of Refugee Studies*, 33(4), 663–666.

Boqa'i, N. (2008). Palestinian internally displaced persons inside Israel: Challenging the solid structures. *Palestine-Israel Journal of Politics, Economics, and Culture*, 15(4/1), 31.

Bouman, M., Lubjuhn S., & Singhal A. (2014). What explains enhanced psychological resilience of students at VMBO schools in the Netherlands? The positive deviance approach in action. Center for Media &Health, Gouda, the Netherlands. http://www.media-gezondheid.nl/beheer/data/cmg.desh26.nl/uploads/Publicaties_en_downloads/PD_Approach_the_Netherlands_CMH_040914_fin.pdf

Cheang, C.J.Y., & Goh, E.C.L.(2019). Why some children from poor families do well - an in-depth analysis of positive deviance cases in Singapore. *International Journal of Qualitative Studies on Health and Well-being*, 13(supl), 156343.

Fight Shimbun Sha. (2011). Miyagi Kesennnuma Hatsu! Fight Shimbun. Kawade Shobo Shinsha. (In Japanese)

Gerrard, B.A., Carter, M.J., & Ribera, D. (Eds.)(2020). *School-based family counseling: An interdisciplinary practitioner's guide.* Routledge.

Gesser-Edelsburg, A., Alamour, Y., Cohen, R., Abed Elhadi Shahbari, N., Hijazi, R., Orr, D., Vered-Chen, L., & Singhal, A. (2021) Creating safe spaces to prevent unintentional childhood injuries among the Bedouins in southern Israel: A hybrid model comprising positive deviance, community-based participatory research, and entertainment-education. *PLoS One,* 16(9), e0257696.

Israeli Mission Around the World. The Bedouin in Israel. https://embassies.gov.il/MFA/AboutIsrael/Spotlight/Pages/The-Bedouin-in-Israel.aspx (accessed April 27, 2022)

Marsh, D.R., Schroeder, D.G., Dearden, K.A., Sternin, J., & Sternin, M. (2004). The power of positive deviance. *British Medical Journal,* 329(7475), 1177–1179.

Pascale, R., Sternin, J., & Sternin, M. (2010). *The power of positive deviance: how unlikely innovators solve the world's toughest problems.* Boston, Harvard Business Review Press.

Pham, P.N., Vinck, P., & Stover, E. (2008) Abducted: Forced conscription and the Lord's Resistance Army in Northern Uganda. *Human Rights Quarterly,* 30, 404–411.

Singhal, A. & Dura, L. (2009). Protecting children from exploitation and trafficking: Using the positive deviance approach in Uganda and Indonesia. Part 4. Life after the LRA: Piloting positive deviance with child mothers and vulnerable girl survivors in Northern Uganda. Save the Children Federation.

Vindevogel S., Coppens K., Derluyn I., De Schryver M., Loots G., & Broekaert E. (2011) Forced conscription of children during armed conflict: experiences of former child soldiers in northern Uganda. *Child Abuse & Neglect,* 35(7), 551–562.

4 The leadership role of the school principal in times of disaster or crisis

Judith E. Giampaoli

Overview

This chapter offers a practical guide to the steps a school principal can take to assure the safety and security of students, staff and families in the event of a disaster. Particular emphasis is placed on preparedness in various forms: (a) creating a comprehensive Disaster Response Plan; (b) preparation of the school community; (c) support of the school community through outreach in response to a disaster and (d) facilitating ongoing mental health supports through a trauma-informed schools and School-Based Family Counseling (SBFC) approach. Examples of actual disaster responses are included.

Preparation-response-recovery

These three words define the major responsibilities of school principals when a disaster or crisis strikes. Emergencies not only disrupt learning but threaten the safety and well-being of students and staff at any school. In my many years of service in education, which has included various administrative roles (principal, assistant principal, program director and dean of students) in inner city schools, I have learned through experience the importance of drawing from a comprehensive plan in times of emergency.

It has been noted that, "Schools experience a wide variety of crises that have the potential to harm the learning environment, mental & physical health and safety of students and educators" (NEA School Crisis Guide, 2018, p. 1). There are natural disasters, such as an earthquake, a wildfire, a pandemic or a flood, that are occurring more frequently across the globe. In addition, there are human-caused crises such as acts of intentional violence, including bomb threats or shootings that can profoundly impact the sense of safety in a school community. There can also be crises more individualized to a particular school, such as the unexpected death of a student or staff member.

Principals play a pivotal role in helping the school community cope with disaster.

> A school's capacity to meet the confluence of needs and mitigate trauma reactions in the event of a crisis will almost always reflect the functionality

DOI: 10.4324/9781003201977-5

of the safety, crisis and mental health resources that were in place before the crises.

(Cowan & Rossen, 2013, p. 5)

Principals who champion school-wide mental health programs can deliver essential supportive services in times of crisis and throughout the school year. Including SBFC practitioners as part of the mental health team will support children and families as they reach out to members of the school community before, during and after a disaster. The principal who recognizes the value of an SBFC practitioner knows the value of the link between the family, community and student success, and recognizes the importance of addressing trauma and stress as fundamental to the preventive measures needed throughout the school year.

The principal must be prepared to lead in all instances. Principals will need to activate their mental readiness to lead by incorporating all of their resources, including their communicational, problem-solving and decision-making skills. They will need to build on the strength of their relationships within the school community to address the emergencies that arise, often without warning.

Preparation

Benjamin Franklin once said, "By failing to prepare, you are preparing to fail." Designing a Disaster Response Plan is the first of many tasks a principal must take to prepare the entire school community for an emergency. However, it must be noted that student stress and trauma exist in schools long before a disaster strikes. It exists throughout all grade levels. The harmful impact of toxic stress on developing nervous systems has been shown to profoundly impede student success. Addressing serious and ongoing stress and trauma in children in our schools can be achieved through the proactive leadership of the school principal in promoting a trauma-informed school environment that includes an environment of safety, connection and compassion. Students can't learn if they don't feel safe and supported in their schools.

The principal can facilitate the development of a comprehensive plan to create a trauma-sensitive school and allocate resources that aim to (1) **Promote** trusting and respectful relationships among students, staff and families; (2) **Provide** ongoing professional development and support for staff related to trauma-informed awareness and classroom practices; (3) **Identify** social-emotional learning programs to help students develop their communication, coping and self-regulation skills; and (4) **Engage** parents by providing learning opportunities related to stress and trauma and its impact on well-being. These efforts will go far in supporting students prior to any disaster that may occur.

Today, a principal doesn't question whether a disaster or crisis will occur but whether the school is prepared to respond. Crises arrive in a variety of intensities and duration. The NEA School Crisis Guide (www.nea.org) provides an excellent step-by-step process for developing a disaster/crisis plan for schools. An electronic version of this guide is available at nea.org/ crisisguide. I found this guide useful in developing the step-by-step plan listed below while also incorporating my own personal experience and suggestions as well.

It should be noted that a Disaster Response Plan may be known, depending on the school district, by various names such as Emergency Response Plan, School Safety Plan, Disaster Response Plan, Crisis Guide or other titles. For the sake of consistency throughout this chapter, I will use the term Disaster Response Plan. They are all similar in that their purpose is to provide schools with a process for managing crises as promptly and effectively as possible, and allowing schools to resume normal functioning.

Designing a Disaster Response Plan is the first of many tasks a principal must take to prepare the entire school community for an emergency. This is not done in isolation, but in partnership with the entire school community. Communication is a critical component of all phases of the development and implementation of the plan.

The following is a summary of steps principals can take to develop the plan. Keep in mind that all schools, while similar in their mission, are unique and, therefore, a Disaster Response Plan needs to meet the needs of your school.

1   Best practices indicate that a principal must **ORGANIZE** and lead a Disaster Response Team of six to eight highly motivated staff members whose skills allow them to serve in key positions during a school crisis. It would be useful to include the school secretary and security personnel as well as support staff such as an SBFC practitioner on the team.

2   It is recommended that the principal **LEAD** the Disaster Response Team. At least one assistant chairperson should be available to step in should the principal be absent.

3   The team should **DEVELOP** a detailed and comprehensive plan for possible disaster/crisis scenarios. The plan should address safety needs before, during and after an incident, in addition to planning for the worst-case scenarios. Also included are staff roles and responsibilities during emergencies and crises, building-specific procedures such as lockdowns and evacuations. **COLLABORATION** will aid in the development of a plan that addresses the unique needs of the school site.

4   Be certain that a complete copy of the Disaster Response Plan has been **DISTRIBUTED** to all faculty and staff, with the understanding that it be kept visible and accessible at all times. Allow time during professional development or faculty meetings to review and discuss procedures.

5   The principal's responsibility is to make certain that **TRAINING** of staff and students on procedures takes place. Everyone must understand their role in a crisis. The principal must ensure that everyone in the school community is familiar with the plan and that staff feel prepared to assume responsibility for the safety of their students.

6   The use of a **STANDARDIZED VOCABULARY** (I Love You Guys Foundation at iloveyouguys.org provides detailed information on Standard Response Protocol) to alert students and staff in an emergency situation allows all to understand the directions and follow the protocol. For example, when the principal announces, "Secure! Get inside. Lock outside doors," students are trained to return to the inside of the building. Adults bring everyone indoors for their safety, lock outside doors, account for students and adults and do their best to remain calm. **PRACTICE** emergency procedures outlined in the plan regularly. The goal is for staff and students to respond as quickly and somewhat automatically to a situation. Drills, such as fire or earthquake drills, are important as are lockdown drills and evacuation drills.

7   **COMMUNICATE** the plan to parents/guardians using presentations, letters/ emails and website newsletters/videos.

8   **REVIEW, REVISE AND IMPROVE** the plan regularly and as situations change. The Disaster Response Plan could be considered a living document that is regularly updated and should outline steps to minimize harm to people and property during any number of emergency situations.

9   **ORGANIZATION** is a key element of all plans. A **WELL-ORGANIZED PROCESS** to reunite children with their families in a timely and safe manner will help to reduce anxiety.

10 It must be said that a Disaster Response Plan alone will not ensure its successful implementation. Building an **ONGOING, TRUSTING RELATIONSHIP** with the school community is essential. Creating those channels of communication provides connection throughout the school year and enhances the principal's ability to lead when a crisis occurs.

It may seem an overwhelming task to complete this process and indeed it is quite challenging. However, as Nelson Mandela once said, "It always seems impossible until it's done." The time and effort devoted to completing the entire process are well worth it and will be invaluable to the safety and security of the school.

Response

Natural Disasters: Earthquakes, Wildfires, Floods, Hurricanes, Tornadoes: Natural disasters, such as earthquakes, wildfires or floods, often require an emergency response from the community-first responders, and are coordinated on a large, all-encompassing scale. When this occurs, principals are required to take direction from school district offices or community response teams. However, the school principal is still responsible for communication with stakeholders, updating them on information specific to their school. In addition, they will need to coordinate with staff and make every effort to normalize school life upon re-opening (i.e., preparing the building, reestablishing the school program and activities for the day when students and staff return to school).

Example: Earthquake

An earthquake struck the San Francisco Bay Area many years ago, devastating large swaths of neighborhoods-collapsed structures, fires, broken water mains and, sadly, injuries and death – a true disaster. One of San Francisco's middle schools was in the heart of the destruction; however, it remained intact. The earthquake struck a little after 5 P.M. and school had ended for the day. No students were present and few teachers were still in the building. The principal, who had just arrived home, was contacted by the Superintendent of Schools and returned to the school site immediately. It was known that the school was designated as a shelter in the event of a catastrophe. By the time the principal returned, City Emergency Response personnel and The Red Cross had assumed command of the school building as an Emergency Evacuation Center, Short Term Emergency Shelter and Feeding Site for citizen's whose homes were destroyed. Generators were brought in to provide electricity to the building, classrooms and the gymnasium where dormitories were established. The yard was being used as a staging area for the distribution of food, water and clothing for residents who couldn't return to their homes.

In the event of such a large-scale disaster, consider the following recommendations:

1 Provide frequent updates to the school community. Communicate what you know, what you don't know and what you are doing to learn more. Thoughtful, frequent communication by the principal reassures staff, students and families and demonstrates that active efforts are being made in confronting the crisis.
2 Be available to address concerns or questions, and call upon the City Emergency Response Team or School District Officials for assistance.
3 Given that control of the building is limited, determine who is the key contact person(s) and communicate with them frequently to receive necessary information, make requests and ask questions.
4 As is the case with many natural disasters, some crises can extend well beyond 24 hours. Determine who can assume leadership responsibilities to assist the principal when a break or time away is needed.
5 Upon students' return to school, provide ways for students and staff to process their experiences, ask questions and express their feelings.
6 Once the school is fully returned to your community, find ways to continue to debrief, support and celebrate, when appropriate. What went well? What could go better next time?

Students remained out of class for a week, and when they returned, things were hardly back to normal. Their gymnasium still housed 40-plus people needing emergency shelter. Also, city workers used a portion of the schoolyard to park trucks and store materials as they repaired roads, sidewalks and power lines. As for the students, many experienced anxiety, were filled with their personal stories of how frightened they were and had missed school and their friends. However, they were happy to be back in school.

Human-caused crises/disasters

Since 9/11, numerous catastrophes affecting entire nations, such as terrorist attacks, have escalated. As a result, most schools are required to have a Disaster Response Plan that specifically addresses attacks, bomb threats or shootings as school personnel carefully consider the safety needs of students while under their supervision.

Example: Terrorist attack

I will never forget the morning of the terrorist attack on September 11, 2001. It was feared the Golden Gate Bridge could be a target of attack and my school, located barely a mile from the bridge, may be in harm's way. City leaders directed us to close the school, immediately evacuate all 1,000 students to their parents and lastly, to release all faculty and staff.

From the very beginning of the school year, we worked to establish a trusting, collaborative relationship with staff, and on that day, they were prepared to follow our directives, despite overloaded telephone lines that required us to pivot and change our plans midstream. They trusted us.

Out of necessity and a limited number of available cellphones, teachers were grouped into teams to address the awesome task of evacuations. Amazingly, within 1.5 hours, all but one student had been released to parents or emergency contacts. Each staff member signed out to confirm that they were all accounted for. The administration remained at school until the last parent(s) arrived to retrieve their child.

As in any serious crisis with the potential for tremendous injury or loss, the principal and staff must do all they can to mitigate the threat and protect students and faculty. Swift and decisive action is needed. Implementing the Disaster Response Plan will give all responsible team members and staff the roadmap for how to proceed.

The following points are recommendations for the prevention of compounding problems when the threat is on a much larger scale than the school site, as in this case, a national threat:

1 Assess the present situation and adjust plans in accordance with your findings and include directives from school and civic authorities.
2 Activate the plan by giving clear directions to all staff and the assignment of roles. Communicate any needed adjustments to all faculty and staff.
3 Continue to communicate as further information becomes known.
4 Monitor the Disaster Response Team activities.
5 Make certain the staging of the Parent Reunification Area is well organized and orderly to minimize confusion and anxiety.

6 In the Disaster Response Plan, be certain to have a method for documenting the names of all students who leave the school and with whom.
7 Once the majority of students have been dismissed, release faculty and staff, making certain all sign out and exit the school building.
8 Administrators are to remain at school until all students have been retrieved by a parent or emergency contact.
9 Confirm that the building has been secured.

Example: Bomb threat

The call came in during the lunch period at my school. "A bomb has been planted on the school campus and is scheduled to go off at 2:00 PM," said the caller. The school secretary, who answered the call, was trained to listen for any details, voice clues for age of caller, background noise, etc. Even though most bomb threats to schools do not result in explosions that cause harm according to the US Department of Justice, each threat must be taken seriously and acted upon immediately.

What is to be done?

1 The principal, as the head of the Disaster Response Team, needs to gather information and assess the present circumstances.
2 Contact law enforcement for immediate support.
3 Activate the Disaster Response Team and notify the faculty.
4 Communicate clearly and simply what steps are to be taken.
"Evacuate! (specify a location)," and follow evacuation procedures.
5 Support police (bomb squad) in their search either personally or by assigned staff.
6 Once the threat is resolved, debrief the community as soon as possible. This would include the students in their classes, the faculty through an after-school meeting and parents through letter/email/auto-dial telephone calls. Provide emotional support utilizing SBFC staff or social workers for any student needing further assistance.

The bomb threat was called in during the students' free time. They were scattered in different locations (i.e., yard, cafeteria, gym and library). The principal was notified and assessed of the situation and recognized the challenges being faced. The principal activated the Disaster Response Team and gave instructions to all staff. They needed to carry out their assigned duties and evacuate in an orderly fashion. The Disaster Response Team assumed their assigned roles. The police were called while the school bell rang with teachers and staff directing all students to the yard to meet their sixth period teacher. There was some confusion among the students since the end of lunch bells were ringing early.

Teachers were informed to take their students to the pre-planned alternative evacuation site (in this case the park next to the school) and account for all students. Any missing students were to be reported to the Disaster Response Team Member assigned the job of accounting for all students and staff. Meanwhile, the principal accompanied the police bomb squad as they carefully examined each room in the building. Since security of the building was carefully monitored, it would have been difficult for someone to have actually planted a bomb on campus; however, all agreed that it was better to be cautious and take the threat seriously.

Fortunately, in this case, the bomb threat was false. When staff and students returned to class, teachers lead discussions regarding the incident. At the end of the day, the faculty met with administrators to debrief as well as make recommendations for how to better implement the evacuation plan. Counseling staff and teachers were alerted to be aware of any student talk about the possibility of a student having called in the bomb threat, as can sometimes be the case. In this situation, a student, who was one of our own and in crisis, was identified. His call for help was addressed with needed family involvement, mental and physical health referrals, and the development of a support plan for his re-entry to school.

Recovery

The role of the principal in leading the way to recovery from a disaster or crisis in the school community is often one of providing support and allocating resources. Be aware of how faculty members, as well as students, react to the crisis. While some may be more resilient, others may need additional support.

Strategies for finding ways to return the school to normal:

1   Acknowledge the personal and professional challenges that teachers and support staff have experienced during the crisis.
2   Provide them with the opportunity to express their thoughts and feelings.
3   Create opportunities for students to ask questions in a variety of settings, such as small groups, classes or individually. Encourage students to express their feelings.
4   Provide students with outlets to share their experiences, thoughts and feelings through curriculum-based activities such as art projects or writing.

    Example: Upon returning to the middle school after the devastating earthquake, a Language Arts teacher organized a school-wide writing project for students to have an opportunity to tell the story of what happened to them during and after the earthquake. He created a book, *Aftershocks: Earthquake Writing*, consisting of a collection of stories, poems and drawings. A copy of the book was distributed to all students.
5   Communicate with parents as to what they can do to support their children. For example, remind them to be available for their children to talk of their experiences, to spend extra time with them and to reestablish their regular routines.

6 Anchor and reinforce the feeling of "We're back together again!" by organizing a celebratory assembly, festival or other event if students have been away from school for some time.

7 As a principal, evaluate your personal response to the crisis. What have you learned? What went well? What improvements would you make?

8 Revisit your Disaster Response Plan and, based on your experience and in collaboration with the Response Team and faculty, make adjustments as needed.

Conclusion

Effective and strong principals who develop a mental readiness to lead will confidently serve as the guide before, during and through times of crisis. They will cultivate a growth mindset as they face challenges, and persevere in planning and implementing a Disaster Response Plan. They will build an atmosphere of trust and cooperation, creating a strong foundation that enables a collective/collaborative response to crises. The principal is the conduit of information from numerous sources and sharing that information with staff helps to maintain the atmosphere of trust. Information is essential to everyone's well-being, as is the sharing of plans that assist the return to some sense of normalcy once a crisis is past. Yes, communication is essential. The principal possesses multiple communication avenues to disseminate information and connect with the entire school community. Traditional avenues of communication can include the following: faculty meetings, the school website, school bulletins, newsletters, auto-dial telephone contacts, and town hall or parent meetings whether in-person or online. Few people can think clearly and logically in a crisis; therefore, it is most important to develop a comprehensive Disaster Response Plan for the sake of everyone's well-being. It can be daunting when a principal examines all of the possible emergency scenarios and the myriad of organizational details involved in getting it right. However, remember, this is a collaborative effort not something done by the principal alone. Staff need to be involved in the ongoing process of developing the plan over time.

Looking beyond the school building, principals can call upon the community, including law enforcement, emergency services and mental health agencies. Equally as important, principals must remain attentive to their own well-being. Principals are so focused on taking care of others in the course of their day; they sometimes do not make room for their own self-care. Building in self-care as part of one's routine is an important addition to personal and professional life. Self-care can lower the risk for depression, burnout, trauma and can decrease anxiety. Examples of self-care include small actions, such as taking deep breaths, taking a five-minute walking break, drinking a glass of water or larger positive lifestyle behaviors such as regular exercise, adequate sleep, healthy eating or pursuing a hobby. As in many other aspects of being an effective principal, leading by example serves oneself and the school.

In conclusion, preparing and responding to a crisis can be a formidable and time-consuming process. Principals are dedicated to making a difference and doing their best to assure that their school community is safe. Ultimately, school principals become the teacher, the parent and the guide as they respond to those in need during times of crisis. In closing, some final words of encouragement for all principals, "Believe in yourself. You are braver than you think, more talented than you know and capable of more than you imagine" (Bennett, 2020).

Resources

Anderson, E., Hayes, S. & Carpenter, B. (2020). *Principal as caregiver of all: Responding to needs of others and self*; CPRE Policy Briefs. Retrieved from https://repository.upenn.edu/cpre_policybriefs/92/
   An examination of how leaders, living among the stressors of a global pandemic, were able to look after their own wellbeing while attending to the wellbeing of their students, staff and community members.
Bennett, R. T. (2020). *The light in the heart: Inspirational thoughts for living your best life*. Roy T. Bennnett.
   Inspirational and motivational thoughts.
Cowan, K. C. & Rossen, E. (2013). Responding to the unthinkable; School crisis response and recovery. *Phi Delta Kappan*, 95(4), 8–12.
   The article outlines the importance of having a comprehensive and coordinated plan that includes prevention, preparedness, response and recovery.
D'Auria, G. & DeSmet, A. (2020). *Leadership in a crisis: Responding to the coronavirus outbreak and future challenges*. McKinsey & Company.
   This article includes five leadership practices to help you respond effectively including making decisions amid uncertainty, demonstrating empathy and communicating effectively.
Keyes, E. & J. (2021, March 25) Standard Response Protocol. The I Love U Guys Foundation. (2021). https://iloveuguys.org/
   This protocol provides consistent, clear shared language and actions among all students, staff and first responders for all disasters. The specific vocabulary for quick and coordinated action develops the muscle memory necessary to respond in moments of crisis.
Lichtenstein, R., Schonfeld, D. & Kline, M. (1994). Special topic / school crisis response: Expecting the unexpected. School crisis response: Expecting the unexpected. *Educational Leadership*, 52(3), 79–83.
   An effective crisis response reflects prevention, intervention and rehearsed reaction. A School Crisis Intervention Model is presented in detail.
National Education Association. (n.d.). NEA's school crisis guide. National Education Association | NEA. https://www.nea.org/resource-library/neasschool-crisis-guide
   The NEA's School Crisis Guide offers a step-by-step outline of what to do before, during and after any school or community crisis such as a natural disaster.
Ritter, K. (2022). Why self-care for school leaders is more important than ever. National Association of Secondary School Principals (NASSP). https://www.nassp.org/2022/01/18/why-self-care-for-school-leaders-is-more-importantthan-ever/

A high school principal shares what he does to reduce stress and feel better prepared to tackle the challenges of being a principal, such as meditation, breathing strategies, sleep, journal writing, etc.

Stough, L.M., Kang, D. & Lee, S. (2018). *Seven school-related disasters: Lessons for policymakers and school personnel*. Education Policy Analysis Archives. https://epaa.asu.edu/ojs/index.php/epaa/article/view/3698

Students are highly dependent on the emergency planning and evacuation decisions made by policymakers and school personnel when disasters occur. This study examined cases of school-related disasters, highlighting how factors of the school intersected with natural disasters and subsequently affected schoolchildren.

References

Bennett, R. T. (2020). *The light in the heart: Inspirational thoughts for living your best life*. Roy T. Bennnett.

Cowan, K. C. & Rossen, E. (2013). Responding to the unthinkable; School crisis response and recovery. *Phi Delta Kappan*, 95(4), 8–12.

National Education Association. (n.d.). NEA's school crisis guide. National Education Association | NEA. https://www.nea.org/resource-library/neasschool-crisis-guide

Part II

School intervention

5 Developing systems for crisis intervention with school personnel

Emily J. Hernandez, Elina Saeki, and Kezia Gopaul-Knights

Overview

The need to address the mental health and well-being of school personnel has never been greater. While there has been a steady increase in mental health awareness and support of students in recent years, current research indicates a profound lack of programs, resources, and interventions to support the mental health and well-being of school personnel during crisis situations. Promoting mental health and well-being is vital not only for school personnel but also for workforce stability and the provision of optimal quality care and safe school systems. This chapter seeks to share information regarding crisis intervention with school personnel within a School-Based Family Counseling (SBFC) lens. For the purposes of this chapter, school personnel refers to anyone working in or supporting a school organization and includes teachers, school-based mental health practitioners, administration, administrative support personnel, and site operational staff. The term "educator" may be used interchangeably with school personnel.

Background

Over the years, the work roles and responsibilities of educators have expanded (Bartlett, 2004). In addition to formal responsibilities associated with teaching (e.g., lesson planning, classroom behavior management, grading, and meetings), educators are informally tasked with supporting students' social-emotional concerns, including addressing bullying and victimization, homelessness, and trauma (Johnson et al., 2011). They are increasingly being called upon to respond to students' crisis needs. These student needs have increased, both in breadth and in depth, during the COVID-19 pandemic. In addition to juggling the responsibility of supporting students' academic, social-emotional, and behavioral well-being, educators are struggling to tend to their own physical and psychological well-being as well (Baker et al., 2021). Educators have reported a decline in their mental health and well-being which are attributed to uncertainty, workload, negative perceptions about the field of education, worry about the health and well-being of self and others, current health challenges, and additional personal and professional roles (Kim et al.,

DOI: 10.4324/9781003201977-7

2021). Taken together, there is a critical need to support educators' mental and emotional health particularly during times of crisis.

School crisis

A school crisis is commonly defined as a sudden, uncontrollable, and extremely negative event that can potentially impact the entire school community (Brock et al., 2009) and can include natural disasters, death of a student or school personnel, and acts of violence. Psychological well-being is often impacted following a school crisis event. When faced with school crisis situations, the literature offers frameworks and programs to support students' physical, social-emotional, and behavioral needs. However, crisis incidents can affect educators as much as they can impact students. For example, teachers may be three times more likely to be victims of violent crimes in school compared to students (Kondrasuk et al., 2005). When crisis situations occur, educators are often underprepared for the potential psychological impact which can negatively affect their well-being. Furthermore, many educators do not receive appropriate support and the negative effects of a crisis are not adequately attended to (Newman et al., 2004). Despite the potential for educators to be exposed to crisis situations in schools, much of the research on crisis intervention has focused on frequently trauma-exposed workers, such as emergency services personnel (e.g., healthcare workers, fire fighters, and police) and disaster workers. There is limited research on support services offered to educators following a school crisis event (Daniels et al., 2007). Given the important role that educators have in providing support to students, it is important to consider the potential impact of school crises on educators and offer critical support.

SBFC model

Crisis intervention with school personnel can be viewed and applied through the lens of the SBFC metamodel and framework. The SBFC metamodel, as described by Gerrard and Soriano (2019), illustrates the primary focus of SBFC to be on the school and the family in the area of prevention and intervention (see Figure 1.1 in Chapter 1). Crisis intervention with educators can be considered a vital construct to be used during a crisis and it aligns with both the school prevention and school intervention quadrants. Utilizing a prevention-focused systems-oriented approach is an important way to build capacity with educators as a foundation for when a crisis does occur.

Procedure

Responding to a crisis is complex and requires a multifaceted approach. In alignment with the SBFC metamodel and framework, the proposed procedure focuses on specific prevention and intervention efforts. The procedural framework is adapted from the National Child Traumatic Stress Network's (NCTSN) "The 3R's of School Crises and Disasters: Readiness, Response, and Recovery", and the "School Mental Health Crisis Leadership" concepts with the Substance Abuse and Mental Health Services Administration (SAMHSA) (National Child Traumatic Stress Network, 2017; Mental Health Technology Transfer Center, 2019). The frameworks have been adapted for the purposes of this chapter to specifically focus on the needs of school personnel. The four stages of the model include Readiness, Response, Recovery, and Renewal. The Four "Rs" reflect the stages through which we understand and process experiences that are crisis-related (Mental Health Technology Transfer Center Network, 2019).

Readiness

The first part of the procedure involves the "Readiness" phase. During this phase, school organizations establish systems and structures to address and respond to crises, emergencies, and disasters. The crisis readiness phase is a continuous cycle of planning, response, and evaluation with the goal of minimizing psychological and physical harm in the development of systems for effective crisis response and recovery. This step is broken down to include a focus on the district/organizational, school-site, and individual levels.

District/organizational level

Prioritization of educator mental health

- Prioritize educator mental health and support in advance of any crisis taking place so that educators, as a main stakeholder, will be involved in policies and procedures moving forward.

Human resources/personnel services

- Human resources and personnel departments should offer benefits packages that include mental and behavioral health components for employees that are easy to access.
- Adopt and implement an employee wellness program and initiatives focused on overall well-being as a base layer of prevention.
- Establish partnerships with effective Employee Assistance Programs (EAPs) to provide immediate short-term support for educators and disseminate information to employees.

Crisis response infrastructure

- Explore and adopt a model for crisis intervention, including procedures which involve educators as one of the primary stakeholders by developing internal and external partnerships for a mobile crisis response team.

- Identify staffing needs to support crisis intervention procedures and work collaboratively for allocation of funding to support and balance decisions related to staffing and support needs.
- Provide a district-wide training for all school staff on mental health/psychological first aid.

District-level crisis response team

- Identify key members and develop a district-level crisis response team that focuses on procedures, implementation, and delivery of services, with plans in place for response to frequent crisis events such as the death of an employee or student, community or school-site violence, psychiatric emergencies, or community natural disasters.
- Develop a procedural manual that is user-friendly and easy to access. The manual should include tools to be utilized during crisis response service delivery, including documentation, templates, and media kits. Provide training and professional development to the district-level crisis response team that includes coverage of the procedural manual.
- Identify school-site level members that should be a part of the school-level crisis response team, then provide training and professional development on the procedural manual.
- Schedule convenings on a quarterly basis of district- and school-level team members for planning and improving the model. This includes debriefing meetings to be held after a crisis event.

School-site level

Prioritization of educator mental health

- All school-site leadership participates in district/organizational-level training to ensure knowledge and awareness of educator mental health/psychological first aid and the procedures for crisis response.
- School-site leadership demonstrates belief systems that value and prioritize educator mental health and foster a school climate that is focused on educator well-being.

School-site level crisis response team

- School-site level leads are identified for participation in the crisis intervention model and to participate in professional development provided by the district. Team members may include out of classroom personnel who are able to respond in times of crisis. The school-site crisis response team serve as leaders for prevention and readiness and provide training and professional development to school staff regarding the site procedures.
- During a crisis, school-site crisis response team members take the lead on crisis response procedures and engage the district/organizational levels as needed.

Individual level

Knowledge and understanding

- Each employee understands and values the importance of educator well-being, through participation in ongoing professional development. Additional training on mental health/psychological first aid is important to learn the basics for crisis response and support to others related to intervening and providing crisis support. All educators hold the responsibility of crisis response as needed and participate in, and advocate for, a positive school climate that fosters educator well-being.
- Educators have knowledge of the resources for supporting employees, including access to mental health benefits and EAPs. It is the professional and ethical responsibility of educators to develop a personal practice of strategies focused on their own mental health and well-being. This includes seeking out assistance to address one's own personal and professional needs for support.

Response

The response phase is the acute phase of the crisis response – the sum total of the school's resources and skills to take decisive and effective action immediately following a crisis. This is the active response phase that is focused on leveraging the systems developed in the readiness phase and implementing delivery of services to minimize harm to all people involved during a particular incident. The focus is short-term and coordination of rapid action and service delivery among all stakeholders and community partners (Wolf-Prusan and Schonfeld, 2020). A variety of tasks are carried out in the response phase, including ensuring physical and psychological safety, assessing the impact of the crisis on those affected, engaging partnerships for crisis support, communicating and disseminating information about the crisis, and providing varying levels of support depending on need.

Communication

- Communicate frequently following a school crisis to provide transparency and predictability for educators, including communicating information regarding procedures, routines, and other pertinent information.
- Organize opportunities for educators to obtain information about the crisis. Dispel any rumors and provide accurate information, address perceptions of ongoing threat or vulnerability, and differentiate the type and amount of information relayed. Considerations include providing just enough information to avoid overwhelming school personnel, using multiple delivery methods (email, in-person, phone), and offering stabilization by being consistently available and predictable.

- Inform educators of the measures being taken to ensure safety (e.g., law enforcement is patrolling the area) and avoid promises that cannot be kept (e.g., "we will be back to normal in no time").
- Recommend that educators minimize their exposure to any media coverage related to the crisis event.

Assess the impact on the community. Ensure physical and psychological safety, in that order.

- Evaluate the impact of the crisis on educators and direct attention toward those who display warning signs or predispositions for trauma.
- Deliver crisis response in a multi-tiered framework to ensure everyone receives support tailored to their individual experience and needs, including individual and collective healing opportunities.
- Assess and return to normal routines as appropriate because concrete and visible signs of safety help people feel safer.

Mobilize crisis response teams

- Execute district and school-wide procedures for handling mental health needs, such as crisis counseling and grief support. School personnel may not be in a position to also provide direct support for themselves and their colleagues when directly impacted by a crisis due to being victims themselves.
- District-level crisis response teams may coordinate the sharing of resources among school-level teams, such as assigning counselors from other schools to a school responding to a crisis.

Engage partnerships for crisis support

- "Outside" mental health practitioners work alongside the school district counselors and other mental health professionals to assist in crisis counseling and determine the most appropriate interventions to provide.
- Contact local mental health agencies, as well as local, state, and national agencies who can provide immediate support to school personnel.
- Districts can partner with EAPs that are focused on providing support to employees. EAPs have the ability to provide immediate support to employees and can provide immediate access to services and resources.

Recovery

Recovery is the ongoing process of restoring the social and emotional equilibrium of the school community and can span from three to twelve months for short-term recovery, and up to five years after a crisis is experienced.

The central recovery process is connectedness and commonality (i.e., finding peer support and resilience). Schools work on the following principles for recovery: (i) empowering survivors and victims of trauma, restoring a sense of control, (ii) mourning and memorialization, and (iii) reconnecting with ordinary life.

Communication

- Continue engaging in transparent communication with educators.

Debriefing

- Provide educators with support, space, and time to process their own emotions about the crisis event. This can happen collectively (e.g., all educators in the school) or separately by grade level or other groupings. Some spaces may need to be held together as a whole and other educators may need more private recovery spaces.
- Disseminate information to educators about best practices in crisis response, so educators will be equipped with tools to support their students as they return to school and normalcy.
- Acknowledge that recovery does not happen all at once and every educator will have different adjustment recovery processes.

Remembrance, mourning, and commemoration

- Schools may facilitate the co-creation of memorials among educators and students, as appropriate. Collaborating on memorial projects can build community and help educators feel like they are moving on from the crisis.
- Prepare for the one-year mark. This is a time when educators are likely to experience a resurgence of feelings associated with the crisis. Mental health practitioners can talk to educators about common feelings that may emerge at the one-year mark, and offer strategies for avoiding reminders about the crisis and coping strategies for working through these feelings.

Follow-up resources and support

- Inform educators about ongoing support services in the school and community, such as crisis support groups. Leverage support from local and state organizations, including county offices of education to support educators through the recovery process.
- Some educators may be unable to handle the "typical" workload following a school crisis. Schools may consider providing flexibility for teachers as they transition to return to normalcy.

Renewal

The renewal phase is the final phase of crisis response and arguably, the most critical and often overlooked of the four-step process. The "Renewal" phase involves healing, making meaning of the event, fostering and building resilience, and determining the need for organizational change. This process is reflective, focused on the bigger picture and is long-term. The completion of this phase can range from a few months to a few years. In renewal, the leadership of the school organization helps in refocusing, promoting resilience, and leading efforts to make changes to current and future crisis response practices (SAMHSA, 2020).

Leadership role

- Convene to plan renewal efforts for educators.
- Examine the need to fund activities related to renewal such as staff retreats, crisis teams, and/or staffing to address shortages.
- Demonstrate a commitment to short- and long-term reflection and practices. This may translate to at least quarterly meetings to review renewal efforts.

Give meaning to the event

- Allow educators to create their own narrative about the event and how it has impacted them. Emphasize that in giving meaning, the loss, hurt, pain, and negative outcomes of the crisis are not minimized.
- Plan specific times to engage leadership, teachers, and related staff in personal and collective narrative formation of meaning. This may be through staff meetings, release time for staff, staff retreats, or through other planned staff only events. Ask:
    - How has the event impacted myself, loved ones, and the community?
    - How have I grown through this traumatic event?
    - What can leadership do in the future to minimize the impact of another traumatic event on educators and the community?

Promote resilience

- School leaders can promote resilience by returning to "business as usual" as soon as it is feasible to do so. Although this can be interpreted as insensitive if people are still dealing with painful memories from the crisis event (Lambiase & English, 2020), the return to normal functioning promotes the resiliency of the school as a whole.
- Create opportunities for educators to continue engaging in mindfulness, self-care, and other mind body activities.
- Connect educators with community resources to further promote healing and resiliency.

Program evaluation

- Leaders reflect on the following questions in the weeks and months following the crisis event and response:
  - What happened?
  - How do we feel?
  - What did we do well in our crisis intervention response?
  - How could we improve our crisis plan?
- Update policies and procedures based on the evaluation and feedback.

Multicultural considerations

In promoting mental health and well-being among educators and providing crisis response services, careful thought must be placed into how services can be delivered in a culturally sensitive manner. Studies on wellness in the educational sector conducted in various countries appear to be in consensus regarding the effects of occupational stress and the lack of resources available to educators (Herman et al., 2020). One of the main distinctions between Western versus Eastern countries is the values of individualism versus collectivism, respectively, and how this impacts the expressed reactions and observable behaviors of educators. The characteristics of these cultures appear to affect workers' occupational and mental health in different ways.

Despite the documented lack of resources and support available during times of crisis, it is important to note that there are culturally significant differences in responses to such experiences. Further, the stigma related to the acceptance of mental health services continues to exist (Sickel et al., 2014). School leadership personnel should acknowledge the barriers that exist to educators' acceptance of mental health services and reduce these barriers. Taken together, it is critical to engage in school crisis prevention, intervention, and postvention efforts while taking into consideration the social and cultural factors that affect educator well-being.

Challenges and solutions

There are many obstacles to navigate when trying to implement the multifaceted components of the proposed procedure. While there will always be challenges in implementing system-wide infrastructure, there are a multitude of solutions that can be put in place when prioritized. First, the prioritization and knowledge of educator mental health and wellness rely on the limited research that is available. This construct has not been prioritized in school systems uniformly and has resurfaced as a main priority recently due to the "COVID-19" worldwide pandemic with increasing educator burnout and compassion fatigue resulting from the massive needs in education at school-site levels. In order to continue to prioritize educator mental health and well-being, more extensive research focused on educator well-being is needed. Other challenges include issues related to budget/funding, limited resources and staffing, varying sizes of the organization, and transitions. In some school districts, there may not be sufficient support and resources for the creation and maintenance of a comprehensive school crisis plan for educators. While funding allocations to support a comprehensive crisis response procedure can be difficult to identify, it is too costly to not have these structures in place. District leaders may need to leverage across personnel and skill sets within their districts and communities to facilitate their efforts. Efforts are also impacted by the size of the organization. In these cases, the establishment of partnerships with community and government-based organizations is critical in order to leverage additional resources and person power when responding to an emergency. Another common challenge faced is the nature of frequent transitions and turnover at school sites and districts. As key crisis personnel transition within or out of a school/district, often that person's knowledge and role in sustaining procedures also transition with them. For these reasons, it is critical to invest time and resources in developing infrastructure within systems so that service delivery is not driven, or collapsed, by these types of personnel changes.

Conclusion

Educators are increasingly exposed to crisis situations to which they must respond. These crisis situations impinge on the well-being of educators and contribute to stress, burnout, and high turnover among other undesirable consequences. Yet, there is no documented crisis intervention response targeted specifically for educators. This chapter acknowledges the importance of attending to the mental health of educators and developing crisis response efforts to help mitigate the negative impact of crises on employees. Drawing upon existing crisis response models, a system for responding to crises is proposed for the educators. Referred to as the Four "Rs", Readiness, Response, Recovery, and Renewal, the model meets the needs of educators and staff and includes prevention and intervention efforts, short-term and long-term responses, and requires support and resources from school leadership. When implemented in a school system, this crisis response effort is likely to intercept widespread threats to educator well-being during crisis situations. The model proposed utilizes a prevention-focused systems-oriented approach in alignment with the SBFC metamodel and framework and is an important way to build capacity with educators as a foundation for when a crisis does occur.

Resources

After a School Tragedy...Readiness, Response, Recovery, & Resources. (n.d.) Retrieved May 16, 2022 Mental Health Technology Transfer Center Network (MHTTC): https://mhttcnetwork.org/sites/default/files/2019-05/After%20 a%20School%20Tragedy_FINAL050919.pdf

This publication was prepared by the Mental Health Technology Transfer Center Network (MHTTC) funded by the Substance Abuse and Mental Health Services Administration (SAMHSA) and provides a general review of the readiness, response, and recovery procedure along with a comprehensive review of resources in the area of grief, loss and bereavement for practitioners working in school systems.

Crisis Response Box: A Guide to Help Every School Assemble the Tools and Resources Needed for a Critical Incident Response. (n.d). Retrieved May 16, 2022 California Department of Education: https://www.cde.ca.gov/LS/ss/cp/documents/crisisrespbox.pdf

The Crisis Response Box is a guide to assist schools in crisis and prevention planning. The Crisis Response Box is an invaluable resource if a critical incident ever arises at your school. It walks you through the steps necessary to assemble a school emergency response plan adapted for your school and community before an event occurs. The Crisis Response Box is an invaluable resource if a critical incident ever arises at your school. It walks you through the steps necessary to assemble a school emergency response plan adapted for your school and community before an event occurs.

Dealing with the Death of a Student or School Staff Member (Video Modules). (n.d) Retrieved May 16, 2022 Coalition to Support Grieving Students: https://grievingstudents.org/module-section/death-school-crisis/

This is a specific module on the website for the Coalition to Support Grieving Students focused on dealing with the death of a student or staff member.

Grief Support Modules for School Personnel. (n.d) Retrieved May 16, 2022 Coalition to Support Grieving Students: https://grievingstudents.org/

*The Coalition to Support Grieving Students was convened by the New York Life Foundation, a pioneering advocate for the cause of childhood bereavement, and the National Center for School Crisis and Bereavement, which is led by pediatrician and childhood bereavement expert David J. Schonfeld, M.D. The Coalition created grievingstudents.org, a groundbreaking, practitioner-oriented website designed to provide educators with the information, insights, and practical advice they need to better understand and meet the needs of the millions of grieving children in America's classrooms.*Recovery from Large-Scale Crises: Guidelines for Crisis Teams and Administrators. (n.d.) Retrieved from National Association of School Psychologists: https://www.nasponline.org/resources-and-publications/resources-and-podcasts/school-safety-and-crisis/school-violence-resources/recovery-from-large-scale-crises-guidelines-for-crisis-teams-and-administrators

This resource was developed by a number of highly experienced school-based crisis responders with the intent of assisting administrators and crisis teams in crisis response and recovery efforts following a large-scale disaster or crisis.

References

Baker, C. N., Peele, H., Daniels, M., Saybe, M., Whalen, K., Overstreeet, S., & The New Orleans Trauma-Informed Schools Learning Collaborative (2021). The experience of COVID-19 and its impact on teachers' mental health, coping, and teaching. *School Psychology Review, 50*(4), 491–504. https://doi.org/10.1080/2372966X.2020.1855473

Bartlett, L. (2004). Expanding teacher work roles: A resource for retention or a recipe for overwork? *Journal of Education Policy, 19*(5), 565–582. https://doi.org/10.1080/0268093042000269144

Brock, S. E., Nickerson, A. B., Reeves, M. A., Jimerson, S. R., Lieberman, R. A., & Feinberg, T. A. (2009). *School crisis prevention and intervention: The PREPaRE model*. Bethesda, MD: National Association of School Psychologists.

Daniels, J. A., Bradley, M. C., & Hays, M. (2007). The impact of school violence on school personnel: Implications for psychologists. *Professional Psychology: Research and Practice, 38*(6), 652–659. https://doi.org/10.1037/0735-7028.38.6.652

Gerrard, B. & Soriano, M. (2019). School-based family counseling: The revolutionary paradigm. In B. Gerrard, M. Carter & D. Ribera (Eds.). *School-based family counseling: An interdisciplinary practitioner's guide* (pp. 1–15). Routledge.

Herman, K. C., Reinke, W. M., & Eddy, C. L. (2020). Advances in understanding and intervening in teacher stress and coping: The coping-competence-context theory. *Journal of School Psychology, 78*, 69–74. https://doi.org/10.1016/j.jsp.2020.01.001

Hernandez, E. J. (2016). Reducing bullying and preventing dropout through student engagement: A prevention-focused lens for school-based family counselors. *International Journal for School-Based Family Counseling, 7*, 1–13. http://www.instituteschoolbasedfamilycounseling.com/docs/IJSBFC%20-%20bullying%20and%20dropout%20-%20final.pdf

Johnson, C., Eva, A. L., Johnson, L., & Walker, B. (2011). Don't turn away: Empowering teachers to support students' mental health. *The Clearing House: A Journal of Educational Strategies, Issues and Ideas, 84*(1), 9–14. https://doi.org/10.1080/00098655.2010.484441

Kim, S., Crooks, C.V., Bax, K., et al. (2021). Impact of trauma-informed training and mindfulness-based social–emotional learning program on teacher attitudes and burnout: A mixed-methods study. *School Mental Health 13*, 55–68. https://doi.org/10.1007/s12310-020-09406-6

Kondrasuk, J. N., Greene, T., Waggoner, J., Edwards, K., & Nayak-Rhodes, A. (2005). Violence affecting school employees. *Education Faculty Publications and Presentations, 125*, 638–647. http://pilotscholars.up.edu/edu_facpubs/2

Lambiase, & English, A. E. (2021). Passing the test: Lessons from a school district's discourse of renewal before, during and after Hurricane Harvey. *Journal of Contingencies and Crisis Management, 29*(1), 36–46. https://doi.org/10.1111/1468-5973.12301

Mental Health Technology Transfer Center Network (2019). *After a school tragedy… readiness, response, recovery, & resources*. https://mhttcnetwork.org/centers/mhttc-network-coordinating-office/product/after-school-tragedyreadiness-response-recovery

National Child Traumatic Stress Network. (2017, February), The 3R's of school crises and disasters: readiness, response, and recovery. Published on National Child Traumatic Stress Network - Child Trauma Home, https://www.tfec.org/wp-content/uploads/Murk_3Rs-ofSchoolCrises.pdf

Newman, K. S., Fox, C., Harding, D. J., Mehta, J., & Roth, W. (2004). *Rampage: The social roots of school shootings*. Basic Books.

Pacific Southwest Mental Health Technology Transfer Center. (2020, June) *School mental health crisis leadership lessons: Voices of experience from leaders in the pacific southwest region*. SAMHSA.

Sickle, A. E., Seacat, J. D., & Nabors, N. A. (2014). Mental health stigma update: A review of consequences. *Advances in Mental Health, 12*(3), 202–215. https://doi.org/10.1080/18374905.2014.11081898

Wolf-Prusan, L., & Schonfeld, D. (2020). *School mental health crisis leadership: Voices of experience from leaders in the Pacific Southwest Region*. Pacific Southwest MHTTC. https://cars-rp.org/_MHTTC/docs/SMH-Crisis-Leadership-Lessons-Guide.pdf

6 How schools can help students cope with the stress of a major disaster

Robyne Le Brocque and Nikki Triggell

Overview

In this chapter, we examine ways in which schools cope with disaster. We also explore how schools can assist students to cope with the stress of a major disaster by examining ways in which accommodations can be made in the classroom.

Background

Disasters impact students, their families, their teachers, the school community, and the wider community, and may result in trauma and distress for all involved. In turn, trauma impacts on the ability of children to engage with learning. Some children will exhibit few or no symptoms of trauma. Other children may experience brief, or transitory, distress. Some children, especially those with pre-existing behavior issues, complex histories, or those highly impacted by the disaster, may experience prolonged symptoms of distress.

The information presented in this chapter comes from research investigating the presentation of posttraumatic responses in children and their families over the past three decades. Following the devastating Black Saturday fires in Victoria, Australia, in 2009, we began to translate our research into possible interventions for children and their families. We have helped support the recovery of communities recovering from fires and floods in Australia and earthquakes in New Zealand and Japan.

We have presented our research and work around the world working with school communities, mental health specialists, and the Red Cross and other organizations assisting communities to recover. Our aim is to build closer connections between the child and their family, the school community, the school-based family counseling (SBFC) practitioner, and community-based pediatric specialist services to facilitate earlier identification of children and families with ongoing distress and connect them to services to provide intervention. When we consider that children are still developing, there is an urgent need to intervene and support children and their families as early as possible.

DOI: 10.4324/9781003201977-8

Our research aligns with the SBFC model. We prioritize both the school and the family to support children recovering from disaster and trauma. We support an integrated approach to mental health and recovery working with the child, the family, the whole-of-school community, and mental health clinicians to provide for the best recovery following disaster. The SBFC metamodel recognizes that a combination of both prevention and remedial intervention promotes well-being and minimizes distress, promotes development, and facilitates learning and academic outcomes. Our work with the Disaster Shock collaboration (https://www.disastershock.com/) has also facilitated the dissemination of trauma and disaster resources around the world. More information on trauma and disasters can be obtained from the Australian Child and Adolescent Trauma, Loss, and Grief Network National (https://earlytraumagrief.anu.edu.au/).

How does disaster impact children?

Exposure to disaster impacts children's mental health putting them at risk of a range of mental health disorders and behavior problems, including posttraumatic stress disorder, depression, anxiety, sleep disturbances and nightmares, somatic disorders, and substance abuse in older children.

How does disaster impact learning?

Disaster impacts learning through the release of stress hormones that impact in a variety of ways on the brain and cognitive abilities. These can impact learning interfering with memory, executive functioning, and attention. Disaster, the resulting stress, and trauma responses can result in changes to the developing brain in children which may become permanent and have long-term impacts. The post-disaster and trauma environment may also be impacted resulting in changes to the family and community.

Stress response

The response to stress or immediate danger is understood to be a protective evolutionary feature designed to engage the body's response to threat. However, this may result in ongoing symptoms of distress in some children. These symptoms, when persistent, can interfere with learning and development.

Symptoms of posttraumatic stress disorder and other stress reactions include disturbances in sleep, nightmares, fear of the dark, and fear of going to sleep; new anxieties such as separation anxiety across all developmental stages, general anxiety, and specific anxiety; irritability and behavior problems; difficulties with concentration and memory; and hypervigilance. Young children may experience regression in previously acquired skills such as toileting or separating from parents. Some children may exhibit avoidance behavior which may be expressed as school refusal.

Children also present with secondary psychological problems that develop after the traumatic event such as somatic complaints and pain. Adolescents are more likely to report depression and increased substance use. Pre-existing issues such as behavior problems, learning difficulties, or autism spectrum disorder may be exacerbated by the trauma experience or the posttrauma environment.

Parenting and family environment

Disaster impacts the family environment. Parents exposed to disaster may also experience the psychological impact of the events and parents are at risk of psychological problems, including posttraumatic stress such as re-experiencing, avoidance, and negative cognition, and other disorders such as anxiety, substance use disorder, and mood disorders.

Exposure to disaster impacts the psychological well-being of parents but also impacts their capacity to manage their family and parenting practices. Changes in parenting behavior will have a flow on effect to their children with the potential to further distress exacerbate their child's reactions.

Disruption in schools

Similar to the impact on parents, teachers, and the school leadership and administration teams are not immune to the impacts of disaster. Teachers and school personnel may have experienced injury and loss within their family and damage and loss of personal property. As a result, teachers and school personnel may experience their own trauma reactions as well as a number of additional challenges. School personnel need to work with traumatized and distressed children and may find that they are called on for additional psychosocial support for children and their families. Indeed, the school often becomes a center for disaster recovery, so teachers may also be responding to the needs of the wider community.

In addition to the psychosocial impact of disaster on the school community, students and their families, teachers, and the wider school community may experience other impacts such as disruption in the academic program, timetables, and schedules, impacts on school infrastructure, and challenges relating to the stability and availability of school personnel.

Disruption in the community

A disaster impacts an entire community and children are closely interrelated within a family, peers, and school, and the broader community context. Families may be displaced. Peers may be absent. Community infrastructure may not be available. Routines are disrupted. These difficulties challenge the coping strategies and resources available to students and their families as well as the school community.

Box 6.1 What to keep in mind following disasters

Despite the aim to return to business-as-usual as quickly as possible, it is important to keep in mind how children react following trauma and disaster.

Most children cope well with trauma and disaster; however, trauma may exacerbate pre-existing behavior and attention problems.

Some children will exhibit transitory symptoms of distress that will resolve quickly over time.

Children with more serious psychosocial problems following trauma may experience problems with concentration, memory, and behavior which may impact learning.

Problems with learning may not be evident for some time and may emerge as knowledge gaps over the following years.

How do these factors impact learning?

Research investigating the trajectories of recovery of children and young people following disasters is emerging and the evidence shows that most students cope well with disasters or have minor problems and recover quickly. Others may experience complex and changing psychosocial reactions.

In the immediate and short term, children may be shocked and withdrawn. Medium- and long-term symptoms may change over time and present as chronic tiredness and irritability. These may be expressed as behavior problems that are difficult to manage in the classroom. Difficulties in concentration impact memory and learning which may not be immediately evident and leave children with significant gaps in foundational learning. Disaster often impacts the ability of the children to even attend school resulting in school displacement or disrupted attendance.

Teachers, dealing with their own stressors, may have less resources to attend to challenges in the classroom and may be under pressure to maintain learning and academic achievement. This is particularly important to consider for significant transitional learning years, such as the final year of primary school and the last year of school before admission into higher education.

Procedure

The disaster response by schools will change over time. In the immediate aftermath of a disaster, the school building and spaces are often utilized by the community to co-ordinate the disaster response. The school may be one of the few spaces with large meeting halls or wide-open spaces to take refuge. When the community begins the recovery phase, services may also be co-ordinated through the school to the wider community. Schools become a priority with the aim to re-establish normal routines and minimize the impact on children and families.

Step 1: Engage language and skills learned in the school resilience and mindfulness programs

Step 2: Screening and Monitoring of Student Distress

Step 3: Modifying the Classroom Environment.

Step 1: Engage language and skills learned in the school resilience and mindfulness programs

Since the 1970s, many schools have implemented some form of resilience program. One example of this is mindfulness and yoga, to calm the body and center the mind in preparation for learning. Other resilience programs are designed to help children to adapt positively despite experiences of significant adversity (Luthar & Cicchetti, 2000). Resilience programs focus on building skills in managing stress, engaging positive coping skills, and building a sense of self-worth and efficacy.

Despite the implementation of these programs and the practice of these skills in many schools across the globe, there is a disconnect between these programs and the strategies used by children, their teachers, and the school community both during and after disaster. The SBFC practitioner can help guide schools to engage these skills when the coping capacity and resources are stretched during extreme events.

Step 2: Screening

Teachers and the school community act in loco parentis – they act in place of the parent when the child is in their care. Teachers may be the only other adults the child is in contact with. This places teachers in a unique position to screen and monitor for mental health challenges emerging post-disaster. In addition to monitoring symptoms, teachers may also have to modify the learning environment to accommodate mental health challenges following disaster.

In the aftermath of disasters and exposure to trauma, schools often prioritize getting back to normal and attempt to begin teaching as soon as possible. This is certainly the priority for children in developmental milestones such as the first year of school, transitioning from early school to high school or secondary school, and for students in the final year of school transitioning into tertiary education.

Prioritizing getting back to normal helps students re-establish their routines and gives them a sense of security in an often unpredictable, post-disaster environment. However, as we discussed above, some trauma reactions may interfere with the child's learning, leading to deficits in achievement. Unfortunately, these may not emerge for some time.

Box 6.2 Screening for posttraumatic stress reactions

A number of easy to use, brief, child trauma symptom screening questionnaires are available through the International Society for Traumatic Stress website (https://istss.org/clinical-resources/child-trauma-assessments). These can be used at regular intervals post-disaster to monitor symptoms and facilitate referral for early intervention.

When getting back to normal, we recommend screening the children for post-disaster psychological distress at regular intervals after disaster. For example, once the normal routine is established, a brief screening questionnaire can be administered to the class. This allows teachers to become aware of any problems that might be emerging and to monitor children who may be particularly vulnerable. A strong, working relationship between the school and SBFC practitioner and community-based services will facilitate referral and early interventions for children experiencing mental health difficulties.

Screening is often used in a stepped-care model which provides Tier 1: Universal psychoeducation; Tier 2: Teacher development and parenting programs; Tier 3: Screening for symptoms of distress; and Tier 4: Targeted interventions for those with significant distress (Le Brocque et al, 2017; McDermott & Cobham, 2014). A number of brief screening questionnaires are available from the International Society for Traumatic Stress Studies (ISTSS: https://istss.org/clinical-resources/child-trauma-assessments). These questionnaires are quick and easy to administer, easy to score, and are free to download. They provide an effective reference point to monitor child trauma symptoms over time. A number of interventions have been trialed and have found success in treating children and their families following disasters such as Cognitive Behavioral Intervention for Trauma in Schools (CBITS) (Jaycox et al., 2012) and Bounce Back (http://bouncebackprogram.org/).

Step 3: Modifying the classroom environment

There are a number of strategies to manage the post-disaster environment. Keeping in mind how trauma may impact on the children's mental health and learning and memory, these strategies help teachers control behavior and help students to gain control over the emotional impact of the disaster. These accommodations include setting clear expectations for classroom and school behavior; building social support; providing safe spaces for a child to withdraw when emotions become overwhelming; providing increased choice about learning and classroom activities; anticipating difficult times and preparing children for situations that may trigger stress reactions; and building on strengths and positives.

Step 3A: Clear boundaries

During times of recovery, it is important for children to return to normal routines and functioning. As part of this, it is important that teachers do not change expectations relating to schoolwork and behavior, rather that they make adjustments, where necessary, to the way they deliver classroom activities.

Acting out and misbehaving is one behavior that children and adolescents may respond to natural disasters and traumatic events. It is important for teachers to set and maintain clear expectations of behaviors and to communicate these to the young person. Generally, young people respond well to clear boundaries and routines which involve firm and clear limits. It will assist young people if behavior expectations are clearly stated (and implemented) with consequences for misbehavior focused on natural consequences with a restorative focus. The emphasis should be on consistent and logical consequences, rather than punitive consequences.

Acting out and misbehaving are common reactions to trauma but also generally a common behavior in young people. Therefore, it is always important to explore the origins of the problem behavior before jumping to conclusions about diagnosis or implementing consequences or discipline strategies. The fact that the young person might be acting out (even a year after the trauma) does not mean that the young person is demonstrating a behavioral disorder (e.g., attention-deficit hyperactivity disorder or conduct disorder).

Even the most disruptive behaviors can be expressions of trauma-related anxiety. It is important to implement consequences when expectations of behaviors are not met. However, the emphasis should be on logical consequences and restorative practice with a trauma-informed lens, rather than

---

Box 6.3 Concentration difficulties

If children are having difficulty maintaining concentration, it may be necessary to reduce the instruction time according to age and development and include multiple short breaks. Physical activity that is brief, such as standing up and shaking out, quick tidying up activities, or changing the desk arrangement in the classroom, can help to stimulate and maintain attention and concentration. Down-regulating activities, such as mindfulness, yoga, breathing exercises, or quiet focus to slow breathing, also support the maintenance of concentration.

Children who are quiet or do not exhibit externalizing behaviors may also be experiencing distress and these children often go unrecognized in the post-disaster classroom environment. Gaps in knowledge due to concentration difficulties and memory processing problems may not emerge until many years later.

Box 6.4 Managing behavior in the classroom

Managing behavior in the classroom – some examples

A child who hasn't completed a homework activity can be asked to remain with the teacher at lunch time to complete homework. A conversation with parent might be beneficial to explore challenges to completion to trouble-shoot difficulties collaboratively.

A child who refused to share with another child is asked to give the toy to the other child and apologize for their behavior.

A young person who has used offensive language may be requested to apologize for the disrespect and be coached in expressing frustration in words that express an "When you ..., I feel..., I would like it if...."

---

unrelated consequences. Responding with care and compassion is more in keeping with trauma-informed teaching pedagogy. The relationships that support the child with boundaries and positive, realistic expectations will guide the child to meet the expectations for behaviors that enhance learning.

Step 3B: Helping students to build a support system

One of the most distressing outcomes following traumatic events and natural disasters is the loss of social support and community. It is important for children and teenagers to build a strong support system. Sometimes, it is important to make sure that they have multiple support sources at school as well as at home.

Teachers can help young people to identify who they can talk to about difficult situations and any problems they are having. Some children may not be aware of supports available such as the SBFC practitioner, school psychologist, student welfare co-ordinator, or youth worker. Teachers may also be able to help students identify other school staff they feel comfortable talking to, should their classroom teacher not be available. For example, they may feel comfortable talking to their sports teacher, the principal, or school nurse. All school staff can be included in the understanding of trauma-informed practice and how to assist when a student approaches for help. The SBFC can play a key role in supporting school staff with this provision for students.

Many schools have a 'buddy' system. Often teachers may implement a buddy system following trauma whereby students are paired with other students to ensure that each student has a support person while at school. Often, this is implemented in the hope that children are not left alone, to facilitate connections between children teaching them social skills, and to provide sources of emotional support to each child. The buddy system may be more appropriate for younger children but teachers might want to think of ways in which teenagers can be encouraged to maintain their own social support systems, perhaps through clubs or sports teams.

Box 6.5 Making connections – some examples

Invite the SBFC practitioner into the classroom to participate in some learning activities. These may or may not be related to the disaster experienced by the school community.

The Librarian may check in with a child if the family has been able to return to their home following the disaster. This may create an opportunity for the child to discuss some of the challenges they are experiencing.

The sports teacher may find a student unable or unwilling to participate in the activity. The student may be engaged to help set up and pack away activities. Use the time they are with the sport teacher to explore what might be happening which may provide support for the child to discuss their worries and concerns.

Box 6.6 Building social support

Some examples for younger children

Allocate a buddy from the same class to accompany the child to the school canteen or bathroom. You may allocate some time in class for the buddies to meet and discuss an issue. This can be problem-based to help solve a problem or a discussion around the class book they are reading or challenges completing homework. Paired activities through curriculum delivery can be effective for learning and facilitates relationships.

Allocate a buddy from the senior classes for a child in a younger class. This creates social connections and facilitates the development of feelings of responsibility and leadership in older children. Once again, allowing students to meet in the classroom for a brief period facilitates these social connections.

Some examples for teenagers

There are many opportunities for teenagers to assume leadership roles within the school. These roles are particularly important following disasters and school trauma. These may be at a class level or across the grades. In some schools, these roles can rotate across the school terms. In others, they may be fixed for the school year such as the School Captain or House Captain roles.

Roles include helping with the disaster response such as compiling lists of replacement belongings needed by families, fund-raising committees, or developing disaster plans. Other roles may include helping with the clean-up and recovery efforts.

Asking individual students to help in any of these roles builds self-esteem and confidence as well as a sense of leadership and mastery.

Although the buddy system might be most useful immediately following the traumatic event, it may still be beneficial to consider for some children over time. Some children have ongoing difficulties, some may not like to be alone, some may require ongoing emotional support, and others may simply enjoy team environments. A buddy or support system might be useful for various classroom activities (e.g., going to the bathroom, relaxation time, and group activities). Over time, buddy systems can be turned into more 'support' or 'companionship/friendship' systems, whereby children are encouraged to use their buddy as sources of emotional or academic support.

Step 3C: Creating safe spaces within the classroom and school

All classrooms can benefit from having safe spaces that are specifically for young people to use when they are experiencing difficulties in the classroom. For some classes, this might be a specific room adjoining the classroom, whereas for others, this might be on seats outside the classroom. Adolescents may even request permission to visit the student welfare co-ordinator or school nurse.

Safe spaces can be used when children or adolescents need some time to calm themselves or self-regulate or if the teacher needs some time to talk to students individually. Placing some comforting children's books or quiet activities such as memory games and puzzles in this space will give children something else to focus on while they take some time out from the demands of the classroom. A comforting environment such as child size chairs, cushions, or soft carpeted areas make the space welcoming and comfortable. Consider decorating with muted soft colors or softer lighting to make the space more calming. Some classrooms provide an enclosed private space like a den or curtained off area.

It may be necessary to set up procedures for the young person to gain permission to leave the classroom or visit the relaxation space. This may be through nonverbal requests (e.g., placing a particular color card on the corner of their desk to indicate to the teacher that they would like some time out, 'relaxation' time, or a space to de-stress and down-regulate).

Step 3D: Provide choices – regain control

Often, during the traumatic event, young people may feel a sense of power-lessness or loss of control. Traumatic events are usually beyond the control of the young person, as are the consequences that follow. One strategy that might be useful is to provide young people with choices or input into some classroom activities. Giving children choices and involving them in decision making can help restore their feeling of control and self-empowerment.

Box 6.7 Involvement in decision making

Ways in which children can be involved in decision making

Providing suggestions regarding fun classroom activities or class rewards.

Choosing between various classroom activities (e.g., books to read, science experiments to perform).

Choosing between assignment topics (for older children, choosing between different essay topics).

Helping to select and organize fund-raising activities.

Box 6.8 Preparing for triggers: example teacher instructions

Example teacher instructions for children aged 5–12 years

"Today the inspectors will be here to test the fire alarms. As you know, the alarms can be very loud.

When was the last time we heard the alarms? That was very scary, wasn't it?

It is going to be very loud again. But we don't have to worry. There is no fire this time. You are safe.

Do you think you are going to be ok when the alarms go off?

What will we do when the alarm goes off?

We know they will just be testing and we are safe."

Step 3E: Prepare children and adolescents for situations which may trigger reactions

Some young people, although generally functioning well, might still be affected by sudden and significant events or triggers. It can be useful for teachers to warn or prepare children for any sudden events. For example, students may need to be warned about upcoming fire drills or testing of sirens. Teachers may also need to let children know if they are about to do anything sudden, like turning off the lights or making loud noises.

For older children and adolescents, it may be useful for teachers to anticipate upcoming events which may trigger responses. For example, teachers may be able to prepare students in advance regarding upcoming assignments or activities that may trigger emotions or memories of the events (e.g., if an upcoming class includes discussion of natural disasters, science class which discusses concepts related to flooding, English class which involves investigation of news/disaster stories). In these instances, some young people might need to be given alternative activities they can participate in.

There is now extensive research to support the inclusion of disaster content in the curriculum to build knowledge and a sense of mastery. In some Australian schools, content on the role of bush fires in regenerating the Australian flora is incorporated into the curriculum. In Japan, students in primary schools investigate how to stabilize structures to make them earthquake proof. Consider how you can integrate knowledge around disasters often experienced in your region into your curriculum, particularly in relation to disaster preparation and resilience.

Step 3F: Anticipating difficult times – planning ahead

It is likely that children and adolescents may re-experience some aspects of the disaster or experience some distress at important milestones. Anniversaries of the event, birthdays of lost family members, and holiday times (Easter, Christmas, Mother's Day, Father's Day) can all be especially difficult for young people and their families. Consultation with the SBFC practitioner is critical for these times.

During these times, it is possible that the young person might demonstrate an intensification of emotional difficulties and problem behaviors. Some children may even develop new behaviors or experience new emotions that cause distress to the young person or class. Where possible, there may be an opportunity to plan ahead and pre-empt these occasions and provide additional support where appropriate. The SBFC practitioner has expertise in this area that will be of assistance for the school community.

For anniversaries, strategies may need to be discussed with other teachers and administrators. Consider consulting with family members to strengthen

---

Box 6.9 Insensitive commemoration

Insensitive commemoration – an example

At the one-year anniversary of devastating fires in Australia, families reported being distressed with the arrival of government officials, the emergency services helicopters, and the media.

The communities felt that they had not been sufficiently consulted on these activities and felt that this was intrusive and insensitive. They expressed anger at the lack of progress for recovery efforts and in settling insurance claims.

The anniversary activities further traumatized the community and were certainly perceived as not providing support at this emotional time.

Box 6.10 How to plan for anniversaries

Consider setting up an Anniversary Committee to consultation with the families and communities impacted by the disaster.

Include children, families, members of the school community, and businesses on the committee.

Consider who else need to be included. For example, some families may have been forced to move away from the area. Can you invite them back for the commemoration? Is there any funding to help bring them home?

Decide on how you would like to commemorate the disaster. Will it be a religious service? Will it be a celebration focusing on the progress in the community since the disaster? Will it coincide with the opening of a new building or commencement of a returning business or service.

Be aware that emotions may be heightened at this time. Provide lots of time and space for the community to come together to support each other.

Teachers may also need to be sensitive to individual students who may require extra support at this time.

If there is no community commemoration, what can your class do to remember the disaster or trauma. Consider making cards and sticking them up on the board. Consider having a ceremony to remember lost friends and families. Can you do an activity such as writing and story or poem to celebrate what you have achieved in the last year.

---

home to school relationships. It is important to consider the wishes of the families affected by the trauma. Far too often, government representatives and ministers arrive with the media at anniversaries of the trauma without consultation with the community which may be distressing for all concerned.

Teachers and schools may plan events to coincide with anniversaries, with an emphasis on survival stories and positive events since the trauma. The growth and rebuilding of a community creates greater cohesion through the shared experience.

Step 3G: Focus on strengths and positives

For many families, there can be a long time following the trauma where the focus remains on the traumatic event, getting their lives back together, and dealing with the problematic reactions that follow. As a result, it can be very easy to focus on the negative things going on in the young person's life, including problems managing emotions and behaviors. Often, little attention is paid to the positive behaviors or coping strategies the young person is showing.

Providing positive acknowledgment or praise for things the young person has done well not only makes the young person feel good about themselves but also demonstrates to the young person what type of behaviors they should

---

Box 6.11 Focus on strengths – little hero

One little girl, five years old, looked out her front door and saw the fire racing toward the house. Her mother was busy trying to get through on the phone to her father.

The little girl was able to tell her mother the fire was close. The little family barely escaped with their lives.

Following these tragic fires in South Australia, the little hero was applauded for raising the alarm for her mother, saving herself, her mother, and her new baby sister.

---

continue to engage in. Acknowledging and recognizing strengths, positive behaviors, and coping strategies can be a particularly important and easy strategy for teachers to practice and implement. This can be as simple as offering praise to students when you notice a positive behavior or personal strength they have developed or demonstrated.

Multicultural considerations

The above strategies have been presented across the world and appear to adapt across many cultures. Our work internationally has found that children may present different symptoms of distress. For example, in South Africa, SBFC practitioners reported diurnal enuresis (daytime wetting) as a significant problem for children living in the informal settlements. In Japan, pediatric psychologists reported school refusal as one of the main challenges for children displaced following the Fukushima disaster. Despite differing presentation of distress symptoms, most of the adaptations to teaching space can be implemented universally keeping in mind cultural and religious appropriateness.

Many resources have been translated into a range of languages such as the Disastershock resources (www.disastershock.com) and the Child and Adolescent Trauma Screen (Sancher et al., 2017). The International Society for Traumatic Stress Studies website (www.ISTSS.org) provides information and resources in multiple languages and also provides contact details for sister organizations operating locally.

Conclusion

Disasters impact children, their families, and the school community in multiple, complex ways and may have a lasting deleterious impact on learning and achievement. The emotional impact may be seen during and immediately after the event; however, the impact on learning may not emerge for some time, even years.

We have explored how schools can help students cope with the stress of a major disaster by describing a number of modifications that can be made to the classroom environment to ensure students remain safe, to help build their social support systems, to create safe spaces for students to take time out from the immediate classroom activity and reinforce their coping capacity, to help to re-establish their sense of control and mastery, build coping skills for dealing with difficult times, and building on strengths.

One of the most powerful activities teachers can do is to monitor student trauma symptoms using quick screening questionnaires available through the International Society for Traumatic Stress Studies (https://istss.org/clinical-resources/child-trauma-assessments). SBFC practitioners also have access to clinical tools to assess and monitor symptoms.

Stepped-care is a hierarchical approach that depends on the needs of the individual and the matching of services to supporting young people after a natural disaster (Cohen et al., 2017; McDermott & Cobham, 2014). This approach provides tiered support to those who need it and prevents overloading mental health.

Targeted early interventions for children and their families may mitigate the effects of trauma and the potential of academic decline. Effective support for students has been shown to enhance the protective balance for adaptive trauma responses and recovery and may mitigate difficulties with social, emotional, and academic functioning of students (Berkowitz et al., 2011; Friedman et al., 2014; McDermott & Cobham, 2014; Goldman et al., 2015).

Box 6.12 A stepped-care approach example

A stepped-care approach after devastating floods

After the floods of 2010/2011 in Queensland, Australia, a stepped-care approach was provided based on evidence that this potentially provides the level of care according to the level of need (McDermott & Cobham, 2014).

At the base of this intervention was communication via podcasts and online information; supported by focused communication to communities most impacted by disaster.

The second tier provided teachers with professional development to understand the trauma response of students and how they could assist.

A parenting program tailored for post-disaster was also offered in this second tier of support.

As it had been established that only a minority of young people would experience severe response to the disaster, children with significant distress identified (via screening) were offered support in the form of cognitive behavioral therapy (Cohen et al., 2017).

We have explored ways in which disaster and experiences of trauma can impact children, their families, and the school community and can impact on cognitive processing, memory, concentration, and learning. We have presented a range of adjustments to teaching practice and the classroom which are designed to support children, their family, and the school community. To implement, these adjustments require minimal effort for teachers and SBFC practitioners; however, it will result in better mental health and well-being during and after these extreme events.

Resources

The Child and Adolescent Trauma Screen https://istss.org/clinical-resources/child-trauma-assessments/child-and-adolescent-trauma-screen-(cats)

The Child and Adolescent Trauma Screen (CATS) questionnaire is a brief, freely accessible screening instrument based on the DSM-5 criteria for Posttraumatic Stress Disorder (PTSD). It is a measure of potentially traumatic events and of posttraumatic stress symptoms (Sancher et al., 2017). The CATS can be administered as a self-report or as an interview and is appropriate for pre-schoolers, children and adolescents. There is a self-report measure (for children aged 7–17 years), and two caregiver versions (for ages 3–6 years and 7–17 years). The interview format may be preferable with younger children or youth with reading comprehension challenges. The CATS has 15 items measuring traumatic events, 20 items measuring DSM-5 PTSD symptoms, and 5 items measuring psychosocial functioning, and can be administered in approximately 15 minutes. It is available in several languages, including German, Norwegian, Spanish, Swedish, Arbabic, Dari, Farsi, Paschtu, Tigrinya, Turkish. More information and access to each version is available through the above link.

References

Berkowitz, S.J., Stover, C.S., & Marans, S.R. (2011). The Child and Family Traumatic Stress Intervention: Secondary Prevention for Youth at Risk of Developing PTSD. *Journal of Child Psychology and Psychiatry*, 52(6), 676–685. https://doi.org/10.1111/j.1469-7610.2010.02321.x

Bounce Back http://bouncebackprogram.org/

Cohen, G.H., Tamrakar, S., Lowe, S., Sampson, L., Ettman, C., Linas, B., Ruggiero, K., & Galea, S. (2017). Comparison of Simulated Treatment and Cost-Effectiveness of a Stepped Care Case-Finding Intervention vs Usual Care for Posttraumatic Stress Disorder After a Natural Disaster. *JAMA Psychiatry*, 74(12), 1251–1258. https://doi.org/10.1001/jamapsychiatry.2017.3037

Early Trauma & Grief Network https://earlytraumagrief.anu.edu.au/

Friedman, M., Keane, T., & Resick, P. (2014). *Handbook of PTSD: Science and Practice*. New York: The Guilford Press.

Goldman, E.E., Bauer, D., Newman, D.L., Kalka, E., Lochman, J.E., Silverman, W.K., Jensen, P.S., Curry, J., Stark, K., Wells, K.C., & Bannon, W.M. (2015). A School-Based Post-Katrina Therapeutic Intervention. *Administration and Policy in Mental Health and Mental Health Services Research*, 42(3), 363–372. https://doi.org/10.1007/s10488-014-0576-y

International Society for Traumatic Stress Studies (ISTSS) https://istss.org/clinical-resources/child-trauma-assessments

Jaycox, L.H., Kataoka, S.H., Stein, B.D., Langley, A.K., & Wong, M. (2012). Cognitive Behavioral Intervention for Trauma in Schools. *Journal of Applied School Psychology*, 28(3), 239–255.

Le Brocque, R., De Young, A., Montague, G., Pocock, S., March, S., Triggell, N., Rabaa, C., & Kenardy, J. (2017). Schools and Natural Disaster Recovery: The Unique and Vital Role That Teachers and Education Professionals Play in Ensuring the Mental Health of Students Following Natural Disasters. *Journal of Psychologists and Counsellors in Schools*, 27(1), 263–268. https://doi.org/10.1017/jgc.2016.17

Luthar, S.S., & Cicchetti, D. (2000). The Construct of Resilience: Implications for Interventions and Social Policies. *Developmental Psychopathology*, 12, 857–885. https://doi-org.ezproxy.library.uq.edu.au/10.1111/1467-8624.00164

McDermott, B.M., & Cobham, V.E. (2014). A Stepped-Care Model of post-Disaster Child and Adolescent Mental Health Service Provision. *European Journal of Psychotraumatology*, 5(1), 24294. https://doi.org/10.3402/ejpt.v5.24294

Sachser, C., Berliner, L., Risch, E., Rosner, R., Birkeland, M.S., Eilers, R., Hafstad, G.S., Pfeiffer, E., Plener, P.L., & Jensen, T.K. (2022). The child and Adolescent Trauma Screen 2 (CATS-2) - validation of an instrument to measure DSM-5 and ICD-11 PTSD and complex PTSD in children and adolescents. *European Journal of Psychotraumatology*, 13(2), 2105580. doi: 10.1080/20008066.2022.2105580.

The DisasterShock Global Response Team https://www.disastershock.com/

7 How to lower stress and strengthen student executive functions during crisis and disasters

Celina Korzeniowski

Overview

This chapter helps school-based family counseling (SBFC) practitioners understand how the emotional distress associated with crisis and disasters impacts children's cognitive and socioemotional development and provides them with strategies for school-based interventions. The key role of teachers in helping children to face emotional distress is highlighted and a set of evidence-based techniques for teachers are detailed.

Background

A disaster, whether natural, technological, or man-made, is an event causing significant disruption to a community, beyond their capacity to cope, and increases people's risk for physical and psychological harm (Berger et al., 2018). Exposure to disasters can have serious and long-lasting effects on children. When children face a disaster, they experience anxiety and concerns related to danger and safety. They fear for their integrity and that of their loved ones. Children may experience behavioral changes, physical symptoms, and emotional distress (Giraudo, 2021; Pfefferbaum et al., 2014a).

Although stress is a natural and adaptive psychophysiological response to a traumatic event which allows people to protect their lives and triggers a coping process, if this response becomes chronic over time, it can significantly impact child health (Gerardo-Luna et al., 2019). The signs and symptoms of emotional stress in children are poor appetite, nervousness, somatizations (i.e. headaches, body complaints, and tiredness), sleeping difficulties or nightmares, regressive behavior, aggressiveness, difficulty paying attention, avoidance of scary situations, withdrawal from friends or activities, and intrusive memories of what happened (National Child Traumatic Stress, 2008).

Children's chronic stress can impair adaptive coping and negatively affect their academic performance, cognitive functioning, and social and emotional development. The literature documents that a significant percentage of children exposed to a disaster present post-traumatic stress disorder (PTSD), anxiety, depression, behavior problems, and grief (Pfefferbaum et al., 2014a). Likewise, it has been observed that children with emotional distress have

DOI: 10.4324/9781003201977-9

lower school performance, higher absenteeism, and a higher dropout rate (Vilaplana-Pérez et al., 2020).

Regarding cognitive development, stress affects the immune and hormonal systems and can raise the risk of neuro-inflammation, increasing the possibility of damaging the Central Nervous System (CNS) and altering cognitive functioning (Kempuraj et al., 2020). In line with this approach, there have been reports of an increase in attention and memory problems, increased irritability and alterations in executive functions (EFs) in children suffering traumatic stress (Abdulah et al., 2021; Schwartz et al., 2021).

EFs are a set of high-order cognitive abilities that control behaviors, emotions, and cognitions which are necessary to achieve goals, solve problems, and provide adaptive responses to novel or complex situations (Diamond, 2013). EFs drive the ability to act with purpose and in a self-regulating manner in the various contexts of social interaction. Self-regulation skills play a key role in facing novel situations, such as a disaster; however, environmental stress can negatively affect them (Hackman et al., 2010).

Thousands of children in the world are currently suffering from emotional stress associated with a traumatic event: the pandemic caused by the coronavirus. The pandemic spread throughout the world, causing millions of illnesses and deaths. The measures adopted to prevent the spread of the virus have generated drastic changes in people's lives.

Children, in particular, have experienced significant changes in their daily routines and activities, as well as long periods of confinement and social isolation. Recent studies have documented the impact of the pandemic on children. At the moment, detriments to the well-being, quality of life, and health of children have been reported, associated with an increase in symptoms of anxiety, depression, as well as an increase in unhealthy lifestyle habits and sleep disorders (Schwartz et al., 2021). Regarding the closure of schools and implementation of remote education, it is estimated that it will generate academic delays and school dropouts (Kuhfeld et al., 2021). Likewise, prolonged confinement has restricted children's peer relationships and participation in group activities, which may impact socioemotional, cognitive, and linguistic development trajectories in children (Cameron & Tenenbaum, 2021). Also, there have been reports of increase in child maltreatment during the periods of quarantine and lockdown (Cuartas, 2020). The COVID-19 pandemic continues to present many problematic consequences for society, and children are one of the most vulnerable populations. In this global scenario, SBFC practitioners need to increase their resources to assist children in order to lessen the impact of the consequences of the pandemic on their integral development.

Family and school are the two institutions that have the greatest impact on the development of children, and consequently, they are areas in which the SBFC practitioner can intervene, strengthening resources to help children in crisis. According to the SBFC metamodel (Gerrard & Soriano, 2020), school interventions can be a key tool to achieve this goal.

Schools provide a natural venue for conducting public health activities such as delivering psychoeducation and social support, assessing and monitoring affected children, and delivering trauma-informed interventions. A trauma-informed school is defined as one where all parties involved recognize and respond to the impact of traumatic stress on children, caregivers, educators, and service providers.

SBFC practitioners play a key role in assisting schools in adopting a trauma-informed approach. SBFC practitioners may infuse and sustain trauma awareness, knowledge, and skills into their school environment. Also, SBFC practitioners will train educators and school personnel to maximize children's physical and psychological safety, facilitate the recovery or adjustment of the child and family, and support their ability to learn and to thrive.

Evidence-based support

In a systematic review of child disaster mental health intervention studies, it was observed that 70.8% of the interventions were carried out at the school site (Pfefferbaum et al., 2014a). At wellness-focused school-based programs, teachers, trained paraprofessionals, and school personnel administered the interventions. The role of the teacher is highlighted for their familiarity with the children and ability to insert the interventions into school activities. Teachers can carry out evaluations, apply interventions to reduce stress, and monitor children, identifying progress and difficulties.

The study reported that school-based interventions have used stress intervention and cognitive behavioral techniques which focused on teaching children coping skills to address anger, loss, fears, and other emotions. Most of the interventions have achieved favorable results, helping children to reduce PTSD symptoms, depression, and anxiety, improving their functioning and behavior problems (Pfefferbaum et al., 2014b).

One of the advantages of the intervention delivered in a school setting is the possibility of using a group format. Group crisis interventions have been reported to have benefits compared to individual ones, including efficiency, reduced costs, access to a large number of children, and the potential to lessen the stigma associated with mental health services and social components of the crisis. For example, Brown et al. (2006) implemented a trauma school-based intervention to help schoolchildren to reduce stress and depression symptoms associated with the terrorist attack on the twin towers that occurred on September 11, 2001 in the World Trade Center, in New York City. The classroom intervention was applied for ten weeks and used the cognitive behavioral therapy approach. Sixty-three children from 8 to 13 years of age participated. Following the classroom intervention, children who continued to meet criteria for PTSD were offered an individualized intervention. The main results indicated that depression improved in children who received the classroom intervention but it worsened in those who received the individualized intervention. The authors reported that the social support inherent in the classroom intervention was essential to improve depression in children.

In sum, school-based crisis interventions are one of the most widely used interventions in assisting children suffering from traumatic stress associated with a disaster or crisis. These interventions show effectiveness in increasing children's coping skills, reducing stress, fostering positive relationships, increasing attendance, promoting children's well-being and engagement with learning, by creating a trauma-sensitive learning environment.

Procedure

In line with the evidence-based crisis intervention delivered in school settings, a pool of strategies and techniques has been selected to help SBFC practitioners support students suffering from traumatic stress. Considering that educators are in an excellent position to help children after disasters, the strategies are designed to be mediated by teachers. A set of strategies to improve stress coping and strengthening self-regulation skills among students are emphasized.

Step 1. **Take care of yourself.** Taking care of others requires taking care of yourself first. Teachers assisting in a crisis have often been exposed to the disaster themselves, so they may experience high levels of emotional distress, anxiety, concerns about their students, as well as symptoms of secondary traumatic stress. Therefore, the SBFC practitioner can provide support and help educators to work through emotional stress, worries, and difficulties using the following strategies:
- Monitoring stress level. Teachers should identify their stress level and gain insight into any areas where they may be struggling.
- Practicing self-compassion.
- Creating a daily routine.
- Using social support as needed.
- Learning about disasters.
- Fostering social connections with loved ones.
- Meditating or going for walks.
- Being a healthy model. When teachers take care of themselves, they are modeling how children can take care of themselves.

Step 2. **Identify students' symptoms of stress.** To identify student stress, a teacher should use teachers' prior knowledge of students' behavior to identify changes in their behavior associated with stress trauma and identify child risk factors – isolation, domestic violence, episodes of depression. Some students may be more vulnerable than others to a disaster (i.e. children from disadvantaged backgrounds) and need further intervention during crisis. SBFC practitioners may help educators to create a checklist of stress symptoms and use it to guide their observation of students' behavior in the classroom and follow-up signs of students' stress to verify their magnitude and duration over time.

Step 3. **Foster a trauma-informed learning environment.** Creating a learning environment that recognizes the emotional consequences of the disaster involves reinforcing a series of actions and strategies that promote support, a sense of safety, connection, and predictability for students.

3.1 *Create a structured and predictable learning environment:* Exposure to a disaster creates feelings of unpredictability and uncertainty. That is why it is important to create a school environment that allows students to regain a sense of stability and foresight. Teachers may help students by:

- *Creating a school routine:* Assist students in the use of a school schedule and calendar, so that they organize and plan their daily and weekly activities. It is important to create rituals to start and end the class to regain a sense of foresight. For example, teachers may share with their students one grateful moment, give a positive message, or practice a mindful activity before or after checking assignments.

- *Maintaining clear and fluid communication:* Students should feel that they can communicate with their teachers with ease. Also, it is important to provide information as clearly as possible, and in student-manageable amounts, using visual outlines, images, and reminders to make it easier for students to get the information.

- *Being flexible*: Adapt the tasks and assessments. Address academic and behavioral issues with empathy and support. During a crisis, students can feel that assignments are more overwhelming. Present instructions in smaller bites, when necessary, and encourage students to ask clarifying questions.

- *Communicating the school's emergency response plan:* After a disaster, students may not want to go to school for fear of a new disaster event and of being separated from their family. That is why teachers have to communicate to students and their families that the school has a plan to handle the disaster. It is important to specify how students' physical and psychological health will be maintained, how the school is going to connect with families, and how any future problems will be handled.

3.2 *Strengthen relationships*: Restricted contact with loved ones and other people is very frequent in a disaster and is one of the greatest stressors for human beings. That is why it is important to (1) let students know that they can discuss their concerns and fears with teachers, counselors, or parents; (2) provide moments when students can enjoy the company of their peers; (3) consider putting students together in small groups to work on projects or activities; and (4) encourage students to connect with their friends and loved ones.

behavior in the classroom and follow-up signs of students' stress to verify their magnitude and duration over time.

Step 3. **Foster a trauma-informed learning environment.** Creating a learning environment that recognizes the emotional consequences of the disaster involves reinforcing a series of actions and strategies that promote support, a sense of safety, connection, and predictability for students.

3.1 *Create a structured and predictable learning environment:* Exposure to a disaster creates feelings of unpredictability and uncertainty. That is why it is important to create a school environment that allows students to regain a sense of stability and foresight. Teachers may help students by:

- *Creating a school routine:* Assist students in the use of a school schedule and calendar, so that they organize and plan their daily and weekly activities. It is important to create rituals to start and end the class to regain a sense of foresight. For example, teachers may share with their students one grateful moment, give a positive message, or practice a mindful activity before or after checking assignments.
- *Maintaining clear and fluid communication:* Students should feel that they can communicate with their teachers with ease. Also, it is important to provide information as clearly as possible, and in student-manageable amounts, using visual outlines, images, and reminders to make it easier for students to get the information.
- *Being flexible*: Adapt the tasks and assessments. Address academic and behavioral issues with empathy and support. During a crisis, students can feel that assignments are more overwhelming. Present instructions in smaller bites, when necessary, and encourage students to ask clarifying questions.
- *Communicating the school's emergency response plan:* After a disaster, students may not want to go to school for fear of a new disaster event and of being separated from their family. That is why teachers have to communicate to students and their families that the school has a plan to handle the disaster. It is important to specify how students' physical and psychological health will be maintained, how the school is going to connect with families, and how any future problems will be handled.

3.2 *Strengthen relationships*: Restricted contact with loved ones and other people is very frequent in a disaster and is one of the greatest stressors for human beings. That is why it is important to (1) let students know that they can discuss their concerns and fears with teachers, counselors, or parents; (2) provide moments when students can enjoy the company of their peers; (3) consider putting students together in small groups to work on projects or activities; and (4) encourage students to connect with their friends and loved ones.

Deep breathing. Focusing our attention on breath helps us feel calm and relaxed. The technique is simple and consists in modeling to students how to breathe slowly and deeply. In the classroom or on the playground, ask students to sit comfortably. Then, breathe slowly in through your nose for three seconds, hold your breath for three seconds, and, then, breathe out slowly for three seconds. Repeat this several times so students get the idea. Then, ask students to breathe with you. You can ask them to count each breath silently or to place their hand on their abdomen to feel the breath in their body. This helps students focus their attention during the exercise. Repeat this exercise with your students for a minute or two. Then reflect with your students on the experience. Talk about how they felt, what they felt in their mind and body, and how breathing has helped them. End the exercise by asking them to draw a picture of the experience or to write a word or phrase that helps them feel calm. Once the students know this technique, teachers can use it to start or end a class, in transitions, or at times when they perceive that students are restless, anxious, or stressed.

Imagining a place of calm and well-being. This technique consists in imagining a place in which we have felt calm and relaxed. Ask students to close their eyes for a few moments and to imagine that place. It could be any place in which they have felt relaxed and calm, which could be the beach, a park, their garden, or their room. Instruct them to use deep breathing while imagining that place. Also, guide their imagination by telling them to focus their attention on some sound or object in the image. Talk to them about how they felt and what they felt in their body and mind. Let them know that this technique can be used when they feel tense or stressed.

Reframing negative thoughts. This technique helps students see something positive in a situation that they consider negative. The teacher can start by taking some negative thoughts of their own and showing them how to reformulate them. For example, "people who get sick from coronavirus die." You can rephrase it by saying, "if people are vaccinated, use social distance, wear masks and sanitize their hands, it is very likely that they will not contract the disease." Encourage students to identify a negative thought and share it. Help them rephrase it. This technique's goal is to show students that their thinking is partially true, but that they have overlooked positive aspects of the situation. This technique helps students reduce their tension and strengthen their sense of hope.

Step 5. Strategies to foster executive functions

Learning to face a crisis implies putting self-regulation capabilities into play. Hence, it is necessary to embed specific activities that foster children's EFs into educational practices.

Improving attention performance. Attention is one of the cognitive functions that is most affected by stress, and consequently, schoolchildren will experience difficulties in focusing and sustaining their attention. Therefore, the following are recommended:

- Observing the students attentional process to identify what captures their attention and what types of activities help them to stay focused longer;
- Varying the stimuli and teaching methods;
- Providing clear instructions;
- Shortening the duration of activities and introducing breaks; and
- Encouraging self-assessment of attention.

Improving inhibitory control. During a disaster, children must learn new rules of behavior and this can be a unique opportunity to promote inhibitory control. Measures could include:

- Placing posters, visual signs, reminders to facilitate the internalization of the new rules; using the role-playing technique to exemplify the new norms of behavior – for example, during the COVID pandemic, a group of students could dramatize the maintenance of social distance and the use of the mask in different scenarios: at recess, in the school canteen, in class, etc., and how children can play an active role in their compliance;
- Fostering initiative: educators are likely to encounter children with difficulty starting tasks, so it is recommended that they use activities that increase motivation. These activities can include playing a game at the beginning of class, doing stretching activities, having a special welcome greeting;
- Carrying out activities that allow students to reflect on their behavior and emotions: self-awareness, self-expression, and self-control techniques can be used;
- Using relaxation techniques.

Improving working memory. Working memory plays a critical role in learning and could be stimulated in the following ways:

- Starting a new topic by updating content learned;
- Practicing mental calculations;
- Using comprehensive reading techniques, such as summarizing the main ideas of the text in a paragraph or making a diagram with the central ideas; and
- Proposing playful activities, in which children must memorize multiple steps or actions to reach the goal.

Improving cognitive flexibility. Cognitive flexibility is an indicator of mental health and a valuable resource in dealing with changing situations:

- Modeling the use of flexibility in times of crisis by adapting tasks, activities, and evaluation to changing circumstances;
- Encouraging children to think of different approaches to problems;

- Training perspective taking;
- Using problem-solving techniques; and
- Using brainstorming and role-playing.

Improving planning and organization abilities. Provide strategies for organizing school activities, planning time, and selecting materials. Suggestions include:

- Creating a monthly or weekly school calendar that helps children visualize deadlines for homework and important school activities;
- Assisting children in the use of the school planner and checking lists;
- Using route maps to diagram for students the stages of the tasks to be carried out, making it easier to see the whole and its parts;
- Encouraging students to carry out projects, with the teacher scaffolding students' planning skills by (a) helping students to identify goals; (b) dividing complex goals into sub-goals that are measurable, achievable, and specific; (c) helping students identify the steps necessary to achieve the goal, manage time, and identify the materials needed for each step; (d) helping them to foresee obstacles to reach goals and to identify the resources to overcome them; (e) helping them to monitor progress in achieving the goal; and (f) outlining the steps to achieve a goal by means of a graph.

Multicultural considerations

Designing crisis interventions requires the multicultural competence of the SBFC practitioner, in order to adjust the intervention to the characteristics of the target community. The cultural practices, values, beliefs, and sociocultural history of the school and families are critical to develop a crisis intervention that can be incorporated into children's daily activities.

If the teacher is responsible for applying the intervention, the SBFC practitioner must be aware of and understand the sociocultural background of the teacher, attend to their race, ethnicity, religious beliefs, cultural background, and gender, so that they can find a simple and inclusive language that allows the SBFC practitioner to transfer the knowledge and strategies to the teacher.

SBFC practitioners must be aware of children's cultural characteristics, such as acculturation, language proficiency, socioeconomic level, and sociocultural history. Also, it is important to understand how children, families, and communities have coped with crisis or disasters. SBFC practitioners or teachers may encourage children to share how their community has dealt with the crisis, what resources they have used to face it, emphasizing that knowing how different communities have recovered from a disaster can help us all with new ideas.

Challenges and solutions

Crisis interventions have proven to be effective; however, some obstacles and challenges may arise in their application.

One of them refers to the school's view on the pertinence of delivering programs that promote mental health among children and staff. Not all institutions include these practices, and consequently, SBFC practitioners must advocate for the role of the school in assisting children who have been exposed to a disaster. SBFC practitioners should highlight the benefits of applying school-based crisis interventions and will play a key role in promoting links between the school and other health institutions specialized in assisting communities in a crisis.

The teacher plays a central role in assisting children suffering from the emotional stress. However, teachers may feel overwhelmed, tired, and stressed. On these occasions, the SBFC practitioner must assist teachers, generate support networks among educators, and request institutional support. Training teachers in the application of new practices in order to create a trauma-sensitive learning environment requires building bridges between mental health and education. To do this, the SBFC practitioner will have to use simple, clear, and culturally inclusive language to favor the transfer of new knowledge and strategies to educators. Teachers must understand the meaning of the intervention, have simple resources that indicate how to implement the strategies in the classroom, and feel supported by the SBFC practitioner when applying the intervention.

Conclusion

Children need to feel supported emotionally, socially, and academically to overcome the emotional stress associated with a disaster in order to thrive and learn. The scientific literature provides evidence of the effectiveness of school-based crisis interventions. In designing and implementing these crisis interventions, SBFC practitioners have a key role in assisting schools to adopt a school trauma-informed approach, by providing evidence-based knowledge and strategies to educators and staff. In line with this purpose, strategies and resources have been provided to help teachers reduce emotional stress and strengthen children's self-regulation skills. Based on their expertise and the cultural characteristics of the target community of the intervention, SBFC practitioners will be able to select those strategies that they consider most useful and can be expected to be stimulated to create new ones.

Resources

Creating, supporting, and sustaining trauma-informed schools: A system framework, by the National Child Traumatic Stress Network, Schools Committee. Los Angeles, CA, and Durham, NC. https://www.nctsn.org/sites/default/files/resources//creating_supporting_sustaining_trauma_informed_schools_a_systems_framework.pdf

This document illustrates the framework of a trauma-informed school and explains what areas are to be addressed when working towards a trauma-informed school.

Disastershock: How Schools Can Cope with the Emotional Stress of a Major Disaster A Manual for Principals and Teachers, by the Disastershock Educator Collaboration Team, Institute for School-Based Family Counseling, University of San Francisco, USA. https://www.disaster-shock.com/educators-disasters

This is an excellent resource providing hands-on, meaningful ideas that can equip schools to cope with disaster-related challenges. It describes coping strategies for school personnel, students, and the school-family community.

How schools can help students recover from traumatic experiences. A tool kit for supporting long-term recovery, by RAND Corporation, Pittsburgh, USA. https://www.rand.org/pubs/technical_reports/TR413.html

This excellent resource provides a compendium of programs for trauma recovery, classified by type of trauma, and explains how to obtain each program's manuals and other aids to implementation.

Psychological first aid for schools: Field operations guide, 2nd Edition, by the National Child Traumatic Stress Network. https://www.nctsn.org/sites/default/files/resources/pfa_for_schools_no_appendices.pdf

This document describes Psychological First Aid for Schools (PFA-S), an evidence-informed intervention model to assist students, families, school personnel, and school partners in the immediate aftermath of an emergency.

Trauma Informed School Strategies during COVID-19, by the National Child Traumatic Stress Network, Los Angeles, CA, and Durham, NC. https://www.nctsn.org/resources/trauma-informed-school-strategies-during-covid-19

This document describes how schools can adapt or transform their practices by using a trauma-informed approach to help children feel safe, supported, and ready to learn during the COVID crisis.

References

Abdulah, D.M., Abdulla, B.M.O. & Liamputtong, P. (2021). Psychological response of children to home confinement during COVID-19: A qualitative arts-based research. *International Journal of Social Psychiatry, 67*(6), 1–9.

Brown, E., McQuaid J., Farina, L., Ali, R., & Winnick-Gelles, A. (2006). Matching interventions to children's mental health needs: Feasibility and acceptability of a pilot school-based trauma intervention program. *Education and Treatment of Children, 29*, 257–286.

Berger, E., Carroll, M., Maybery, D. & Harrison, D. (2018). Disaster impacts on students and staff from a specialist, trauma-informed Australian school. *Journal of Child & Adolescent Trauma, 11*, 521–530.

Cameron, L. & Tenenbaum, H.R. (2021). Lessons from developmental science to mitigate the effects of the COVID-19 restrictions on social development. *Group Processes & Intergroup Relations, 24*(2), 231–236.

Cuartas, J. (2020). Heightened risk of child maltreatment amid the COVID-19 pandemic can exacerbate mental health problems for the next generation. *Psychological Trauma: Theory, Research, Practice, and Policy, 12*, 195–196.

Diamond, A. (2013). Executive functions. *Annual Review of Psychology, 64*(1), 135–168.

Gerardo-Luna,G.,Zambrano-Guerrero,C.,Ceballos-Mora,A.&Ojeda-Rosedo,E. (2019). Relationship between risk perception, stress and coping to extreme risks in a student community located in a volcanic threat zone. *Psicología desde el Caribe, 36*(2), 207–227.

Gerrard, B.A. & Soriano, M. (2020). School-based family counseling: The revolutionary paradigm. In B.A. Gerrard, M.J. Carter & D. Ribera (Eds.), *School-Based Family Counseling: A Interdisciplinary Practitioner's Guide* (pp. 1–15). New York: Routledge.

Giraudo, S. (2021). How to identify when students are stressed. In Disastershock Educators Collaboration Team (Eds.), *Disastershock: How Schools Can Cope with the Emotional Stress of a Major Disaster a Manual for Principals and Teachers* (pp. 19–23). San Francisco: Institute for School-Based Family Counseling.

Hackman, D.A., Farah, M.J. & Meaney, M.J. (2010). Socioeconomic status and the brain: Mechanistic insights from human and animal research. *Neuroscience, 11*(9), 651–659.

Kempuraj, D., Selvakumar, G.P., Ahmed, M.E., Raikwar, S.P., Thangavel, R, Khan, A., Zaheer, S.A., Iyer, S.S., Burton, C., James, D. & Zaheer, A. (2020). COVID-19, mast cells, cytokine storm, psychological stress, and neuroinflammation. *The Neuroscientist, 26*(5–6), 402–414.

Kuhfeld, M., Soland, J., Tarasawa, B., Johnson, A., Ruzek, E. & Liu, J. (2020). Projecting the potential impact of COVID-19 school closures on academic achievement. *Educational Researcher, 49*(8), 549–565. https://doi.org/10.3102/0013189X20965918

National Child Traumatic Stress (2008). *Child Trauma Toolkit for Educators.* Los Angeles, CA, and Durham, NC: National Center for Child Traumatic Stress.

Pfefferbaum, B., Sweeton, J., Newman, E., Varma, V., Nitiéma, P., Shaw, J., Chrisman, A. & Noffsinger, M. (2014a). Child disaster mental health interventions, part I. *Disaster Health, 2*(1), 46–57.

Pfefferbaum, B., Sweeton, J., Newman, E., Varma, V., Nitiéma, P., Shaw, J., Chrisman, A. & Noffsinger, M. (2014b). Child disaster mental health interventions, part II. *Disaster Health, 2*(1), 58–67. doi: 10.4161/dish.27535

Schwartz, K.D., Exner-Cortens, D., McMorris, C., Makarenko, C., Arnold, P., Van Bavel, M., Williams, S. & Canfield, R. (2021). COVID-19 and student well-being: Stress and mental health during return-to-school. *Canadian Journal of School Psychology, 36*(2), 166–185.

Vilaplana-Pérez, A., Sidorchuk, A., Pérez-Vigil, A., Brander, G., Isoumura, K., Hesselmark, E., Sevilla-Cermeño, L. … Fernández de la Cruz, L. (2020). Assessment of posttraumatic stress disorder and educational achievement in Sweden. *JAMA Network Open, 3*(12), 1–14.

8 Group counseling in schools following a crisis or disaster

Reshelle Marino and Wendy D. Rock

Overview

This chapter can help school-based family counseling (SBFC) practitioners understand how to facilitate family group counseling after school and assist students and their family members to cope with grief and loss, for example, in the aftermath of a natural disaster or following the death of a member of the school community. A four-step approach to implementing group sessions with students and their parent(s)/guardian(s) is detailed. Challenges and barriers are also explored.

Background

Disaster and crisis can impact a school community at any time. To respond appropriately and effectively, schools should make plans in advance. A crisis or disaster may take the form of a weather event such as flood, fire, tornado, hurricane, or earthquake; the death of a student or teacher; or even the extreme of a school shooting or terror event. These incidents can cause students to experience stress and grief, impact their sense of safety, and can have negative effects on their academic achievement and social and emotional development.

Small group counseling is one intervention SBFC practitioners can use to respond to the social and emotional needs of students following a crisis or disaster. Small group counseling allows for reaching a greater number of students, given the time constraints in a school setting. These small groups can address the effects that crisis and disaster cause, including stress and grief, and can help students regain a sense of safety, hope, control, and connection.

The SBFC model is particularly useful for addressing crisis and disaster in the school setting. Utilizing a multidisciplinary approach and involving caregivers in the provision of group counseling will benefit students and further increase their resilience in the aftermath of a crisis. Social support and community connectedness offer protective factors following a traumatic event. By involving the family in small groups following a crisis or disaster, the family can better support the student at home with coping skills and provide a sense of safety and connection that goes beyond the school building. In addition,

DOI: 10.4324/9781003201977-10

caregivers may be directly or indirectly impacted by the crisis or disaster themselves and involvement with the SBFC practitioner's small group counseling intervention not only supports their child's resilience and healing but can also support the caregivers' well-being. If a caregiver is being supported, it further supports the child's healthy development.

Procedure

While most SBFC practitioners (e.g., school counselors, social workers, and psychologists) are trained in crisis prevention and intervention, oftentimes they are tasked with managing multiple duties and roles within the school. There may be overlapping roles of SBFC practitioners, which can lead to role confusion. SBFC practitioners can best be utilized if they are able to ascribe to the definition of their nationally recommended role. For example, according to the American School Counselor Association (ASCA), a school counselor's role is to "design and deliver school counseling programs that improve student outcomes. They lead, advocate and collaborate to promote equity and access for all students by connecting their school counseling program to the school's academic mission and school improvement plan" (ASCA, 2021, p.2). Likewise, school social workers (SSW) "provide a focused reach to support all students specifically in areas of social-emotional learning and mental health needs, and are uniquely trained to integrate the school, community, and family context into interventions and resource referrals" (School Social Work Association of America [SSWAA], 2021, p.1). The reader may also consider the role of a school psychologists who "provide direct support and interventions to students; consult with teachers, families, and other school-employed mental health professionals (i.e., school counselors, school social workers) to improve support strategies" (National Association of School Psychologists [NASP], 2014, p.1). Facilitating small groups for short-term counseling is an appropriate duty for SBFC professionals regardless of their specific discipline; in fact, any SBFC practitioner would be an ideal person to provide such services. For the purposes of this chapter, the authors will describe how an SBFC practitioner can provide group counseling services to students and their families following a crisis or disaster.

Step 1: Needs assessment

Since a crisis or disaster is not a planned event, it may behoove the school to offer prevention services to all students year-round through classroom lessons, small groups, and other supports like media campaigns or schoolwide events (e.g., mock crash events and active shooter drills). In addition, schools should have in place an emergency operation plan, with input from multiple stakeholders, including SBFC practitioners, so they are prepared in the event of a crisis or disaster. Following a crisis or disaster, the first step is for the SBFC practitioner to disseminate a brief needs assessment to school personnel, students (as developmentally appropriate, e.g., fifth grade and older), and students' families. The needs assessment would provide an overview of the role of the SBFC practitioner and explain the services offered. Questions such as the following may be considered: (1) Have you been impacted by the recent crisis/ disaster? (2) What specific concerns do you have related to the recent crisis/ disaster? (3) Are you interested in attending a small group to gain support following the crisis/disaster? Once the SBFC practitioner disseminates and collects the completed needs assessments, the students and families in need of services can be identified. Next, the students and families would need to be screened for appropriateness of the group counseling sessions (Gladding, 2020).

Step 2: Screening

The maturity, readiness, and composition of membership play a major role in determining the success of a group (Riva et al., 2000). The goal of the small group counseling intervention after a crisis or disaster is to help students and their families reduce their stress response and prevent the development of long-term problems. The overarching goal of screening is to determine whether a particular group is right for a particular individual at a specific time (Gladding, 2020). The SBFC practitioner can contact the parent/guardian who indicated a willingness to be a member in a group session and identify the parent's needs, expectations, and commitment; challenge myths and misconceptions about group counseling; and convey information about the group process (Gladding, 2020). Assuming the parent/guardian is deemed suitable for the group, the SBFC practitioner can proceed to meet with the student individually. The SBFC practitioner will want to gain assent from the student by reviewing the aforementioned as well. Once all parent(s)/guardian(s) and students have agreed to be a member of the group, and are deemed a good fit for the group, the SBFC practitioner can send home the details about the meeting in the form of a flier or letter.

Step 3: Planning

The planning process will be dependent on the total number of participants. For example, one student may have one parent/guardian that wishes to participate and another student may have two or more. This will need to be taken into consideration. On average, a group runs well with 12 individuals; therefore, the SBFC practitioner will need to divide the groups up accordingly. Due to the sensitive nature of crisis/disaster groups, it is suggested that the groups are offered after school hours. The after-school group can meet in a confidential setting somewhere in the school building which administrators approve.

As an example, if 20 families are selected, the SBFC practitioner could offer the group to four families on a Monday, four families on a Tuesday, four families on a Wednesday, four families on a Thursday, and four families on a Friday. The group would meet for 1½ hours depending on the developmental level of the members. The SBFC practitioner could then send home a detailed flier or letter notifying the families about the start date of the group, location, time, and the number of weeks they will meet. It is recommended that the group meet at least six weeks. This length of time would allow for a group to run each of the four quarters in a school year. The flier should also detail any resources that will be used in the group, including any books, handouts, videos, or software, for example. Parents(s)/guardian(s) should be provided an opportunity to review any resources or materials before they are introduced in the group. It is important to note that ongoing needs assessments should be given to families throughout the year since impacts from the crisis or disaster may continue and needs may change throughout the school year. The SBFC practitioner may want to also consider a friendly reminder call to the participants the day before the group is scheduled to begin.

Step 4: Facilitating the group

Setup

In a room large enough for four families, arrange chairs in a circle and have families sit next to each other. The SBFC practitioner will also sit in the circle with families.

INTRODUCTIONS

The SBFC practitioner can begin the group with introductions and an icebreaker activity. This provides an opportunity for group members to learn each other's names and begin to build trust and rapport. An example of an icebreaker activity is to bring a bowl of colored candy (i.e., M&Ms, Skittles, Starbursts, ensure no one has an allergy in advance). Have each member of the group take some candy from the bowl but they are not to eat it. For each color of candy, have a "get to know you" question; for example, for red "What is your favorite food?" for yellow "If you had a superpower what would it be?" Go around the circle and have each member of the group introduce themselves and answer questions based on the color candies they picked. At the conclusion of the activity, group members may eat their candy.

ESTABLISHING GROUP NORMS

The SBFC practitioner should follow introductions with setting group norms and allow the students and their caregivers to learn the group process. Begin by describing the purpose of the group. Ask for questions from participants and provide answers as needed. Review confidentiality, the limits of confidentiality in a group setting, and the exceptions to confidentiality. Co-create group rules with group members. Examples of group rules may include, one person speaks at a time, respect yourself and each other and keep phones off and out of sight.

Group structure

It is important to create a group structure. This structure should include a topic each week. For example,

week 1: introductions, group purpose, and norms, introduce the topic
week 2: impacts of crisis and disaster
week 3: safety
week 4: difficult emotions
week 5: healthy coping strategies
week 6: creating a memory box, closure, and termination

These topics can be explored using handouts, videos, general discussion, and/or literature. Literature can help students identify and discuss feelings that can feel scary and overwhelming by relating to situations or characters in a story.

Process

A book that can be utilized for group sessions for ages 12–14 is "Be the One: Six True Stories of Teens Overcoming Hardship with Hope," by Byron Pitts. For group sessions with older teens, "Chicken Soup for the Soul: Tough Times for Teens: 101 Stories about the Hardest Parts of Being a Teenager," by Jack Canfield, Mark Victor Hansen, and Amy Newmark, is appropriate for ages 15–18. "When Someone Very Special Dies," by Marge Heegaard (1996), is a book that is appropriate for ages 6–12 and is written to guide children in processing their grief. While this book is targeted for younger children, it can be adapted to older children if the group leader uses language and guides the drawing activities based on the developmental and chronological age of the students participating in the group. We will use it as an example for leading a first-grade group following a crisis or disaster. The book has easy to understand language for children and has pictures to explain how death is a part of living. The SBFC practitioner can have one book they read aloud to the group, or if funding is available, have a book for each child or for each participant. The parent would be instructed to assist their child in completing the drawing activity in the book if they have one or on plain paper. Encouraging the parent(s)/guardian(s) to share the book provides a great sense of connection between parent(s)/guardian(s) and the child. The SFBC practitioner can elect to cover a certain number of pages per week in the group, depending on how many weeks the group will meet. It is important to consider where each student is in their grieving process. Some students will be more willing to share and others might not yet be at that point. The SBFC practitioner should encourage the group members to respect and support each other as they will all likely participate in the group at a different level. A check-in and a check-out each group session allows for the members to close out the group prior to going home. The SBFC practitioner would keep the books or drawings each week until the group terminates and then the family would keep their completed book or drawings. If group counseling notes are kept, they should be secured and kept on file as per school policy.

EXAMPLE OF MODEL DIALOGUE (SESSION FOUR USING THE HEEGAARD BOOK, WITH 1ST GRADE STUDENTS AND THEIR PARENT(S)/ GUARDIAN(S))

SBFC PRACTITIONER: Last week we talked about all kinds of feelings. What color best represents how you are feeling today? Tell us a little about how you are feeling.

JACOB: Red

SBFC PRACTITIONER: How does red represent how you are feeling, Jacob?

JACOB: Because my baby sister colored in my book.

SBFC PRACTITIONER: So red is like anger, you are mad that your sister drew on your book (Provide a reflection. Go around and give each student and their parent an opportunity to share).

SBFC PRACTITIONER: This week we are going to talk about feeling better. What is something that makes you feel good?

CHELSEA: I feel good when my grandma takes me to the park.

CHELSEA'S MOM, BETH (SMILING): My mother watches Chelsea and her sister on Saturday mornings, they always have a good time together.

SBFC PRACTITIONER: Chelsea, I can tell you really enjoy spending time with your grandma at the park. Beth, it sounds like it brings you joy to know they are having fun together. (Offer reflection to participant responses, give a few participants an opportunity to share).

SBFC PRACTITIONER: What causes you to feel frightened? Draw a picture and share it with the group. (Give participants time to draw a picture). Sam, can you tell us about your picture?

SAM: My picture is a tornado, like the one in my neighborhood last month. It was really scary. We had to hide in a closet.

SBFC PRACTITIONER: That must have been very frightening to you. What else is in your picture?

SAM: My mom, my dad, and our cat Buster. We were in the closet together.

The group talks about how drawing a picture of something scary can help it feel a little less scary. Following the model above, the exercise continues. Participants draw pictures of things they worry about and discuss the importance of sharing their worries with others. They finish the prompt, "Sometimes I feel different because…" and identify three things they like about themselves. The last activity is to draw a picture of something they are good at with a discussion about how everyone is good at something and no one is good at everything.

SBFC PRACTITIONER: What is one thing you want to remember about our time together today?

JACOB: I want to remember that I can write a poem when I feel angry. I am a good writer.

SBFC PRACTITIONER: You are good at writing, and it helps you feel less angry (continue to encourage participants to share their takeaways and provide reflections).

Closing

It is up to the SBFC practitioner to decide when the specific group members need to have an appropriate termination to the group and the group process. Families might have different ideas on how they wish to terminate. One idea would be to create a memory box. Instruct the group members to fill a box with memories of their loved one. The memories could be items that once belonged to the loved one, pictures, letters, or any items that provide memories. The purpose would be to say goodbye and find closure to the death. This activity can be utilized for other types of crises or disaster; for example, if homes have been lost as a result of a weather event, the memory box could hold memories of the home. The SBFC practitioner instructs the students to write a note detailing the memories in the box which they also share with the group. This makes a nice keepsake for the families. If the families need additional support, resources and/or referrals should be provided. It is important for the SBFC to check in on the students periodically throughout the year and share any concerns with their families.

Multicultural considerations

The SBFC metamodel offers a systemic and holistic approach to counseling students in schools. This is important as it can work well for both individualist and collectivistic cultures. The SBFC practitioner should ensure that equitable and just considerations remain at the forefront of all planning and practices associated with providing the family group counseling services to the students and their families. *The Multicultural and Social Justice Competencies* can serve as a guide for the SBFC practitioner (Hipolito-Delgado et al., 2015). Although not an exhaustive list, factors to consider are the following: (1) developmental level of each student and family member; (2) transportation and financial wherewithal to attend the groups after school hours; (3) cultural considerations; (4) confidentiality and its limitations; and (5) readiness to enter into a group counseling experience. It is tantamount that the SFBC practitioners espouse a culturally competent lens in which to conceptualize the group members. It would behoove the SBFC practitioner to have knowledge of systemic theories of counseling so that all world influences can be considered. This is especially important following a crisis or disaster as different religions, racial and ethnic groups, for example, may have different traditions and beliefs in their response, particularly if death is involved.

Challenges and solutions

Providing small group counseling in the school following a disaster or crisis is not without challenges. One ethical concern is the impact of the disaster or crisis on the person providing the service. While the SBFC practitioner is responding professionally to the crisis event, they may also be dealing with a personal reaction. SBFC practitioners must be in tune with how the crisis or disaster has impacted them, attend to any impairment they may be experiencing, and determine if they are able to provide services safely and effectively. One strength of the SBFC metamodel is the interdisciplinary approach. Collaborating with other SBFC professionals can be a source of support for a practitioner who needs to focus on their own needs.

Another challenge is to overcome social and cultural barriers to counseling, especially families that are very private, distrust mental health professionals, believe seeking counseling will bring shame on their family, or a variety of other reasons that attaches a stigma to counseling services. As previously addressed in the multicultural considerations, a strength of the SBFC metamodel is its systemic and holistic approach which includes the family rather than focusing on the individual. The family is a resource that is engaged in the process. The SBFC practitioner must be familiar with the cultures and norms of the students and families in the school, and this will inform their approach.

A third barrier to implementing this intervention is the time constraint in a school setting. SBFC practitioners must be creative in their approach to providing group counseling services. Times may need to be set before or after school to avoid the disruption to instructional time. Sometimes, SBFC practitioners may be able to conduct group sessions during lunch although this can be difficult if students need to eat while participating. In addition, some may not want to miss the opportunity to socialize with peers. Some teachers may be willing to give up some instructional time if the SBFC practitioner collaborates with them and plans in advance. Pointing out that the group can help students increase focus in class following a disaster or crisis may be a reason a teacher would be willing to give up some of their class time. It is also possible if students have enrichment or elective classes, or even a study hall or recess, these times may be ideal for the creative and flexible SBFC practitioner to schedule group sessions. It is important to keep an open mind and collaborate with other education professionals, especially teachers and administrators, to find the best time for your group.

Finally, not all SBFC practitioners will have training in group counseling, grief or crisis counseling. It would be important for the SBFC practitioner to collaborate with another mental health professional in the school trained in these areas to assist in providing these groups.

Resources

Below are resources for helping families in the aftermath of a traumatic event.

The American School Counselor Association (ASCA) https://schoolcounselor.org/

ASCA has resources that can be of benefit to SBFC practitioners including resources for after a school shooting, anti-racism, COVID-19, crisis and trauma, natural disaster, racial violence, and for responding to suicide: https://schoolcounselor.org/Publications-Research/ Publications/Free-ASCA-Resources.

The Center for Disease Control (CDC) https://www.cdc.gov/childrenindisasters/ children-disaster-help.html.

The Center for Disease Control (CDC) provides tips for parents and caregivers in supporting their children in the aftermath of a crisis or trauma. This site includes an explanation about why children are at risk for mental health concerns following a crisis and provides information on how to help children cope.

Mental Health America https://www.mhanational.org/coping-disaster

Mental Health America provides a list of common reactions children may display following a disaster and suggestions for helping them cope.

The National Child Traumatic Stress Network https://www.nctsn.org/

The National Child Traumatic Stress Network offers a smartphone app designed to help parents talk to their children following a disaster with suggestions on how best to support their child. It comes in both an Apple and Android version. Apple: https://apps.apple.com/us/ app/id1069028637 and Android: https://play.google.com/store/apps/details?id=nctsn. helpkidscope&hl=en.

The Red Cross and the Federal Emergency Management Agency (FEMA) https://www.redcross.org/ and https://www.fema.gov/

The Red Cross and FEMA have a resource for helping children cope with disaster: https://www.redcross.org/content/dam/redcross/atg/PDF_s/Preparedness_ Disaster_Recovery/General_Preparedness_Recovery/Emotional/Helping_ children_cope_with_disaster_-_English.pdf

The Substance Abuse and Mental Health Services Administration (SAMHSA) https://www.samhsa.gov/

SAMHSA offers a variety of resources. One helpful resource for parents is Tips for Survivors of a Disaster or Other Traumatic Event: Managing Stress: https://store. samhsa.gov/product/Tips-for-Survivors-of-a-Disaster-or-Other-Traumatic-Event-Managing-Stress/SMA13-4776?referer=from_search_result.

Another helpful resource from SAMHSA is Tips for Talking With and Helping Children and Youth Cope After a Disaster or Traumatic Event: A Guide for Parents, Caregivers, and Teachers: https://store.samhsa.gov/product/tips-talking-helping-children-youth-cope-after-disaster-or-traumatic-event-guide-parents/ sma12-4732?referer=from_search_result.

For the SBFC practitioners working with youth who are impacted by crisis or disaster, SAMHSA's guide titled Psychosocial Issues for Children and Adolescents in Disasters discusses theories of child development in the context of disaster, crisis, and trauma. The guide offers case studies, practical suggestions, and a resource guide: https://store. samhsa.gov/product/Psychosocial-Issues-Children-and-Adolescents-Disasters/ ADM86-1070R?referer=from_search_result.

The U.S. Department of Education https://www.ed.gov/

The U.S. Department of Education offers tips for helping students recover from traumatic events: https://www2.ed.gov/parents/academic/help/recovering/index.html.

Books

Canfield, J., Hansen, M. V., & Newmark, A. (2012). Chicken soup for the soul: Tough times for teens: 101 stories about the hardest parts of being a teenager. Chicken Soup for the Soul Publishing. https://www.chickensoup.com/book/tough-times-for-teens

Teens will find comfort and inspiration in these stories, written by other teens just like them, who overcame their challenges and found happiness and meaning in their lives. Great advice and inspiration from people who really care.

Pitts, B. (2017). *Be the one: Six true stories of teens overcoming hardship with hope.* Simon & Schuster.

Emmy Award–winning ABC News chief national correspondent and Nightline coanchor, Byron Pitts shares the heartbreaking and inspiring stories of six young people who overcame impossible circumstances with extraordinary perseverance.

References

American School Counselor Association (2021). *The role of the school counselor.* https://schoolcounselor.org/getmedia/ee8b2e1b-d021-4575-982c-c84402cb2cd2/Role-Statement.pdf

Gladding, S. (2020). *Groups: A counseling specialty* (8th ed.). Pearson.

Heegaard, M. (1996). *When someone very special dies: Children can learn to cope with grief.* Woodland Press.

Hipolito-Delgado, C., Ratts, M., Singh, A., Nassar-McMillan, S., Butler, K., & McCullough, J. (2025). *Multicultural and social justice counseling competencies*, retrieved from https://www.counseling.org/docs/default-source/competencies/multicultural-and-social-justice-counseling-competencies.pdf?sfvrsn=20

National Association of School Psychologists. (2014). *Who are school psychologists? Helping children thrive: In school, in home, in life.* https://www.nasponline.org/assets/Documents/About%20School%20Psychology/Brochures/who_are_school_psychologists_flyer.pdf

Riva, M. T., Lippert, L., & Tackett, M. J. (2000). Selection practices of group leaders: A National survey. *Journal for Specialists in Group Work*, 25, 157–169.

School Social Work Association of America. (2021). *Who are school social workers?* https://www.sswaa.org/_files/ugd/426a18_98102fe3074e4529a17602419d-f0be59.pdf

9 Using Solution-Focused Brief Therapy with students who have experienced trauma

Carol E. Buchholz Holland

Overview

The focus of this chapter is to describe how to use Solution-Focused Brief Therapy (SFBT) with students who have experienced trauma. It includes a brief overview of this counseling approach. In addition, it provides a case example which illustrates how this approach can be applied during an initial counseling session with a student who is dealing with trauma.

Background

When working with clients who have experienced trauma, many traditional counseling approaches take the stance that it is necessary for clients to share detailed descriptions of their past traumas and to process these traumas in depth so that therapeutic healing can take place. While engaging in problem-solving activities, these counseling conversations often concentrate on the past. However, Solution-Focused Brief Therapy (SFBT) takes a different stance about how to work with individuals who are dealing with trauma. SFBT emerged in the early 1980s when Steve de Shazer, Insoo Kim Berg, and their colleagues at the Brief Family Therapy Center in Milwaukee, Wisconsin used an inductive manner to identify effective therapeutic techniques and determine what worked in therapy sessions (Berg & Steiner, 2003). They concluded that it was more effective for mental health practitioners to help their clients identify and co-construct solutions instead of concentrating on how to resolve their clients' problems. This paradigm shift from problem-solving to solution-building had a major impact on the focus of conversations during counseling sessions. In SFBT sessions, attention and energy are redirected to efforts designed to create rich descriptions of the clients' preferred futures and to identify what possible solutions may already exist in their lives instead of concentrating on the clients' problems. Identification of clients' existing strengths, resources, and past successes help build the foundation for developing solutions.

SFBT practitioners also believe that asking a client to provide a detailed description of a traumatic experience or having the client reflect on painful aspects of the trauma is not always helpful. In fact, a client might become

DOI: 10.4324/9781003201977-11

overwhelmed or even retraumatized if therapeutic conversations focus primarily on their past traumas. In addition, clients are more likely to become engaged in a counseling session that focuses on their positive traits instead of their deficiencies (Sklare, 2005). Engaging clients in the counseling process is especially important when working with someone who is in crisis.

How SFBT can be used to build levels of hope

Since clients who have experienced trauma often feel hopeless, helpless, or out of control, they greatly benefit from counseling conversations which highlight and build their resilience and protective factors such as hope. Hope is a powerful healing ingredient for people who have experienced trauma and SFBT is well equipped to help people foster hope.

Snyder (2000) developed *Hope Theory* which hypothesizes that hope consists of three interactive components: *goals, pathway thoughts, and agency thoughts*. All three parts must be addressed when working on building hope. Snyder viewed *goals* as "the object of hope" and asserted that "without goals there is no hope" (Kondrat & Teater, 2010, p. 5). The second component, *pathway thoughts*, pertains to "the perceived ability to produce plausible routes to goals" (Snyder, 2000, p. 9). The more routes or pathways a person can conceptualize, the more options a person has for achieving their goals. Having more available options also means that a person has a better chance of avoiding potential barriers to achieving their goals (Kondrat & Teater, 2010). The third component is *agency thoughts* and agency can be viewed as a person's belief that they will be able to achieve their goal. Agency thoughts develop from a person's past experiences that involve successfully achieving goals. Recognizing *past successes* helps people expand their agency thinking. If a person feels that they have a better chance for achieving their goals, they are likely to also feel more hopeful. SFBT is a good fit for helping a person build hope because it (1) encourages goal formation, (2) identifies a person's past successes and exceptions which can then be used as *pathways* to achieve a goal, and (3) increases a person's sense of *agency* through the identification of their past successes.

How SFBT fits within the school-based family counseling metamodel

SFBT is a good fit for work with students who have experienced trauma. In addition, SFBT fits within the school-based family counseling metamodel for several reasons because both:

- are strength-based;
- are collaborative;
- engage individuals in counseling process;
- are culturally sensitive;
- help students and families identify their own resources;

- emphasize respect, caring, and humility;
- promote student success and wellness; and
- are action-oriented (Gerrard, Carter, & Ribera, 2020).

Box 9.1 provides examples of Solution-Focused Brief Therapy evidence-based studies.

Box 9.1 Solution-focused brief counseling evidence-based studies

Bannink, F. P. (2008). Posttraumatic success: Solution-Focused brief therapy. *Brief Treatment and Crisis Intervention*, 8(3), 215–225. https://doi.org/10.1093/brieftreatment/mhn013

Beauchemin, J. D. (2018). Solution-focused wellness: A randomized controlled trial of college students. *Health & Social Work*, 43(2), 94–100. https://doi.org/10.1093/hsw/hly007

Eads, R., & Lee, M. Y. (2019). Solution focused therapy for trauma survivors: A review of the outcome literature. *Journal of Solution Focused Practices*, 2(1), 47–65.

Franklin, C., Moore, K., & Hopson, L. (2008). Effectiveness of solution-focused brief therapy in a school setting. *Children & Schools*, 30, 15–26.

Gingerich, W. J., & Peterson, L. T. (2013). Effectiveness of solution-focused brief therapy: A systematic qualitative review of controlled outcome studies. *Research on Social Work Practice*, 23, 266–283. https://doi.org/10.1177/1049731512470859

Procedure

Solution-focused practitioners realize the importance of language and they use carefully crafted questions as tools to facilitate the identifications of clients' strengths and solutions (Berg & Steiner, 2003). Solution-focused questions and Socratic questioning are the main tools/techniques of this approach. The following fictional case example is provided to illustrate the use of the solution-focused approach with a student who has experienced trauma.

Case example: Anna

Anna is a 15-year-old student who was involved in a school bus accident on her way to school three months ago. Her school bus driver and one student were killed in this accident when a truck t-boned her school bus on a very foggy morning. Although Anna only suffered from minor physical injuries, she has been struggling with trauma reactions such as intrusive thoughts, sleep problems, anxiety, and depression since this accident. Anna's mom encouraged her to meet with an SBFC practitioner due to her ongoing trauma reactions so Anna set up an appointment for herself.

Below is a description of steps taken during Anna's first session with the solution-focused practitioner:

Build rapport with the student and create a safe therapeutic environment

When working with a student who is in crisis or is trying to overcome a traumatic experience, it is important to develop rapport and to find a way to join with them. Henden (2008) stressed that the first ten minutes of a session was a critical period in the development of a counseling relationship. A student could either become engaged in the counseling process or could begin to withdraw internally. One simple way of helping engage a student is to take a few minutes to encourage problem-free talk with them. For example, a practitioner could ask the student: *"What is your favorite activity to do on the weekends?"* or they could look for other clues about what is important to the student such as a school activity or a pet. It is imperative not to rush into talking about the student's problem before some level of rapport has been established. In addition, the student needs to feel a certain level of safety and trust with the practitioner before asking about the student's concerns.

Ask for a brief description of the student's concern

After taking a few minutes to engage in problem-free talk, the practitioner then pivots and asks the student to briefly describe what prompted them to schedule a meeting with the practitioner (if they self-referred). When working with individuals who have experienced trauma, solution-focused professionals ask them to disclose "only what is necessary for healing" (Dolan, 1991, p. 142). This stance is a departure from many traditional approaches which believe that it is necessary to gather detailed information about client trauma. However, solution-focused practitioners are interested in helping their clients identify what would immediately benefit the clients instead of spending time focusing on the causes of their problems (Fiske, 2008). When they are successful in communicating this, solution-focused practitioners are more likely to see clients who (1) open up more freely; (2) engage in the counseling process; and (3) return for follow-up sessions (Fiske, 2008).

One way to help the student focus and provide a brief description for their concern(s) is to ask them the following question:

Practitioner: "Anna- What would be most helpful for me to know about the reason you decided to schedule a meeting with me?"

In order to clarify the student's primary concern, the practitioner might also ask:

Practitioner: "What concerns you the most about this situation?"

Both questions are respectful because they allow the student to maintain a sense of control and to decide what information they feel is most important to share. Helping a student maintain a sense of control is especially important when working with someone who is feeling powerless or helpless.

Informally assess student's safety level

After listening to the student providing a brief description of their problem(s), it is important to gather basic information about the student's current emotional state and then informally assess the student's level of safety especially if the student has experienced a trauma. Since some students may struggle to choose descriptive words to convey their personal pain, they may find it easier to use a number on a scale to represent how they are feeling. This basic number can provide a great deal of information and can help prompt a meaningful conversation between the student and the practitioner. In addition, it might be easier for students to be more honest about how they are feeling if they are asked to pick a number for how they are feeling.

Here is an example of a scaling question that a practitioner might ask:
Practitioner:

> So I'm curious Anna- on a scale of 0 to 10, with '10' being that you are 'feeling great today' and '0' being the complete opposite, where would you put yourself on that scale today? Where would you have put yourself on that scale yesterday (or last week, etc.)?

Here is a helpful follow-up question to ask:
Practitioner: "So you feel that today you are a '6' on this scale. What tells you that you are at a '6'? How is your '6' different from when you might be a '5' on this scale?"

It is helpful to ask the student to scale not only how they are feeling today but also how they have felt in the past. Getting two or more numbers provides a great deal of information without requiring the student to provide a lengthy answer. If the numbers are different, they can be used for further comparison. These differences can also highlight possible solutions which will be discussed later in this chapter.

After asking the initial scaling question, the practitioner can then ask a second scaling question which can be used for a quick assessment. Here is an example:
Practitioner:

> Anna- It sounds like you are going through a tough time right now. Whenever I talk with a student who shares with me that they are struggling, I need to see if they are safe. So I'm now going to change the scale and this time the '10' represents that you have 'strong thoughts of hurting yourself' and '0' represents that you have 'no thoughts of hurting yourself'. Based on this new scale, where would you put yourself on it today (yesterday, last week, etc.)?

Instead of using the phrase "thoughts of hurting yourself," the practitioner may decide to use the phrase "thoughts of suicide." If the student indicates any risk of suicidal ideation, the practitioner will need to shift the focus of the conversation toward helping the student identify coping strategies to decrease the intensity or even eliminate their suicidal ideation. However, in Anna's case, she is not experiencing any suicidal ideation.

Engage the student in a "coping dialogue" if the student is in distress or is not ready to start the goal formation process

Typically, in a non-trauma-related counseling session, the next step in a solution-focused conversation would be to help the student identify their goals for counseling. However, not all students who have experienced trauma may be ready at this point in the session to start the goal formation process. Instead, the practitioner may sense that it would be more beneficial for the student to engage in a *coping dialogue*. During a *coping dialogue*, the practitioner asks the student *coping questions*.

Coping questions help identify helpful actions that the client has taken in the past to cope with their problem(s). These actions can also be viewed as *"pathways"* for reaching the client's goal. In addition, coping questions help uncover small yet undeniable successes the client has experienced while dealing with their problems (De Jong & Kim, 2008). For example, a practitioner might ask a student who is struggling to make it to school the following question:

Practitioner: "Anna- What helped you get out of bed this morning and make it to school on time?"

Solution-focused practitioners also assist clients in identifying their *microsuccesses* which are especially important when a client is overwhelmed or feeling defeated (De Jong & Kim, 2008). Identifying client's *microsuccesses* can help them build upon them and experience more success over time which, in turn, can help build a client's confidence and sense of *agency*.

Practitioner: "Anna- What is one small thing you have done in the past couple of weeks that has helped you feel a little bit better? What else?"

This coping question encourages the student to explore coping skills that they already possess and to identify times when the student successfully dealt with a difficult time. In other words, the practitioner is directing attention to the student's *past successes*.

A practitioner might also ask a scaling question designed to elicit information about the student's current coping ability such as:

Practitioner: "Anna- On a scale of 0 to 10, with '10' being 'very strong' and '0' being the complete opposite, how strong do you think your coping skills are right now?"

If the student struggles to identify any past successes, it might be an indication that the student potentially needs more intensive care or monitoring. Helping a student develop a longer list of coping strategies or *pathways* and helping the student increase their sense of *agency* are crucial steps in building *hope*.

Acknowledge, validate, and normalize student's feelings and reactions to their trauma

If a student has experienced trauma, it is especially important to acknowledge, validate, and normalize the student's feelings and their trauma reactions.

ACKNOWLEDGE

Students who have experienced trauma may feel isolated or overlooked. Many are hoping to find someone who is genuine and has some understanding of their pain. When a student's suffering is acknowledged in an authentic manner during a counseling session, the student is more likely to feel understood and more likely to engage in a therapeutic relationship. The statement listed below is simple yet an effective way to acknowledge a student's struggle with their trauma.

Practitioner: "Anna- From what you have told me about the accident, you have given me a pretty good idea about how difficult it has been for you."

VALIDATE

It is also important to validate a student's feelings and thoughts related to their trauma. For example, a practitioner might state:

Practitioner: "Based on everything that you have shared with me about the accident, it is understandable that you are anxious about riding on a school bus again."

By validating the student's response to the trauma, the practitioner hopes that the student's feelings of shame about their struggles with coping are reduced.

NORMALIZE

Normalizing a student's stress reactions after a trauma is an important part of helping a student who might be feeling as if they are losing control over their life or are losing their mind. Providing a student with brief psychoeducation about normal trauma reactions is very helpful in a session. In addition, making a statement such as *"A traumatic stress reaction is a normal response, by normal people, to an abnormal circumstance"* can be very comforting to a student who might otherwise feel that they are reacting to their trauma in an abnormal way.

Begin the goal formation process with the student

When it is time to start developing goals, it is helpful to ask a *miracle question* which is a hallmark of SFBT (De Jong & Berg, 2008). The miracle question prompts a student to imagine and describe what their future will look like when things are going better in their life. Here is an example of a *miracle question* that might be used with a person who experienced a trauma:

Practitioner:

> Imagine *tonight while you are sleeping, a miracle occurs. The miracle is that the trauma reactions you have been experiencing since your accident are gone. Because you are sleeping, you don't know that this miracle has taken place. So when you wake up tomorrow morning, what will be the first sign you notice that will tell you this miracle has happened? What else?*
>
> > *What will you be doing? What will you be doing differently? What else?*
> > *How did you make that happen? What did you do differently to make that happen?*

It is also helpful to ask a *relationship question* such as "*What will other people notice you are doing after the miracle has occurred?*" Asking a *relationship question* encourages a student to take a 3rd person perspective. Changing the perspective often helps increase creativity because it allows things to be viewed from a safe distance.

Sometimes, it might be in the student's best interest to encourage them to scale down their miracle especially if they have recently experienced a major trauma or disruption in their life. De Jong and Berg (2008) recommended tailoring the miracle question to fit each client's situation. For example, the miracle might involve smaller changes such as being able to sleep better at night or being able to focus better in their classes. By focusing on smaller "miracles," the student will hopefully find this more manageable and will be more hopeful that they can achieve them. It is also helpful to share the SFBT phrase "small change can lead to bigger changes" with students because it emphasizes the value of taking small positive steps toward a goal.

After asking this miracle question, the solution-focused practitioner is encouraged to get as many details as possible about "what" the student is *doing*. The richness of these details provides valuable information that can be used to assist the client in developing their goals which, in turn, helps build hope.

Assist the student in identifying exceptions

A basic assumption of SFBT is that no problem is constant and the intensity and/or frequency of a problem fluctuate. One effective method for utilizing hope and building upon it is to assist a student in identifying *exceptions* (times when the problem is not occurring, is less frequent, or less severe). After asking the miracle question, it is helpful to look for *exceptions*. For example:

Practitioner: "Anna- I'm curious to know if a small part of your miracle has happened or if a small part of your miracle is happening today. Tell me more about the last time you felt a little better since the accident.

What were you doing differently when you felt a little better? What else?

How did you make that happen?

How did you decide to do that?

What did you discover by doing that?

What would happen if you tried that again?"

These follow-up questions serve the purpose of amplifying the exceptions. Murphy (1994) described the "5-E method" which was designed to recognize and use exceptions that exist in students' lives. The 5-E method involves (1) eliciting times when the problem is absent, less intense, or less frequent; (2) elaborating on the conditions and features of these times; (3) expanding these identified exceptions to other contexts; (4) evaluating these exceptions using pre-established goals; and (5) empowering the client to maintain positive change over time (Murphy, 1994). Since exceptions are often overlooked, solution-focused practitioners need to be very intentional in identifying and amplifying these "micro-solutions" (Sharry, Darmody, & Madden, 2002, p. 392).

Provide compliments to the student

Providing compliments to students is an effective method for highlighting and reinforcing students' strengths and resources. The compliments should be reality-based and specific. SFBT uses two different forms of compliments – direct and indirect (Fiske, 2008). A direct compliment is a positive reaction from a solution-focused practitioner in response to something a student has shared in the session. For example:

Practitioner: "Wow, Anna! I'm sure that must have been difficult for you to take the school bus home and yet you were able to overcome your fear of riding on the bus again."

An indirect compliment involves using a question to invite the student to describe what they did and how they were able to do something that challenged them. For example:

Practitioner: "Wow, Anna, how did you manage to get the courage to ride the bus again even though you were really afraid to do it?"

An indirect compliment could also be blended with a relationship question such as:

Practitioner: "What would your parents appreciate about how you handled taking the bus home last week?"

Provide bridging statements and identify tasks during the session wrap-up

After the solution-focused practitioner has given compliments to the student, they may use a *bridging statement* which can be linked to therapeutic tasks. Here is an example:

Practitioner: "Anna- Today you mentioned that you felt a little better and more relaxed when you helped walk dogs at the animal shelter. Would you be interested in making time this week to do that again?"

In addition to using bridging statements, the practitioner encourages the student to help summarize the student's goal, coping skills, and past successes that were mentioned during the session. This collaborative process is a valuable part of the session and practitioners need to be mindful about allowing enough time at the end of this session for this wrap-up. The format of this initial session is designed to encourage the student to use their coping strategies, to empower the student, and to help the student become more hopeful about having the ability to overcome their trauma.

Multicultural considerations

SFBT is inherently a culturally sensitive approach. However, there are a few aspects of this approach that may need to be adapted based on a student's culture.

Focusing on a student's strengths may not be congruent with the student's culture

For some students, focusing on strengths may be contrary to their cultures' values such as humility. Instead of focusing on identifying the student's *strengths*, the culturally sensitive conversation can be shifted to identifying available *resources* within the student's life such as strong personal relationships, spiritual beliefs, or school activities. In addition, it may be difficult for the student to hear *direct compliments* from the solution-focused practitioner. One alternative would be to use *indirect compliments* which encourage the student to identify actions he/she took that were helpful. For example, a practitioner could utilize an indirect compliment by asking: *"Wow- How did you complete all of your assignments on time?"*

Making the miracle question culturally sensitive

In certain situations, it may not be appropriate to ask the *miracle question* as it was originally worded. Using the word *"miracle"* may feel too religious for some students. However, there is an easy fix for this. Instead of encouraging a discussion about the student's miracle, the practitioner can ask the student about what they would be doing after they wake up and start having a *"really awesome day."* Even though the question's wording is a little different, similar information can be gathered from both versions of the miracle question.

Challenges and solutions

When working with younger clients, it is important to use interventions that are developmentally appropriate. Even though SFBT is a good fit for use with children and adolescents, its techniques and questions sometimes need to be adapted for this population. Since children are concrete thinkers, they initially might need additional assistance in identifying and applying exceptions to their lives since exceptions are an abstract concept.

Below are a few examples of how to enhance solution-focused activities for younger clients who have not yet reached the formal operations developmental stage.

- Children naturally communicate through play so it is helpful to incorporate it into counseling sessions. In addition, Berg and Steiner (2003) recommend using creative solution-focused activities because they can help unleash children's resources.
- De Jong and Berg (2008) recommend drawing activities because drawing can slow down the conversation and provide the child or adolescent an opportunity to think. In addition, drawing helps make thoughts and ideas more concrete, and easier to share.
- Using white boards during a counseling session is a helpful tool which encourages the client and the practitioner to co-create visual representations of the client's goals and solutions.
- Games such as Jenga, Pick-Up Stick, or Sorry can be turned into solution-focused activities with the simple addition of solution-focused questions.

Conclusion

Solution-focused practitioners have access to a wide array of effective therapeutic questions and tools which promotes the collaborative solution-building process with their students. In addition, the solution-focused approach facilitates the "hope building" process which is an essential part of the healing process. By building hope and identifying their strengths and resources, a student is more likely to shift from being a *trauma survivor* to a *thriver*.

Resources

Bannink, F. (2014). *Post traumatic success: Positive Psychology & Solution-focused strategies to help clients survive & thrive.* New York: W.W. Norton & Company.
This book provides numerous examples of how to assist clients overcome trauma and grow from their traumatic experiences.
Bannink, F. (2015). *101 solution-focused questions for help with trauma.* New York: W.W. Norton & Company.
This book provides useful examples of solution-focused questions that can be used when working with clients who have experienced trauma.
Metcalf, L. (1995). *Counseling toward solutions: A practical solution-focused program for working with students, teachers, and parents.* San Francisco, CA: Jossey-Bass.
The author provides practical examples of how to use the solution-focused approach with students, teachers, and parents in school settings.
Selekman, M. (1997). Solution-focused therapy with children: Harnessing family strengths for systemic change. New York: Guilford Press.
This book provides creative and developmentally appropriate methods for adapting the solution-focused approach to use with children.

Web site

Dr. Linda Metcalf's web site: https://solutionfocusedschool.com/
Dr. Metcalf provides excellent free solution-focused resources and training webinars on her web site.

YouTube video

Arnoud Huibers' interview with Insoo Kim Berg
https://www.youtube.com/watch?v=kWifZOBuxIU
In this YouTube video, Arnoud Huibers interviews Insoo Kim Berg who helped develop the solution-focused approach. Talks about not needing to know the problem when helping client find a solution.

References

Berg, I. K., & Steiner, T. (2003). *Children's solution work*. New York: W.W. Norton.

De Jong, P., & Berg, I. K. (2008). *Interviewing for solutions* (3rd ed.). Belmont, CA: Thomson Brooks/Cole.

Dolan, Y. (1991). *Resolving sexual abuse: Solution-focused therapy and Ericksonian hypnosis for adult survivors*. New York: Norton.

Fiske, H. (2008). *Hope in action: Solution-focused conversations about suicide*. New York: Routledge.

Gerrard, B. A., Carter, M. J., & Ribera, D. (2020). *School-based family counseling: An interdisciplinary practitioner's guide*. New York: Routledge.

Henden, J. (2008). *Preventing suicide: The solution-focused approach*. West Sussex, England: John Wiley & Sons.

Kondrat, D. C., & Teater, B. (2010). Solution-focused therapy in an emergency room setting: Increasing hope in persons presenting with suicidal ideation. *Journal of Social Work*, 12(1), 3–15, DOI: 10.1177/1468017310379756

Murphy, J. J. (1994). Working with what works: A solution-focused approach to school behavior problems. *School Counselor*, 42, 59–68.

Sharry, J., Darmody, M., & Madden, B. (2002). A solution-focused approach to working with clients who are suicidal. *British Journal of Guidance & Counselling*, 30(4), 383–399.

Sklare, G. B. (2005). *Brief counseling that works: A solution-focused approach for school counselors and administrators* (2nd ed.). Thousand Oaks, CA: Corwin Press.

Snyder, C. R. (2000). *Handbook of hope: Theory, Measures, & Applications*. San Diego, CA: Academic Press.

Part III
Family intervention

10 Un Respiro de Vida, a breath of life

Giving wings to farmworker families during the COVID crisis

Belinda Hernández-Arriaga and Juan Carlos Ruiz Malagon

Overview

Farmworkers are one of the most vulnerable populations in the United States. At the same time, they are the backbone of our economy and our country. During COVID and natural disasters, farmworkers continued in the field, supporting the country, while their families suffered compounded disparities. Understanding best practices to provide direct support to this community is necessary to support their well-being. Ayudando Latinos A Sonar is a California nonprofit that has been on the front lines of working with Latino families in a rural Northern California community. Through their story, we understand the impact of going out into the fields to bring cariño (care), advocacy and support to farmworkers and their families during crisis.

Background

The COVID-19 pandemic led to a global emergency due to the contagious and deadly nature of the virus. This emergency brought upon shelter-in-place mandates, extended lockdowns as well as guidelines to limit social interactions (Chicas et al., 2022). Although this was the case worldwide, governmental guidelines deemed certain individuals "essential" at the start of the pandemic. Within the United States, agricultural workers were included in the designated group of essential personnel. There are an estimated 2.5 million farmworkers with a larger majority of them being foreign-borns and more than half lacking any form of documentation (Hernandez and Gabbard, 2019; Tippett, 2020). It is estimated that more than 68% of farmworkers are either from Central America or Mexico, which creates implications for racialization and systemic exclusions due to the legacies of racism within the United States.

Compared to other workers who were deemed essential, farmworkers face an increase in limited occupational protections in addition to facing language barriers, lack of access to social resources and adequate educational and legal services (Liebman et al., 2021; Ramos, 2018). In spite of farmworkers contributing to the 1.109 trillion dollar industry of agriculture, they were faced

DOI: 10.4324/9781003201977-13

with unique challenges of survival in relation to both health and social realms (Devadoss and Luckstead, 2008; National Center for Farmworker Health).

Amid the pandemic, existing social and health injustices only were heightened due to the legacies of systemic racism found within the United States (Bailey et al., 2017). COVID brought an unfamiliar wave of crisis to the world, but not so unfamiliar for farmworker communities who have endured decades of exploitation and exclusion from governmental support. For farmworker families, their experiences during COVID have been physically, emotionally and economically challenging. While most of the country went into quarantine, our farmworkers went out into the fields every day to provide food, nutrition and health for our country. They were in the direct line of exposure to COVID, many who did not start out with personal protection like face masks, face shields, goggles and hygiene protection. Instead, they worked long hours, side by side and with rigor to make sure that our country was taken care of. The crisis of COVID hit their families economically and physically as some lost their jobs, falling ill to COVID, many who do not have access to medical insurance. Their children had an increase in exposure to COVID as a result of parents having to continue working in the fields. Farmworker children grappled with school inequities living in remote areas with minimal wifi as well as the economic and physical hardships that plagued their families. As the COVID pandemic swept through the United States, the physical and emotional sacrifice of our farmworker community was heroic as they pushed through difficult and life-threatening work conditions to keep harvesting food for our communities. Their families endured a pandemic crisis vulnerable and exposed with minimal resources, unable to quarantine. As essential workers, they continued strong, even in the face of death and tragedy with COVID in the fields and in their homes.

While farmworkers battled COVID, a Northern California Coastal community of farmworkers faced a second threatening crisis of the CZU Lightning wildfire, burning over 86 acres (cite). Families were displaced, losing work and housing in the midst of the pandemic.

Farmworker children were challenged with attending online classes, displaced from home and with minimal access to technology and resources. Fleeing their homes with minimal belongings and already in fear, the trauma they endured was compounded by the natural disaster that plagued them. A crisis response organized by the Latinx led nonprofit organization of Ayudando Latinos A Soñar, also known as ALAS, www.alasdreams.com, is presented as a model of trauma and community response. ALAS embraces the SBFC metamodel that underscores community intervention as key to the well-being of families and children in schools (Gerrard & Soriano, 2018). What we have learned at ALAS is that community partnerships with farmworker families are critical and necessary as extending support and direct care. As Latinx writers, we introduce the work of ALAS through the lens of scholars, SBFC professionals and community organizers.

As a first author, I identify as a Latina Licensed Clinical Social Worker, Educator and Founder of ALAS in the rural community of Half Moon

Bay, California. Second author identifies as a Latinx public health scholar, first-generation and low-income college student and from a farmworker family from Central Mexico. This chapter gives a "cariño" (care) perspective of the accompaniment and crisis response work organized by ALAS. Lessons learned on working with farmworker families during crises are necessary as we embrace and elevate them as key pillars of our country.

According to testimonios shared with ALAS from the local Latino farmworker community of the North Coast in San Mateo County, they report working alone in the fields for thirty years with no outreach or services provided directly to them onsite. During our initial visits with them, they repeatedly stated that "In thirty years no one has helped us with any services, no one has come to visit us or meet us here on the farms". One senior farmworker shared during ALAS' Farmworker Fridays, "In all my years as a farmworker on the Coastside, no one has even offered us a coke to drink, nothing". Coastside Farmworker families have been an underserved community, facing mounting challenges of inequity and disparities that are evident in the economic challenges they are plagued by, the educational barriers their children navigate, complicated housing situations and the devastation of the COVID pandemic. The reality of the isolation they have lived through pushed ALAS to create urgent programming that addressed the crisis and instituted long-term support.

ALAS has committed to embed itself in spaces where there are families facing disparities and isolation as well as engage in systems like schools, churches, city and government to provide programming, outreach and advocacy. Farmworkers receive resources for medical enrollment that otherwise they would be challenged to access. Children receive I.E.P. advocacy by ALAS staff to increase educational equity and resources. Victims of crime receive accompaniment by our ALAS mental health team and overall we position ourselves in spaces to advocate and provide ongoing support where needed. In summer of 2021, as children suffered isolation from the pandemic, ALAS hosted its first ever summer camp for five weeks to sixty children, the majority from farmworker and essential working families. The emotional healing that happened as a result of the camp was significant. The City of Half Moon Bay and the County of San Mateo have recognized our work and program as a trusted agency in the community.

Procedure

While businesses were forced to shut down during the pandemic, ALAS opened the doors to accompany farmworker families. All of the ALAS programs discussed in this chapter were developed out of a direct response to COVID and the wildfires. ALAS was motivated by a sense of urgency and cariño (care) to enact a culturally centered impactful crisis response. What was most important during this crisis was to go out into the community to take the resources. The ALAS team pivoted to emergency response, with all staff motivated to be there for the community. The first priority to address was the economic and food disparities that were scarce. The irony of farmworkers harvesting our food but not having enough food for their families is heartbreaking but true.

Basic needs during crisis

Food support was one of the most important responses to the crisis of COVID and wildfires. The trauma of what farmworkers were living through was complicated by economic disparities that included loss of wages, loss of employment, COVID infection, health challenges and quarantine. Before the team could address the emotional challenges, ALAS heard from the community how critical it was for them to get access to healthy food. ALAS organized several food initiatives to include a home delivery program, a food pantry and a warm meal program.

ALAS' staff and community volunteers delivered food to the homes of those ill with COVID and or in quarantine. Instacart or Doordash was not an option for the many families that were isolated and in fear. ALAS used the generous donations of philanthropy groups, city and county officials and the community to supply food directly to the homes of those in the farms and community. ALAS learned the complexities of COVID and transmission in shared housing spaces. This reality posed another complication of families not being able to cook in shared kitchens due to risk of exposure. With numerous calls coming in, ALAS sent staff out daily with cooked meals to families. Each step of the way, ALAS listened to the concerns of the community and what was needed.

The second food program initiated during the crisis was setting up a whole foods pop up food pantry. ALAS worked with local farms, food delivery programs and mobilized donations from across the community to set up a drive through the food pantry. Creating a COVID-safe food pantry, ALAS developed a car drive up procedure with 250 cars, feeding over 1,200 individuals each week. Many in the community who wanted to support local farm workers found an opportunity to give back and came out to volunteer, collect food supplies and share resources. One of the most important considerations in setting up the ALAS food pantry was taking into account what the community needed to eat and be healthy. The pantry focus was sharing whole healthy foods that the community consumed, including fruits, vegetables, milk, eggs, rice, beans, oil, maseca and more. ALAS gave each car a food card to use for their additional grocery needs and made the process very simple. There were no complicated forms to complete or questions about status or work income. The food pantry operated on a trust basis and as a result witnessed large numbers of farmworker families utilizing the program. One teen shared, "we are only eating right now because of the ALAS food pantry".

One positive outcome of the pantry that stood out during COVID and the wildfire response was the direct outreach ALAS was able to do each week during the pantry. ALAS engaged those coming to the food pantry as an opportunity to share information about COVID and critical resources of support. The food pantry became an emergency portal of communication. ALAS staff passed out flyers for COVID vaccine clinics, shared county announcements and provided COVID education and resources for mental health and medical support. Most importantly, we were able to hear how the community was doing and what they needed during this time. The food pantry became a base of communication during the crisis and an opportunity to share PPE with the community. We gave out masks, hand sanitizer, gloves and even face shields. For students, we checked in about wifi hotspots and assessed for educational challenges they were having. The food pantry provided a good communication portal for us to understand weekly what the community was suffering. Two years later, the food pantry continues forward as a result of the continued pandemic and economic crisis.

The next food program ALAS began was the Farmworker Friday lunch program. This program was born out of a Taqueria calling to offer lunch to farmworkers during the pandemic. From this day forward, Farmworker Friday's was born. An important part of this lunch program is that the community becomes a part of donating and supporting this cause. Individuals and companies that want to make a difference sponsor a meal for farmworkers and their families. This bridge of connection from the community to the farms was a key foundation of support. For the farmworkers, it was and continues to be a positive source of support to see others appreciate their work and contribute to their well-being.

Un Respiro de Vida masks

When COVID hit, there were no masks available to the farmworker community. While the numbers were rising, a panic broke out among those in the field of how they would stay safe, given the close proximity of their work together. Several of the ALAS staff, including a Mental Health Clinician and our Arts Director, Zenón Barron, brought together mothers from ALAS to sew masks for the community. In the first months of COVID, ALAS mothers made over 15,000 masks. They worked non-stop to make masks to be delivered to the farms.

Fabric and donations were donated from across the country. There was an outpouring of community invested in showing their care for the farmworker community. In addition to masks made, ALAS received an outpouring of donated masks once they became available. At every food pantry or community contact made, ALAS made sure to give masks, hand sanitizer, donated face shields and any PPE supplies.

Vaccine education and support

One of the early concerns presented to ALAS staff was the assumption that the Latinx community would not get vaccinated. In hearing from the community, the opposite was true, they wanted to be protected, safe and be able to go to work and return to their families. The community shared how scared they were to be infected as it forced a shutdown to their overall well-being, especially to those living in shared housing. To be proactive and get education to the community, ALAS launched the first Latinx testimonio video for the community. Senior farmworkers volunteered to be the first to be vaccinated with San Mateo County and ALAS' support. We worked with them to share their stories of the importance of staying healthy for their families and shared it widely across social media. ALAS staff also went to meet with families on the farm as well as all farmworkers to provide vaccine information. As a result of building trust, staff partnered with the County and other groups to co-facilitate vaccine clinics at the farms. Work was done to enroll them and support the vaccine and booster process. The Latinx community responded with lots of enthusiasm and a large number were vaccinated; others received COVID education, reducing the spread of COVID to others on the Coastside.

El Jardin summer camp

To support the youth, ALAS developed a summer camp on site at the farms to provide reading and activity for the youth. Children at the farms were struggling to connect to wifi and attend online school. Many students had challenges with completing homework at home due to language and technology challenges. However, another key stressor that was identified was the emotional fatigue of what COVID presented in their lives. The sudden departure from school, the health and economic challenges of COVID, and many being locked up in shared housing for long periods of time, concerned our ALAS team. University of San Francisco (USF) School of Education faculty partnered with ALAS to bring education and tutoring straight to the farms for the first summer program in the fields and online. Every week children were smiling, excited and reported the positive impact of having teachers and community come out to be with them.

Keeping safe with all the PPE, it was significant to note that USF committed to making a difference while also going out during a time when others were sheltering in place. With safety in mind, the ALAS and USF team understood the critical importance of getting education out to a vulnerable population that had minimal access to online learning.

Following the first year of education in the fields, ALAS wanted to impact a larger group of children getting ready to go back into school in the Fall and launched a bigger El Jardin summer camp. Together with USF educators, artists, youth counselors and ALAS staff, El Jardin was an immersion into the arts focused on healing and educating in a way that built community and fun. Below is a sample of the core activities offered in the camp program:

Mondays, Wednesdays, Fridays

Class 1   Capoeira
Class 2   Hip Hop
Class 3   Voz & Guitar

Class 4   Arts & Crafts
Class 5   Cajon
Class 6   Sewing

Tuesdays, Thursdays

Academics: math, science and reading

Soccer included every Tuesdays and Thursdays for big muscle movement and development. The soccer program is led by coaches and youth camp counselors.

Youth that participated in the camp shared how much they loved being back with friends and engaged in learning. Several youth stated that during COVID, they felt as if they were stuck in cages and now were free. The emotional crisis of COVID was glaring as children seemed to come back to life as they immersed themselves in the activities and cariño that was shared with them at El Jardin. ALAS has committed to continue this camp every year with the same goal of bringing arts and culture front and center to the farmworker community.

Our veggies are Moonraised

In our visit to the farms, we felt the cold foggy air come upon us. Farmworkers shared that they spent many mornings cold, starting their day early at 5 am with little protection. ALAS decided to begin a Hoodies for Farmworkers program. With permission from local Latino youth, we worked with them to transform their slogan of "We Are Moonraised" to "Our Veggies Are Moonraised". Hundreds of green hoodies along with gallons of drinking water were given out by the ALAS Farmworker team. Farmworkers shared that having warm clothing meant so much as they worked long days in the field. With an outpouring of support during COVID, community members and corporate sponsors contributed donations of rain boots, jackets, knee pads, PPE, gloves, sanitizer and other equipment that helped with their job. ALAS made an Amazon Wish List organized by farmworkers. With donations, they were able to get direct support and save their income for rent and basic necessities for their families. Listening to what the need was and finding creative ways to increase resources for this community has been an important part of ALAS' crisis response.

Mental health in the fields

One of the most important areas of support given during COVID and the wildfire crisis was mental health support. For ALAS, it was important to rethink office visits as it was a time of quarantine. Telehealth was not an option for everyone as the majority did not have access to technology or wifi. Families shared the increased stress and isolation their children were experiencing.

Many children and families reported feeling overwhelmed, fearful and anxious. ALAS also was supporting many families with grief and loss of loved ones. With the increasing urgency to provide support, ALAS' mental health team went out to the farms to offer direct support and provide group counseling for children and mothers. We found that this was a critical life line for many that felt very alone and unsure of what was happening in the world around them. As School-Based Family Counseling practitioners, it was critical for us to be able to create space for healing and wellness. So many needed to process grief, isolation, fear, illness and sadness. Our crisis response not only addressed the emotional domain but also focused on physical health and well-being.

Cultural consciousness and humility

ALAS centers the community as its core tenet in order to celebrate identity and cultural pride. In doing so, our programming is reflective of the vision and mission to work for social wellness through multicultural practices, mental health care, as well as collective support for education, immigration and advocacy. ALAS' commitment to their community, especially their Latinx/e population, is rooted in cultural, social and linguistic consciousness. This enables a social justice lens to be applied that is race-conscious and policy-informed in order to effectively serve community members through familial relationships rather than a hierarchical approach. *Familismo* has enabled ALAS to build trust with their Latinx/e-community through unconditional support, acceptance, warmth, protection and loyalty (Calzada et al., 2013; Patrón, 2021). In essence, *familismo* provides ALAS the opportunity to protect its community members against physical and emotional stress through the support networks it has developed over the years (Marin and Marin, 1991). This focus on family is a hallmark of the SBFC approach.

Through these support networks and community *familismo*, staff has been able to embody cultural humility due to their commitment to self-reflection and self-critique regarding the power dynamic that exists in advocacy work (Tervalon and Murray-García, 1998). ALAS centers a constructive process to have staff consistently bring forth their cultural identities and backgrounds in order to build recognition and respect for those they serve who may have different cultural priorities and practices (Tervalon and Murray-García, 1998). Cultural competence is challenged in all the programming conducted at ALAS; rather, the space centers lifelong learning regarding privilege, positionality, identity and community. This has enabled ALAS to successfully advocate for the community and lead programming that address systemic injustices and barriers, especially for farmworker communities.

Challenges and solutions

Challenges during this time were the glaringly dangerous COVID infection. It was clear that every day that passed ALAS was out in the community, far from being quarantined. The commitment of the staff was admirable and concerning all at the same time due to the reality that they could become infected with COVID. Staff members were given the opportunity to stay at home; however, many in our team choose to put themselves on the front lines for crisis support. They committed to change, even when the vaccine had not been made available. Other challenges included COVID exposure, getting PPE that was scarce and meeting the increase in demand from the community. As families got sick and the pandemic worsened, ALAS had to increase staff to get supplies and warm meals out to isolated and quarantine families. As a team, ALAS had to do remote meetings, but worked in isolation. On a daily basis, ALAS was on the front line of COVID working on behalf of the community and giving it their complete devotion.

Conclusion

ALAS embodies familial relationships in all their advocacy work, especially with the farmworker population. As a community organization, ALAS believes that in order to support a community, you must transcend boundaries established within the professional realm. Activist accompaniment provides individuals who have been most oppressed and excluded to take agency over their activism and provided raw emotions (Tomlinson and Lipsitz, 2019). ALAS works toward developing and maintaining long-term relations with the community in order to establish interpersonal *conocimiento* (Hernandez-Arriaga and Argenal, 2022). In doing so, we are actively engaging with them in order to live and experience the conditions the community faces rather than separating ourselves. By incorporating emotional presence in the work conducted within the community, humanization is reestablished in order to create sensory connectors in community narratives. Through these community narratives, ALAS responded effectively and rapidly to crisis situations such as the COVID-19 pandemic. In situations of dire need, ALAS has established trauma-informed services in order to address the most pressing disparities being faced. ALAS is able to address complex issues due to the emotional connection and trust that has been developed over the years. *Familismo* truly guides the nature of work and response ALAS has; all efforts are approached with cultural consciousness and with the mission to disrupt cycles of injustices.

References

Bailey, Z. D., Krieger, N., Agénor, M., Graves, J., Linos, N., & Bassett, M. T. (2017). Structural racism and health inequities in the USA: Evidence and interventions. *Lancet (London, England)*, *389*(10077), 1453–1463. https://doi.org/10.1016/S0140-6736(17)30569-X

Calzada, E. J., Tamis-LeMonda, C. S., & Yoshikawa, H. (2013). Familismo in Mexican and Dominican families from low-income, urban communities. *Journal of Family Issues*, *34*(12), 1696–1724.

Chicas, R., Xiuhtecutli, N., Houser, M., Glastra, S., Elon, L., Sands, J. M., McCauley, L., &Chicas, R., Xiuhtecutli, N., Houser, M., Glastra, S., Elon, L., Sands, J. M., McCauley, L., & Hertzberg, V. (2022). COVID-19 and agricultural workers: A descriptive study. *Journal of immigrant and minority health, 24*(1), 58–64. https://doi.org/10.1007/s10903-021-01290-9

Devadoss, S., & Luckstead, J. (2008). Contributions of immigrant farmworkers to California Vegetable production. *Journal of Agricultural and Applied Economics, 40*(3), 879–894. https://doi.org/10.1017/s107407080000239x

Gerrard, B., & Soriano, M. (2018). The role of community Intervention in school-based family counseling. *International Journal for School-Based Family Counseling, 11*, 1–11.

Hernandez, T., & Gabbard, S. (2019). Findings from the National Agricultural Workers Survey (NAWS) 2015–2016: A demographic and employment profile of United States farmworkers. *Dep Labor Employ Train Adm Wash Dist Columbia.*

Hernandez-Arriaga, B., & Argenal A. (2022). Todos Somos Humanos, Danos Una Oportunidad. In C. Magno, J. Lew, & S. Rodriguez (Eds), *(Re) Mapping Migration and Education* (pp. 158–175). Brill Publications.

Liebman, A. K., Seda, C. H., & Galván, A. R. (2021). Farmworkers and covid-19: Community-based partnerships to address health and safety. *American Journal of Public Health, 111*(8), 1456–1458. https://doi.org/10.2105/ajph.2021.306323

Marin, G., & Marin, B. V. (1991). *Research with Hispanic Populations.* Sage Publications, Inc.

Patrón, O. E. (2021). Complicating traditional understandings of familismo: Precariousness in the lives of queer Latino men in college. *Journal of GLBT Family Studies, 17*(1), 30–48.

Ramos, A. K. (2018). A human rights-based approach to farmworker health: An overarching framework to address the social determinants of health. *Journal of Agromedicine, 23*(1), 25–31. https://doi.org/10.1080/1059924X.2017.1384419

Tervalon, M., & Murray-García, J. (1998). Cultural humility versus cultural competence: A critical distinction in defining physician training outcomes in multicultural education. *Journal of Health Care for the Poor and Underserved, 9*, 117–125.

Tippett, R. Counting Farmworkers in the 2020 Census. Carolina Demography, 16 April 2020. www.ncdemography.org/2020/04/16/counting-farmworkers-in-the-2020-census/.

Tomlinson, B., & Lipsitz, G. (2019). *Insubordinate spaces: Improvisation and accompaniment for Social Justice.* Pennsylvania.

11 Conjoint family counseling with grief and loss

Michael J. Carter and Emily J. Hernandez

Overview

This chapter will focus on using a school-based family counseling (SBFC) approach when working with issues related to grief and loss with families. Initial experiences of grief and loss for families usually involve a crisis state of functioning for family members. Learning of the loss of someone or something that one loves can create conditions for crisis. When a family is in crisis, there is a temporary period of reduced functioning in the family system and specifically for individual family members. Families in crisis find that their usual ways of coping or problem solving do not always work; and as a result, they feel vulnerable, anxious, and overwhelmed. Grief and loss may manifest itself differently in members of the family depending on a variety of factors. While grief and loss directly impact each person in the family, it also impacts the family system as a whole. For this reason, an SBFC approach utilizing conjoint family counseling is recommended for working with families experiencing grief and loss. This approach can help within the context of school settings to increase the level of functioning in children that have experienced losses in their family which can indirectly affect their availability for learning. The proposed counseling procedure can be conducted directly in school settings by experienced SBFC practitioners as needed.

Background

Grief is a universal response to the loss of a loved one or some type of significant life change. While these responses are universal in nature, there is variability in the ways that people process and experience grief and loss on a personal level. Having a general knowledge of grief and an understanding that it is a natural non-linear process that can be difficult to navigate, it can be helpful to many going through it. Our grief reactions can vary based on a number of factors, including our personality, current circumstances, social context, external influences, life experiences, previous experiences with grief and loss, developmental age, internal coping skills, cultural practices, and the type and magnitude of the loss. While most individuals are resilient in the grieving process and do not require specialized support, some will struggle

DOI: 10.4324/9781003201977-14

more depending on these factors and may develop prolonged or complicated grief reactions.

The current Coronavirus pandemic has exacerbated grief and loss for many because of the circumstances related to the pandemic and interruptions in grieving routines and rituals. Further, the longevity of the pandemic along with increasing uncertainty, stress, and anxiety surrounding the events and life changes related to living in a pandemic has collapsed the coping mechanisms that people have in place to get through short durations of high stress or crisis situations. This has contributed to increased stress, anxiety, depression, and burnout. For many experiencing grief and loss during the pandemic, what would be normally referred to as normative or uncomplicated grief has evolved into complicated grief due to the prolonged exposure, complex variables, and interruptions to the grieving process related to the pandemic.

Understanding the differences between bereavement and grief are important. Bereavement refers to the period of time of mourning and grief following the death of a loved one. There is no specific timeline for this period of bereavement. Grief is the emotional, cognitive, functional, and behavioral reactions a bereaved person might experience as a result of that loss (Zisook & Shear, 2009). Both bereavement and grief contribute to a sense of crisis for the person or family.

The basic framework for understanding what one goes through after the loss of a loved one is the Kübler-Ross' stages of grief. The five stages, Denial, Anger, Bargaining, Depression, and Acceptance, are a part of the framework that help understanding, and learning to process and live with, the loss in our life (Kübler-Ross & Kessler, 2014). The stages have evolved since their initial introduction and researchers have now included an additional stage of generativity, following the stage of acceptance. It is important to remember that there is no typical response to a loss, since there is no typical loss. The way a person processes grief and loss is unique to the person. It is as individual as our lives. Another important understanding regarding the stages is that they are non-linear and individuals may cycle through them differently, and this includes the repeat visiting of stages. Coping with grief and loss is a process that will take time and for many may never be fully resolved. Through the understanding of the stages over time, one can experience the grief less intensely and develop healthy coping mechanisms to process the loss.

How grief and loss affect families

As indicated above, while grief and loss may affect families and individuals in many different ways, it clearly constitutes a crisis situation despite its different manifestations. The extent and the severity of the effects of this crisis on different family members depend upon their unique temperament, specific Individual Life Cycle stage, and their role in the family.

In addition, there are specific factors about the family that further impact the unique experience of grief for each family member during a crisis. These factors are related to the Family Life Cycle stage that the family is currently involved in, which depends upon the age of the children and the family dynamics caused by their different developmental stages. Briefly, the stages of the Family Life Cycle (Karpel & Strauss, 1983) are Onset of Marriage or Committed Relationship, Birth of the Child, Individuation of the Child, Individuation of the Adolescent, Departure of the Children, and Aging and Death of Parents.

Karpel and Strauss (1983) also wrote about an analysis of the different Dimensions of the family, including the Factual Dimension, Individual Dimension, Systemic Dimension, and the Ethical Dimension. These Dimensions constitute many of the most important factors regarding families that can be assessed through individual and group interviews along with observations and analysis by the SBFC practitioner. This analysis leads to an assessment of the most important issues currently affecting the family, including cultural and historical factors, which then leads to specific treatment goals and specific steps to reach each goal.

Treatment involves conjoint meetings with the whole family present and other meetings with subsets of the family, typically related to the family subsystem (i.e., Spousal, Parental, or Sibling) that is being addressed. Another important aspect of this work involves the use of "Dyad Work", where two family members work directly with each other to focus on and improve communication through Active Listening Techniques and mutual perspective taking with facilitation by the SBFC practitioner (Hernandez, Ribera & Carter, 2019). Following a significant loss, these conjoint processes can help families to grieve together and increase the mutual support that often results in the family growing closer together rather than further apart.

Connection to SBFC model and framework

Conjoint family intervention with grief and loss falls largely in the area of the family and school intervention quadrants if you are viewing the construct through the SBFC metamodel and framework. The SBFC metamodel, as described by Gerrard and Soriano (2019), illustrates the primary focus of SBFC to be on the school and the family in the area of prevention and intervention. Working with families experiencing crisis involves an intervention focus utilized with the goals of providing immediate stabilization to the family system. For families with children, this is directly connected to the school focus and may also involve collaboration with the schools and school intervention. The proposed procedure in this chapter is systemic in nature and also falls within the prevention quadrants of the SBFC model (see Figure 1.1 in Chapter 1) (Gerrard & Soriano, 2019).

Procedure

This procedure is an SBFC approach on how to do grief counseling with families that are in crisis. Since grief reactions can be experienced and processed by members in the family differently, it will be important to work with the families as a whole and to work with the family subsystems separately at times. The following procedures include a conjoint family process to address grief and loss in a family system.

First step: 1st meeting with parents alone

The process begins by working with the parental subsystem before talking with children. It is important to use a wide definition of parents and to determine who are the active parents in the family's structure. Typically, this includes both biological parents, the mother and father, but often deviates from this traditional model. It is important to understand that the primary parental figures may be step-parents, extended family members, and partners who do not have a formal step-parent designation. For the following discussion, the term "parents" will be used to include all of these different types of primary parental figures.

The first step is to talk with both parents together about the loss and determine which parental figure was most affected by the loss (i.e., the parent who has a closer relationship to the deceased). Once this has been determined, the SBFC practitioner assists the parents to begin to share what happened to the deceased. It is critical for the clinician to understand the importance of working with the parents to begin their grieving process as soon as possible so that they can be better prepared to assist their children in their grieving process, which is often more complicated and delayed. While it is sometimes easier to assist parents in "scheduling" their grieving, it is much harder to predict when children may experience their grief. Consequently, parents must be prepared to notice and assist their children's experiences of grief during a wide variety of possible times and places. Parents are typically much more worried about their children, so it may be necessary to get a clear affirmation from the parents about their understanding of this process.

Specific talking points and areas to explore during this first meeting with the parents include:

- Acknowledge that the loss has an impact on their family.
- Validate the experience by explaining that this is a significant life event affecting their family.
- Explain that everyone grieves in their own way and in their own time.
  - Emphasize the importance of respecting each person's differences in how they are affected and grieve as they may be in different stages of the grieving process.

- Ask the parents to share more about what happened.
  - Gather specific facts about the death and what has happened before and after with them and their family.
  - Distinguish between progressive illness death (PID) and sudden death (SD). For PID, ask specific questions about the type of illness, the length and treatment of the illness, and length of hospice care. For situations related to SD, gain as much information as possible about the incident, including what happened before and after the death. It is important to be very respectful of the fact that they may not know, or have as much information about, the details at this time.
- Explore with the parents their perspectives on how each person in the family is dealing with the loss (feelings, behaviors, etc.).
- Ask about the cultural and religious/spiritual factors that may be important to the family. During this discussion, be respectful of the specific way each of them may believe or utilize their religious/spiritual orientation or embrace their own cultural expectations (e.g., they may attend services but not really believe in the spiritual aspects of the religion or gain comfort from the traditional rites related to loss).
- Explore the existing support systems and structures in the family.
- Provide psychoeducation regarding the grieving process and the stages of loss.
  - Teach about the stages in the "DABDAG" model (Denial, Anger, Bargaining, Depression, Acceptance, and Generativity) and that they may cycle through these in different ways as it is a non-linear process.
  - One of the most important aspects to impress upon the parents is that while it is natural to have strong feelings throughout each of the stages of the grieving process, it is important to be aware of engaging in a negative thought process regarding these feelings because it can lead to getting "stuck" in that stage.
- End the session by providing a summarization of what was shared in the session and validating all their feelings as being natural and appropriate to such a significant loss.
- Establish expectations for the next meeting which will include meeting again with the parents only.

Second step: 2nd meeting with parents alone

The second meeting begins by meeting with both parents to assess how they have been doing since the first session and whether or not they have any questions regarding aspects that were discussed. It is explained that the next step will be to have individual sessions with each parent regarding their own unique experiences of grief. The SBFC practitioner then meets with each parent individually for about 20–30 minutes each and then reconvenes with both of them to finish the session.

Specific talking points and areas that can be explored during the individual meeting with each parent separately include:

- How did the person find out about the death?
- Where were they at that time?
- Who was with them when they found out?
- What were their feelings at that moment?
- Did they have the time and a place to fully experience their feelings?
- How have their relationships with the other parent, their children, and others been affected during this time of grieving?
- How have they been doing since the loss? Explore the following:
  - Main areas of life functioning during this time; amount and quality of sleep, consistency and nutritional value of eating, and general activity level.
  - Attendance at employment and whether they have taken days of bereavement from their job. If they have attended work, what has been their level of ability to attend to critical responsibilities, interactions with co-workers, and any grief expression during work hours. It is also important to explore whether or not they have a safe space at work to be alone when necessary.
    - For most adults and children, it is natural to experience a reduced level of functioning and a lower quality of production in their work or school during the first few weeks of their return. It is important to encourage the parent to express this reality to their supervisors or their children's teachers, who may not understand that this is a natural consequence of the grieving process.
    - For some people however, going to work may provide a respite from the overwhelming feelings of grief. While this may be true, it is still important to ensure that the person is scheduling enough time in their daily life to allow time for grieving.
- Provide closure to the individual parent meeting by validating their experiences, thoughts, and feelings. In addition, remind them that each person grieves in a different way and the importance of recognizing and respecting their feelings.
- Explore coping mechanisms to relieve any pressure built up by feelings of grief. This may include helping the parent to schedule daily time after the children go to sleep to allow themselves to cry or journal about their loss.
- This process should then be repeated with other parent.

After the brief individual sessions with each parent, bring them back together and have them share with each other where they are in their grieving and facilitate their active listening and acknowledgment of each other's feelings. Remind them of the importance of sharing their grief with each other versus isolating, in order to best support each other now and in their work together with their children. Lastly, assess their readiness to begin focusing treatment on the children.

Because the parents will still be grieving, this focus on the children needs to be a concurrent process of meeting their needs as well as their children's.

Third step: First whole family meeting

The third step involves meeting with the family as a whole. After meeting together with the parents and other adults and interviewing them individually, a meeting with the whole family, including the children, is convened. This meeting is to provide the children with support and a context for the loss and process of grieving. It begins by providing the children with the same perspective as the adults described above in Step #2 but the focus and information provided are with an approach that is modified to the developmentally appropriate range of the children's ages.

Specific talking points and areas that can be explored during the whole family meeting with include:

- Acknowledge that there has been a loss that has impacted their family.
- Validate their experiences by explaining that this is a significant life event that affects their whole family.
- Explain that everyone grieves in their own ways and in their own time.
  - Emphasize the importance of respecting each person's differences in how they are affected and are grieving as they may be in different stages of the grieving process.
  - Have the parents explain that they have already been working with the SBFC practitioner about this loss and have met together and individually with the SBFC practitioner, so now it's the children's turn to do the same. Emphasize that what is talked about in these meetings will be confidential unless someone's safety is at risk.

Meeting with the children individually

At the beginning of each individual meeting with the children, it is important for the SBFC practitioner to help the child understand the nature of the meeting and their role in it. When interviewing children, the following may help in this regard:

> *I'm going to ask you some questions about you and your family. There are no wrong or right answers to these questions, but what's important is that you try to be honest about what you think and feel. What we talk about will be confidential, except if something comes up that might involve someone getting hurt. If that happens, we will talk about it so that no one will get hurt. I want to remember what you say, so I will be writing down your answers. Do you have any questions?*

One process used to get to know the child before exploring their experience about the loss is to explore the various areas of the child's life. This "circle of life" encompasses current and past functioning in health, school, financial concerns, living arrangements, friends, immediate and extended family, personal goals, and recreation.

As the interview questions are being asked, there are often opportunities to go beyond the respondent's immediate answer to survey deeper aspects of the issues relating to the question. The child may be open to this exploration but the SBFC practitioner must be mindful about the level of rapport and not push the child too early in the evaluation process.

After getting to know the child through the "Circle of Life", the interview continues with a focus on the child's experience of the loss.

Specific talking points and areas that can be explored with the child regarding the loss include:

Asking: How did the child find out about it?

- Who was with them when they found out?
- What were their feelings at that moment?
- How have they been dealing with this loss so far?
- How does the family deal with someone talking about the deceased?
- How comfortable does the child feel about talking about the loss with any family member and with whom?
- How does the family deal with someone crying about deceased?
- How comfortable does the child feel about crying in front of any family member and whom?
- Is there anything else that the child thinks the SBFC practitioner needs to know about the child or their family?

After the child answers all of the questions, the SBFC practitioner then says:

> *"Now that you are finished, is there anything that you have talked about that* you do not want me to share with your parents?" If the child indicates that any responses should not be shared, then the SBFC practitioner should circle those answers and not share them with the parents or others.

Once all the interviews are finished with the children, the SBFC practitioner brings the whole family back together before ending the session. At this time, the SBFC practitioner summarizes what has happened so far and provides feedback on where the family is in the grieving process and what the next steps will be. These next steps will include continuing to meet with the family, both individually and as a group, to work through and address individual and family issues and concerns regarding the loss and how grief is being manifested with each person.

Fourth step: Continue conjoint family counseling sessions

The fourth step includes a continued course of treatment in working with the family within a conjoint format, with individual sessions as necessary.

A minimum of six to eight sessions is recommended beginning with weekly sessions, then alternating with longer intervals between meetings to assist with maintenance and ongoing support.

The remaining sessions should focus on creating opportunities for the family to share their feelings in a space where each person can feel heard and supported no matter where they are in their own grieving process. If somebody is not comfortable in sharing their own feelings, it is important to remind them that every family member needs to be there to listen and provide support for each other. There are important issues to consider when working with the family over the next few sessions.

Important considerations to work through during the grieving process

As the SBFC practitioner continues to work with the family, it is important to keep in mind the developmental stage and individual needs of each child, including taking into consideration any areas of special needs with the children. One of the main considerations is whether to include children under five years in all of the family meetings. For children under five, they may be overwhelmed by the emotions of other family members and might distract from the group process because they are too young to fully understand and participate in the deeper levels of awareness and processing of grief. There are additional treatment areas below to consider.

Common patterns related to becoming "Stuck" in a stage of grief

Throughout the process of working through the stages of grief, a person may seem to become "stuck" in one stage for a considerable period of time lasting from weeks to months and even throughout their lifespan. Signs of this are often behavioral and affective in nature with extended periods of time spent perseverating on the same theme. When this is observed, the SBFC practitioner must explore the thoughts underlying these symptoms to identify any signs of negative, repetitive thought processes that may cause the client to become "stuck" in that stage, which often hinders their ability to progress through the stages of grief, now and in the future. Some common patterns are described below with some examples of how SBFC practitioners can respond to these situations.

Addressing feelings of guilt and regret

During the stages of Anger and Betrayal, it is common for a person to start to feel guilt and regret over things that they would have done differently if they had known the person was going to die. While this initial thought may be a natural response, continued focus on unreasonable guilt can intensify feelings of sadness and turn into long-term depression that can lead the person to become "stuck" in this stage of the grieving process.

If this occurs, it is important to reflect to the client that this is happening and the importance of learning how to deal with this in a constructive manner to promote healing. While guilt can be a useful emotion in order to remedy situations that are within our control, it can be very destructive when guilt is irrational or perseverated upon when nothing can be done to remedy the situation. In this case, it's important to "clean out the guilt" as soon as possible so that the grieving process can continue. First, the SBFC practitioner will validate and acknowledge that it is natural to have these feelings. After doing this, the SBFC practitioner then explores the thinking involved in the guilty feelings and provides a reframing of the situation in a more realistic and constructive view. For example, people will often say that if they had known that a person was going to die, they would have done something differently (e.g., spent more time with them) and now feel guilty. An effective reframing response might be: "But isn't it also true that *you did not know then* what you know *now*? So, do you think it's fair to feel guilty *now* about what you didn't do *then* when you didn't know they were going to die?" Another important question in response to this might be: "If you feel that the person you lost loved you, do you think they would want you to feel guilty now over something you had no control over?" It's also important to note that this process of "cleaning out unreasonable guilt" often requires gaining verbal confirmation from the client of this truth so that they will remember it later if the thought recurs.

Addressing the "Anger-Betrayal Loop"

A common pattern often observed when a person becomes "stuck" in a stage is related to the person cycling through the stages of Anger and Betrayal in a repetitive pattern. This "Anger-Betrayal Loop" is often related to the feelings underlying the expression of Anger and the thoughts involved in the feelings of Betrayal. Expressions of Anger are often the result of three main feelings: fear, frustration, and sadness. These are sometimes experienced separately and often in combination. Feelings of Betrayal are often related to beliefs concerning the causes of death and the ability of a person or deity to prevent this from happening. These beliefs may be related to a doctor, government, or universal powers, such as God. For example, it's not unusual to hear someone at a funeral express their Anger at mistakes that may have been made by medical staff in the care of the person who died or others they think could have prevented the death. At the same time, the person may believe that God has betrayed them in taking a loved one from them, despite their religious or spiritual practice. This pattern is problematic because it leads to thoughts of Betrayal reactivating feelings of Anger which then reactivates a sense of Betrayal which then reactivates Anger and so on and so on, resulting in a process of emotional paralysis that can last for years.

Wound analogy

The above experiences often result in prolonging the painful nature of grieving for many years. While the person may be able to continue functioning on many levels, their emotional functioning is often severely impaired and they can become highly vulnerable to maladaptive ways of relieving their emotional pain. These adaptations can include engaging in substance abuse and other addictive behaviors or having frequent angry outbursts that potentially can ruin their interpersonal relationships with those closest to them. In responding to these types of situations, it is often useful to engage in a discussion of how these emotional wounds are similar to physical wounds that are experienced in our bodies. If a physical wound becomes infected, it can cause more pain and loss of functioning, even to the point of death. To treat a physical wound, the diseased tissue must be cleaned out, which may cause the wound to bleed again, and then antibiotic ointment is provided in order for the wound to heal. An emotional wound can also become infected and lead to similar consequences. Similarly, the emotional experience must be revisited for catharsis and cleaning out of guilt, which may cause more tears, but then constructive context and support (See Feelings of Regret and Guilt above) are provided in order for the wound to heal. This healing process is gradual and non-linear but the person can still move forward while recovering by reestablishing healthy routines to the extent possible. It's important to remind them that, "You're going through the Motions, although you haven't yet gone through all the Emotions".

Warning signs of harm to self and others

Throughout the course of treatment with the family, it is always important to continually assess for safety as needed with all family members. Due to the individual nature of grieving, some members of the family may struggle more than others. If there are any observed or reported warning signs related to harm of self or others, the SBFC practitioner must do their due diligence in ensuring safety as required.

Multicultural considerations

An individual's experience of the stages of grief is often affected by the nature of their cultural and historical backgrounds. For example, in many patriarchal cultures, there are gender-related expectations of what feelings are appropriate for women or men to acknowledge and express, which are embedded during the process of their socialization beginning in childhood. A traditional theme is that men are allowed to express Anger but are not allowed to express sadness or fear. This can be a significant problem because men may not allow their children to cry in their presence for fear that they themselves may become emotional and start crying. Conversely, women are often allowed to express sadness and fear but are discouraged from expressing Anger. While these traditional mores are definitely changing, they are still quite prevalent throughout a variety of cultures and personal histories. Therefore, it's important to remind everyone that feelings are important and should not be suppressed or family members apologize for expressing them.

Challenges and solutions

The proposed procedures present challenges that may impact the ability to facilitate all aspects of the procedure. First, the procedures require the SBFC practitioner to have basic training in facilitating conjoint practices. The majority of grief work is done on an individual level and through support groups. Utilizing conjoint practices to facilitate grief work in families can be difficult due to the intensity of emotions, roles each member plays in the family, and the specialized skills required by the SBFC practitioner to navigate the grief healing process with the family as a whole. While this requires specialized skills in conjoint family counseling, the healing effects of the process are curative for the family. SBFC practitioners should regularly work with families to continue building on these skills and engage in continuing education to specialize in working with families as a system. Another challenge includes the existence of stigma to mental health, particularly in families and in different cultures. Addressing mental health stigma is a larger issue and this stigma can lead to resistance on the part of families to participate. Psychoeducation, trust, and rapport are critical to working with families experiencing stigma and resistance to getting support. Lastly, access to services is a challenge. Due to the limited number of practitioners that engage in family counseling work, it can be difficult for families to gain access to this type of service. In addition, many mental health benefits through insurance do not provide reimbursement to practitioners for family counseling and thus adopt a more Eurocentric model of treatment focused on the individual and diagnoses. It may also be difficult for families to have the financial means to pay for access to practitioners that can provide conjoint treatment if their insurance does not cover the service. Similarly, to financial access, is understanding how to navigate a mental health system and know what services are needed and how to obtain them. For these reasons, it is critical that SBFC providers that work in settings, such as school systems, learn how to provide conjoint services so that they can engage with families through these systems to provide services and healing to the students and families that they serve.

Conclusion

This chapter focused on using an SBFC conjoint family intervention approach to working with families in crisis related to dealing with grief and loss. Working with grief and loss issues is complex for practitioners and even more complex for families navigating this experience. This approach uses conjoint family counseling processes to work with the family together to provide support during the family crisis. The proposed procedure is a 6–8 session model for addressing grief and loss with a family using conjoint family counseling practices. The procedure also covers other important clinical areas of attention for assessment during the sessions with the family. SBFC practitioners are uniquely positioned to create opportunities for healing for the family system as a whole especially during times of crisis related to grief and loss which can assist in moving the family from loss to resilience.

Resources

Website

Mental Health Technology Transfer Center Network, Substance Abuse and Mental Health Services Administration (SAMHSA). (n.d) Responding to COVID-19 Grief, Loss and Bereavement Resources. Retrieved from https://mhttcnetwork. org/centers/global-mhttc/responding-covid-19-grief-loss-and-bereavement
An excellent website featuring a list of informational resources related to grief and loss.

Books

Kübler-Ross, E. (1973). *On death and dying.* Routledge.
Seminal work by Dr. Kübler-Ross and recommended reading for any practitioner doing work in the area of grief and loss.
Neimeyer, R. A. (Ed.). (2015). *Techniques of grief therapy: Assessment and intervention.* Routledge.
This book offers a set of innovative approaches to grief therapy to address the needs of the bereaved. Providing both an orientation to bereavement work and an indispensable toolkit for counseling survivors of losses of many kinds, this book belongs on the shelf of both experienced clinicians and those just beginning to delve into the field of grief therapy.
Worden, J.W. (2003). *Grief counseling and grief therapy.* Springer.
Worden incorporates emerging theories and cutting-edge research into this fully revised edition which includes: a chapter on the mourning process discussing the personal and social difficulties that shape mourning with detailed guidelines for approaching special types of grief including suicide, sudden death and miscarriage. Grief Counselling and Grief Therapy is an essential resource for everyone working with the bereaved, from those just entering the field, to seasoned practitioners.

References

Gerrard, B. & Soriano, M. (2019). School-based family counseling: The revolutionary paradigm. In B. Gerrard, M. Carter & D. Ribera (Eds.) *School-based family counseling: An interdisciplinary practitioner's guide.* Routledge.
Hernandez, E. J., Ribera, D., & Carter, M. J. (2019). Family intervention: How to build collaboration between the family and school using conjoint family counseling. In B. Gerrard, M. Carter & D. Ribera (Eds.) *School-based family counseling: An interdisciplinary practitioner's guide.* Routledge.

Karpel, M. & Strauss, E. (1983). *Family evaluation*. Gardner Press.

Kübler-Ross, E. & Kessler, D. (2014). *On grief & grieving: Finding the meaning of grief through the five stages of loss*. Scribner.

Zisook, S. & Shear, K. (2009). Grief and bereavement: What psychiatrists need to know. *World Psychiatry*, 8, 67–74. https://doi.org/10.1002/j.2051-5545.2009.tb00217.x

12 Couples in crisis

A poststructuralist approach

Jeff Chang

Overview

In this chapter, I propose a framework for conceptualizing crisis intervention with couples. School-based family counseling (SBFC) professionals are often called upon to consult with parents subsequent to school-based crises. At other times, because of their availability and familiarity to parents, SBFC professionals may be called upon for brief crisis intervention with parents regarding an event outside of the school. Most crisis intervention literature focuses on individual clients in crisis. The framework I propose provides guidance to SBFC professionals on incorporating the interpersonal interactions within couples into their crisis intervention efforts. Situating myself in a poststructuralist approach to therapy, I have drawn on solution-focused and single-session therapy, the IPscope, and narrative approaches to therapy. I conclude with a composite case example.

Background

Definition of crisis

Yeager and Roberts (2015, p. 13) suggest that individuals are in crisis when they:

1 Perceive a precipitating event as being meaningful and threatening.
2 Appear unable to modify or lessen the impact of stressful events with traditional coping methods.
3 Experience increased fear, tension, and/or confusion.
4 Exhibit a high level of subjective discomfort.
5 Proceed rapidly to an active state of crisis—a state of disequilibrium.

Most sources on crisis intervention focus on individuals (Dass-Brailsford, 2010; Kolski & Jongsma, 2014; Miller, 2011; Sandoval, 2013). Couples therapy sources (Carson & Casado-Kehoe, 2011; Dattilio, 2010; Harway, 2005; Nelson, 2020) tend to treat crisis intervention as an afterthought, typically focus on crises like infidelity (Peluso, 2007) or intimate partner violence (Shipway, 2004), and focus mainly on ongoing treatment, not crisis response. When a crisis affects a school community, the parental subsystem's functioning, and

DOI: 10.4324/9781003201977-15

particularly their decision-making, may also be impaired. School-based family counseling (SBFC) practitioners can help the parental subsystem regain their equilibrium and make sound decisions on behalf of their children. Viewed through the SBFC metamodel, supporting couples in the aftermath of a crisis falls in the *family intervention* quadrant.

Complexity with couples

Besides the defining characteristics of crisis described by Yeager and Roberts (2015), when couples present in crisis, the interactions between them add another level of complexity. Taibbi (2018) suggests that couples tend to be *highly focused on content*. Each partner has a version of precipitating events to which they might be wedded. This can extend to each individual working to convince the therapist of the truth of their respective accounts, what Taibbi (p. 8) refers to as *playing courtroom*. Finally, following Doherty et al. (2015), Taibbi calls our attention to differential commitment to the relationship—*leaning in vs. leaning out*. These factors make crisis intervention with couples more complicated than intervening with an individual.

Procedure

From a poststructuralist perspective, I rely on the literature and practices of single-session and walk-in therapy (Slive & Bobele, 2011), narrative therapy (Madigan, 2019; Morgan, 2000), and the IPscope (Tomm et al., 2014). While single-session and walk-in therapy provides the core of the procedure, narrative therapy and the IPscope inform the process. While these therapeutic practices depend on different theoretical roots, their shared poststructuralist assumptions provide a common base for integration (Chang, 1998; Chang & Nylund, 2013; Chang & Phillips, 1993).

Single-session and walk-in therapy

According to Slive and Bobele (2011), single-session and walk-in therapy borrows from approaches such as solution-focused brief therapy (SFBT; Chang, 2021; de Jong & Berg, 2013, de Shazer, 1988), the strategic approach developed at the Mental Research Institute in Palo Alto, CA (MRI; Fisch et al., 1991; Watzlawick et al., 1976), narrative therapy (Madigan, 2019; Morgan, 2000), and other brief collaborative approaches (Keeney & Ray, 1993). Slive and Bobele (2011) provide a general procedural outline for single-session interventions. These may be done in sequence, but in practice are more likely to be intertwined tasks.

Step 1: What does the client want?

Slive and Bobele (2011) recommend asking about how the practitioner can be of help today: "The first step is learning what the client wants. The remainder of the session is about giving that to the client" (p. 45).

Step 2: Developing a contextual understanding

What has impelled the couple to seek help now? Has the acting out of their adolescent son finally resulted in school suspension? Has their middle school child lost their teacher to cancer? Did their teenager being verbally bullied escalate into a physical assault? In the aftermath of a flood the previous year, has their kindergartener become fearful of rainstorms? *Why now?*

Step 3: Inquire about client resources

SBFC professionals create a context for clients to experience their strengths, solution behavior, and resources (Slive & Bobele, 2011). How has the couple managed to avoid being totally overtaken by the crisis? What do they do that works, even somewhat? How they have "hung in"? What helpful characteristics make a difference? Solution-focused therapists (ref) call these *exceptions* (de Shazer, 1985; Korman et al., 2020) and narrative therapists call these *unique outcomes* (Madigan, 2019; Morgan, 2000).[1]

Step 4: Ask about attempted solutions

The MRI approach (Fisch et al, 1991; Watzlawick, et al., 1976) suggests that there are times when *the problem is the attempted solution*—problem-solving efforts may be backfiring, exacerbating the problem.

Step 5: Utilizing client motivation

Thinking in terms of *visiting relationships, complainant relationships,* and *customer relationships* (de Shazer, 1988) may be useful in understanding clients' receptivity to our intervention. It is also helpful to "keep an ear peeled" for implied statements of client values or what they might treasure or long for. Narrative therapists have called this the *absent but implicit* (Carey et al., 2009).

Step 6: Think small

Focus on the smallest changes possible in the immediate future (today or tomorrow). Thinking small can help practitioners "take pressure off themselves and… not make the error of promoting more than the client wants" (Slive & Bobele, 2011, p. 47).

Step 7: Compliments/commendations

Compliments or commendations are useful as a prelude for suggestions or homework. These are based on client descriptions of what they are doing that is helpful, or as Insoo Kim Berg (1994) calls them "evidence-based compliments." This highlights solutions and/or strengths that have escaped the clients' notice. Compliments can surprise clients who expect to be blamed or criticized and increase receptivity to the practitioner's suggestions.

This approach to single-session work largely parallels traditional crisis intervention approaches like Roberts and Ottens' (2005) seven-step crisis intervention model. I have found these conceptual frames helpful as I move through these seven steps:

The IPscope

The *IPscope* (Tomm et al., 2014)—"IP" standing for *interpersonal patterns*—is an approach to conceptualizing human functioning developed by Dr. Karl Tomm and colleagues at the Calgary Family Therapy Centre. The IPscope views humans' experiences as embedded in the interpersonal patterns (IPs). In effect, an IP is the smallest unit of systemic functioning—the coupled behaviors in an interaction between two individuals (see Figure 12.1).

Some IPs have beneficial "healing" or "wellness" effects. This depends on the specific coupled behaviors and the meanings the participants ascribe to them. For example, a *wellness interpersonal pattern* (WIP), as seen in Figure 12.2, would likely be experienced by the participants as supportive.

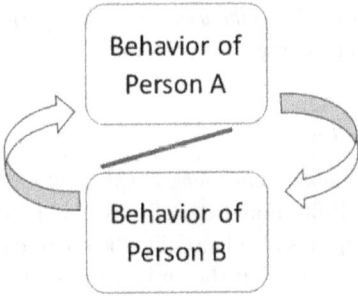

Figure 12.1 Coupled behaviors in an Interpersonal Pattern (IP)

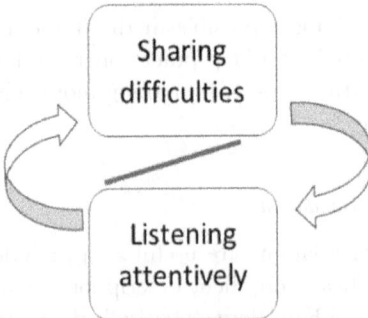

Figure 12.2 A hypothetical Wellness Interpersonal Pattern (WIP)

Some IPs have detrimental effects on the participants. These *pathologizing interpersonal patterns* (PIPs) are vicious cycles that invite participants into negative emotions and behavior and tend to reduce connection. For example, as seen in Figure 12.3, one partner's criticizing could be coupled with the other's defending, with the likely effect of pushing participants apart.

A healing interpersonal pattern (HIP) is a subcategory of a WIP, one meant to be an alternative or antidote to a PIP. For example, a couple in crisis might enact a PIP as seen in Figure 12.4.

An SBFC professional might seek to highlight an alternative HIP as seen in Figure 12.5 as an antidote to the PIP in Figure 12.4.

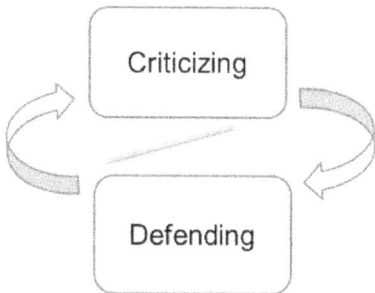

Figure 12.3 A hypothetical Pathologizing Interpersonal Pattern (PIP)

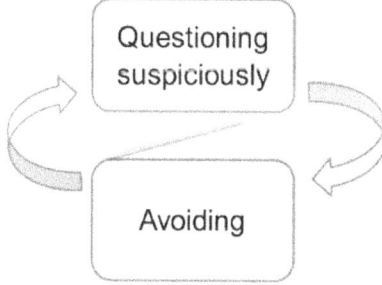

Figure 12.4 A hypothetical Pathologizing Interpersonal Pattern (PIP)

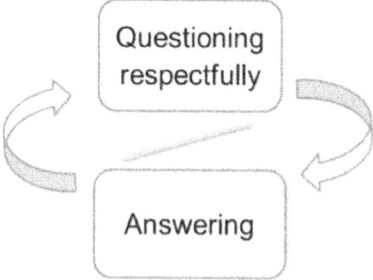

Figure 12.5 A hypothetical Healing Interpersonal Pattern (HIP)

A telescope or a microscope enables us to see something different than the unaided eye. Similarly, the IPscope permits us to see something other than Western culture's default to individual explanations. However, unlike a telescope or microscope, what we see through the IPscope is not "real"; we are not seeing what is "really wrong" the couple. Distinguishing PIPs, WIPs, and HIPs permits us to make pragmatic distinctions that may help us make sense of a couple's intersections.

Two other kinds of IPs are worth mentioning. *Deteriorating interpersonal patterns* (DIPs) are a kind of PIP that occurs when progress is slipping. DIPs typically occur when a precipitating event disrupts the stability of a WIP, which precipitates a crisis; or when a couple has made some progress, one or both may still be hypervigilant or awkward practicing new behaviors, leading to the feeling of "walking on eggshells." *Transforming interpersonal patterns* (TIPs) are usually initiated by SBFC professionals, inviting clients to describe their preferred outcomes, or to think about a situation differently. The purpose is not to correct unhelpful beliefs as suggested in cognitive therapy (Beck, 2020) but to invite reflection on whether the assumptions are useful.

The IPscope provides a useful frame for viewing couples in crisis. The event precipitating the crisis overwhelms the couple's stable WIPs, increasing their fear, tension, and/or confusion, facilitating a state of disequilibrium. Couple-oriented crisis intervention requires SBFC professionals to recognize the PIPs that are initiated, inquire about more helpful coping (WIPs and HIPs), and facilitate TIPs to bring about change.

Narrative practices

Narrative therapy (Madigan, 2019; Morgan, 2000) relies on the idea that cultural discourses specify how we ought to live our lives in ways that are largely unexamined and therefore invisible. Clinical problems are largely about how we interface with these cultural specifications. Narrative therapists deconstruct them, clarify clients' preferences in relation to them, and support clients to act accordingly.

Narrative therapy is known for *externalizing the problem*. SBFC practitioners refer to the problem by a specific name (e.g., in the historic published account, White [1984] referred to encopresis as Sneaky Poo). This can be a way to playfully refer to a problem and question the client about how it influences, interferes with, troubles, or tricks them. When partners are at odds, externalizing conversations can join them against a common enemy in a common project. More than just a clever technique, externalizing conversations deconstruct the idea that problems are inherent to individuals and uncover the cultural discourses that support problems.

Reauthoring conversations start with descriptions of times when the client is acting in accord with their values. Thickening these descriptions can assist the client to move toward a new identity that incorporates and highlights the changes on which the client is embarking.

Case example: Myra and John[2]

To illustrate a poststructuralist-informed approach to crisis intervention with a couple, I provide the example of Myra and John. Myra (44) called my office at about 4:30 p.m., asking to come in with her husband John (43) as soon as possible. She stated that their son Wyatt (16) "got suspended from school today for getting in a fight. He came home at lunch time, we got into it, and he hit me. Now he's in lock-up. We need to figure out what to do. Is there any way you could see us in the morning? He has a bail hearing at 2:00 p.m."

Fortunately, my calendar was open.

On their arrival, Myra looked haggard and worried, John looked taciturn.

JEFF: (after introductions and administrative requirements) I know there's some urgency about this time today because of court this afternoon. What's the result you would like to see out of today's session?

I already know some of the contextual elements (Why now?), namely that Myra and John's son Wyatt was incarcerated the night before after assaulting Myra, but I need to know more.

MYRA: Well, as I told you on the phone, our son hit me last night.

JOHN: Yeah, he shook her like a rag doll and then just slugged her.

JEFF: That sounds terrible. I imagine you must have all kinds of thoughts and questions about this. What would you like the main focus of this meeting to be?

In keeping with Slive and Bohele (2011), I focused almost right away on what the clients want.

MYRA: Well, we need to decide what to do today. Wyatt has a bail hearing this afternoon, and we are not on the same page at all.

JEFF: Would you mind starting out by telling me about the incident?

MYRA: Well, Wyatt had been sent home from school when he got suspended. I got a call from the vice-principal in advance. So by the time he got home, I knew what was going on. I was so mad that when he came in the door, I laid into him. I told him how irresponsible he was, how disappointed I was, and how I was ashamed of him. I was so furious.

I know I probably should not have said what I did, but he just looked at me like a crazy person. He shook me and called me a bitch and then punched me in the face. I was so shocked I didn't know what to say and I told him to just get out. And he did. And then I called John to come home from work.

JEFF: What happened next?

JOHN: Well, I was home within ten minutes. Myra seemed OK physically, but she was pretty shaken up. And we had all the doors locked and Wyatt forgot his key and he started knocking on the door, then banging on it, then he started kicking it. I called 911 and the cops were there in a couple minutes, and they hauled him away.

MYRA: I couldn't believe they were taking him away!

JEFF: And what did the police have to say?

JOHN: Wyatt's being charged with domestic assault. Because of this, we don't have the choice of pressing charges or not. The police don't want victims just letting their family members off, but I think it's the right thing to charge him.

MYRA: I don't know if it is or not, but the police told me that have no choice— that he would be charged. But now we have to decide whether to post bail.

JOHN: And I am totally against it. He needs to sit and think about what he's done, and know that we just won't let him get away with this – like he has everything else (glaring at Myra).

MYRA: I don't know that I can do that.

JOHN: There is no choice. We have to. You've done nothing but coddle him and you see where that's ended up. And you have no appreciation for the time I have put into trying to smooth things out between the two of you, trying to help you two get along.

MYRA: All that did was help him figure out how to play me and undermine me, but that's in the past. I know he'll get even worse if he stays in jail.

Some PIPs are coming into focus. I distinguished a PIP occurring in session that I show in Figure 12.6: John trying to impose his position on Myra, while Myra explains, to no avail, why she does not think his suggested course of action will be best for Wyatt.

John and Myra have not told me much about their history, but they have hinted at some of their historic interpersonal interactions surrounding Wyatt's problems. John experiences that he tried to help "smooth things out" between Wyatt and Myra, but she interpreted this as undermining her (Figure 12.7).

JEFF: So you are at odds about this and you've got a very tight deadline. So the main focus of our meeting today is for you two to make a decision about posting bail.

MYRA: Yes and I don't think we will ever agree on this.

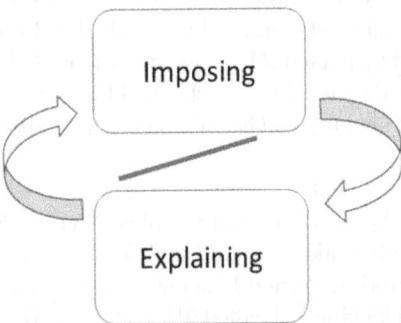

Figure 12.6 The first Pathologizing Interpersonal Pattern (PIP) identified by Myra and John

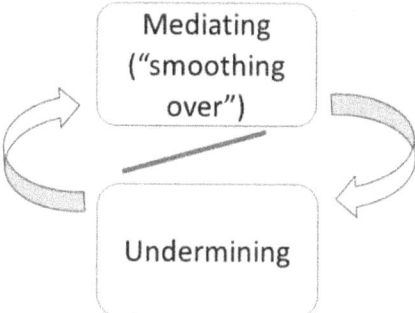

Figure 12.7 The second Pathologizing Interpersonal Pattern (PIP) identified by Myra and John

JEFF: Well, I hope I can help. Can you two tell me about a time when you made a difficult decision together?

JOHN: Well, the one that comes to mind for me was when we decided to move here. I really enjoyed my job in [another city] and it was a hard decision to move here. That was when Myra's mom was diagnosed with cancer and we really needed to be back here. I hated leaving that job, but it was important for the family—not just us, but the extended family as well.

JEFF: So for you it's about supporting the family—connection.

JOHN: Yes, for sure.

JEFF: One thing I am curious about is—What went into that decision?

MYRA: Well, I know that John made a big sacrifice and I appreciated it. And I know he was just starting to achieve some recognition in that job, and getting raises and getting lots of pats on the back, and more responsibility in his different positions. I'm sure they were disappointed when he left. I think he lost five years of progress in his career. But you know, I appreciated it so much—that he made that sacrifice.

JEFF: So, John, you were thinking about the well-being of the family, and Myra, you appreciated the sacrifice that John made. John, I am wondering how you knew that Myra appreciated your sacrifice.

JOHN: Well, she told me. And I said, really it's nothing. I mean it wasn't really nothing, but it was something that I was willing to do because I knew it was important to do for Myra, and also because it turned out that—because Myra's mom did end up passing—and Myra got to support her mom as her life ended, and she got to be her for Reg—that's Myra's dad. And also, Wyatt did get to spend those last months with Jeannie—that was Myra's mom's name. And Wyatt often talks about his grandma. He was only eight then, but he remembers a lot about her.

MYRA: And I know that there were some parts of moving here that John did not like and has never liked, but he just does not complain about it or hold it against me.

JEFF: He does not hold it against you, and even more, he appreciated what you did, and this was a major decision that you made together. Tell me more about how you arrived at the decision.

MYRA: Well I felt terrible about making John leave his job. And he bent over backwards to tell me and tell me that it was OK, that he knew I needed to be with my mom in her last few months.

JEFF: So you knew that, above all, John supported you.

MYRA: Yes. Yes, I did.

JOHN: And I appreciated that she appreciated what I did.

JEFF: So it sounds like you were in a pattern that worked in this case—can I call it *mutual appreciation*? You both were aware of the motivation behind your choices. Myra, you were very clear about the fact that John was very motivated by his commitment to family, and John, you very much appreciated that she did not take your sacrifice lightly.

> *I noted a WIP in which John and Myra had engaged earlier. Myra appreciated John's sacrifice in moving, connected as it is to his commitment to family. In turn, John appreciated Myra's appreciation (Figure 12.8). I thought at the time that this could provide an entry point to the process of making this important decision.*

JEFF: Well, it's clear that you both care very much for Wyatt and want what's best for him and for each other. Despite the differences you've had about how to manage situations with Wyatt, family is very important to you. Are these things that could factor into how you make this decision?

MYRA: Yes, but I'm so worried about him. And we totally disagree with each other about what to do.

JOHN: We certainly do.

JEFF: It seems to me that, whatever you end up doing, the decision will be tough for one of you to swallow. What aspects of your relationship can you keep in mind as we think out loud about how to go forward?

> *As Slive and Bobele (2011) suggest, I am asking about client resources. I consider Myra and John's previous success making a difficult family decision about moving to Calgary to care for Myra's terminally ill mother an exception or unique outcome. Of*

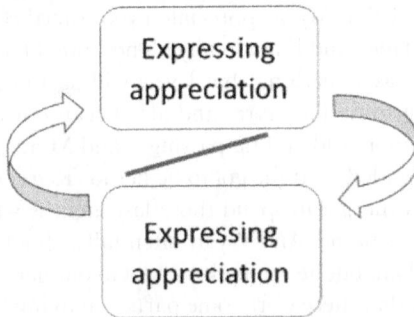

Figure 12.8 A Wellness Interpersonal Pattern (WIP) identified by Myra and John

course, if it is not salient to John and Myra, if it's not a difference that makes a difference (de Shazer, 1988), pointing this out is not useful. In this case it was.

JOHN: Well, our conversation so far has reminded me about how important this family unit is to me. Talking about the move here, Myra talked about how much she appreciated moving here, and really, it was a no-brainer. So that just brought it all back.

MYRA: And I was just thinking that about that whole period in our lives. The word that comes to mind is "generous." John was so generous during that time.

> *This was a new distinction that Myra made. I saw this as the absent but implicit—Myra missing and longing for John's generosity.*

JEFF: That's an interesting word. John, does this resonate for you?

JOHN: It's nice to hear, but I never really thought of it that way. It's just what I do. It does not seem like making an effort in any way.

JEFF: OK. Myra, I'm curious. Tell me about John's generosity.

MYRA: Oh, there are so many examples. Back to when my mom had died, my dad was pretty much paralyzed by grief. He really could not do anything. Their house was already kind of falling apart, because Dad had not done any of the upkeep. And he became even more unable to take care of things. John just jumped in and fixed everything. He was really kind to my dad, too. He didn't come in there taking charge.

JOHN: Well, it didn't really seem that complicated. I'm a practical guy and Reg couldn't do it, and I like hanging out with him. I just suggested we do some of the stuff around the house. It was cool to see because I was still working through the day, and then I would pop over dinner or after work. He started saying "Say, Myra and Wyatt are doing something. Just come over after work and I'll make something". I mean, he was not the greatest cook, but he wanted the company. So we'd have a steak or something—he never made veggies—and then we'd pull up some carpet, or lay some tile, or fill some dents in the wall, or something like that.

JEFF: It sounds like you developed a very strong connection with Reg. Myra, what are some other examples of John's generosity? How does John's generosity come out?

MYRA: Well, there's a lot… (Myra cites several examples)… And one time he was just so generous with Wyatt. Wyatt was in a fight with another boy at school—he was suspended from school. I expected John to be really upset. But he was so kind to Wyatt, and so understanding. It seemed like the other boy was taunting Wyatt—not that there is any justification for violence—but John was so understanding, and I know he was angry when he first learned that Wyatt was suspended.

JEFF: John, what was going on for you then? How did you mobilize your generosity?

JOHN: Well, I was mad at first. This was about three years ago when things started to go south. But he seemed so hurt and lost that day, and I just felt like I had to support him.

In a reauthoring conversation, John, Myra, and I conversed about several examples of how John enacts generosity. We co-constructed detailed accounts of how John was generous with Wyatt.

JEFF: When is it hardest to access generosity when dealing with Wyatt?

JOHN: Oh, that's easy. When he abuses Myra, I go into a rage. After all she's done for him and how she has put herself out, I can't stand it. I can't even think straight. I just see red.

JEFF: So how does Rage get in the way of generosity?

JOHN: Oh, interesting. I just can't stop thinking about how Wyatt is so abusive of Myra. In my way of thinking—the way I was raised—you treat your mother with respect. You almost revere your mother.[3] So, all I can think of is this, and it totally wipes out any generosity.

JEFF: So Rage blocks you from exercising generosity? How does Rage do that?

JOHN: Well, Rage just keeps saying, "How can you put up with that? You don't mistreat your mother that way. There must be consequences."

I've been externalizing the problem. John has adopted externalizing language, too.

JEFF: And when Rage is on board, how do you act toward Wyatt?

JOHN: Well, I very nearly slugged him yesterday. I've gone chest-to-chest with him and called him out… But bigger picture, when Rage is on board, I forget about how much I love him.

JEFF: Rage interferes with your generosity and gets in between you and Wyatt.

In a noncrisis interview, I might focus more on the effects of Rage on the relationship between Wyatt and John.

JEFF: How does Rage get in between you and Myra, John?

Because the focus here is on the process of joint decision-making, I want to support the WIPs we noted earlier, first by discussing the impact of Rage on their relationship.

JOHN: I can be so blinded by Rage that I forget that Myra is doing her best to care for Wyatt. Also, everything she does that is not 100% in agreement with me I take personally. She disagrees but I take it as a personal affront…

JEFF: … when Rage gets a hold of you.

JOHN: Exactly!

JEFF: Does that square with your experience, Myra?

MYRA: Well, yes. I never thought about it this way, but yes, Rage gets between us very badly. I feel very demeaned when John disagrees with me so vehemently. He says he takes it personally. I take it very personally. I know he's not himself, but it still hurts very much.

JEFF: So Rage gets John to take things personally. Rage invites him to interpret your disagreement as personal affront, and then Rage blinds him to your care and love for Wyatt—only gets him to see what he calls "coddling" and cuts him off from his generosity.

MYRA: That's a good summary. That's about it.

JEFF: So John, what would it take to approach this conversation being in touch with your sense of generosity?

JOHN: Well, I could just keep in mind that Myra does have Wyatt's best interests in mind. She really does only want to best for him and I know it's hard for her to be firm because she thinks she's failed him as a mother.[4] And I could stay focused on being generous toward Wyatt, although it will be hard.

John, Myra, and I then have a conversation about some practical aspects of how John will stay connected with his generosity and how Myra can both stay connected with her appreciation for John's generosity and her strengths as a mother. Being aware of potential PIPs that could arise and being anchored in the WIP of expressing appreciation coupled with expressing appreciation, John and Myra discussed a plan for bailing Wyatt out of jail, expressing their love for him, and setting realistic limits (not trying to control Wyatt, and working to maintain WIPs between them as a couple), they were able to agree on a plan to deal with Wyatt going forward.

Multicultural considerations

Using a poststructuralist approach invites clients to question their relationship with the cultural discourses that are most influential on them. In this composite case example, I have not specified the ethnicity or cultural background of each partner. Myra's reported sense of failure as a mother and John's sense that mothers should be revered are manifestations of patriarchy. Inviting the couples to question these social constructions transcends culture.

The approach to crisis intervention with couples described here sidesteps the typical Western construction of problems as residing within people. The IPscope values what goes on between people as much as what goes on within people. Narrative practices connect clinical problems with cultural stories. Both these approaches may be more congenial to those from collectivist cultures. Importantly, those from individualistic Eurocentric cultures may benefit from therapeutic conversations that interrogate typical Western discourses.

Challenges and solutions

One challenge in brief crisis-oriented work is the tendency to become overwhelmed at the extent of the problems with which clients present. My time working in single-session walk-in service taught me that any session can be the one and only or last session. As Slive and Bobele (2011) suggest, *think small*. Asking clients what they would like to accomplish in one session orients the SBFC professional to a realistic goal, which usually entails asking the client what they would find useful.

Intervening with a couple in crisis brings its own challenges. Each partner has different views of the nature of the crisis and how to solve it. As Taibbi (2018) suggests, they may play courtroom, trying to convince the SBFC practitioner of their particular truth. It is essential to avoid aligning with either partner's view. Research on the working alliance in couple and family therapy indicates that *shared sense of purpose* is the most important contributor to the alliance (Escudero & Friedlander, 2017). Inviting clients to think in terms of IPs or externalizing the problem can help join the partners in a shared sense of purpose. Focusing on the IPs between the partners, as opposed to the content, is essential.

Conclusion

Crisis intervention with a couple requires SBFC professionals to attend to the patterns of interaction between the partners. Thinking in terms of IPs and using narrative practices can decrease the likelihood of aligning inappropriately with one partner and increase the possibility of developing a shared sense of purpose. In this way, SBFC professionals can support parents to make sound decisions to promote stability on behalf of their children when school crises or disasters occur.

Notes

1 Some may be interested in discussing this issue theoretically: "Exceptions to what?" "What's unique about unique outcomes?" As Hoyt (editor's endnote in Chang, 1998, p. 270) quips, "Clients prefer both."
2 This case example is a composite and all client names are pseudonyms.
3 The cultural discourses that invite men to place women on pedestals might seem contradictory to attitudes that sponsor abuse toward women. Actually, both are supported by patriarchy. A full discussion of this is outside the scope of this session and this chapter, but could be the focus of ongoing counseling.
4 In ongoing therapy, I might take the opportunity to interview Myra and John about the cultural discourses of what it means to be a good mother and how those discourses influence them both.

Resources

Greene, G. K. (2016, February 2). A solution-focused approach to crisis intervention, part 1 Video]. YouTube. https://www.youtube.com/watch?v=WuDVwdh-iXg

Greene, G. K. (2016, February 2). A solution-focused approach to crisis intervention, part 2 [Video]. YouTube. https://www.youtube.com/watch?v=JtvNjGi5C7A

This simulated crisis intervention interview goes through specific steps, illustrating the questions and interventions used in a solution-focused approach to crisis intervention.

Greene, G. K., & Lee, M.-Y. (2015). How to work with clients' strengths in crisis intervention: A solution-focused approach. In K. Yeager & A. Roberts (Eds.). *Crisis intervention handbook: Assessment, treatment, and research* (pp. 69–98). Oxford University Press.

This comprehensive chapter provides additional detail to elaborate in the videos by Greene (2016). The chapter describes how to use solution-focused therapy to tap into the strengths of clients in crisis, steps for structuring a solution-focused/strengths-based approach to crisis intervention, how to consistently engage clients in "change talk" and not stay stuck in "problem talk", guidance for co-constructing goals with clients that include a problem-free future, and instructions for developing a collaborative relationship.

Hoyt, M. F., Bobele, M., Slive, A., Young, J., & Talmon, M. (Eds.) (2018). *Single-session therapy by walk-in or appointment: Administrative, clinical, and supervisory aspects of one-at-a-time services*. Routledge.

This comprehensive resource on single-session therapy describes the clinical aspects of single-session work, its empirical basis, the worldwide reach of single-session therapy, supervisory aspects, and new directions.

Hoyt, M. F., & Cannistrà, F. (2021). Common errors in single-session therapy. *Journal of Systemic Therapies, 40*(3), 29–41. http://dx.doi.org/10.1521/jsyt.2021.40.3.29): 29.

In this tongue-in-cheek article, the authors, proponents of single-session therapy, cite "some ways to avoid successful single session therapy": insisting that therapy be only one session; disbelieving that therapy could be only one session; lowering hopeful expectations; not clarifying a specific goal for the session; disregarding real-life issues; insisting on one model of therapy; ignoring context and working against the client's culture; aiming for total resolution, as opposed to a single-session goal; and neglecting implementation, supervision, and administrative support.

Slive, A., & Bobele, M. (2011). *When one hour is all you have: Effective therapy for walk-in clients.* Zeig, Tucker, & Theisen.

Comprehensive book on single-session and walk-in therapy describing the practical and empirical case for single-session work, and providing examples of single-session work international.

Young, K. (2020). Multistory listening: Using narrative practices at walk-in clinics. *Journal of Systemic Therapies, 3*, 34–45. https://doi.org/10.1521/jsyt.2020.39.3.34

After describing the growth of single-session therapy in Ontario, Canada, this article describes a narrative therapy approach to single-session services.

White, M. (1984). Pseudo-encopresis: From avalanche to victory, from vicious cycles to virtuous cycles. *Family Systems Medicine, 2*, 150–160. https:/doi.org/10.1037/h0091651

References

Beck, J. S. (2020). *Cognitive behavior therapy: Basics and beyond* (3rd ed.). Routledge.

Berg, I. K. (1994, April). *Brief therapy with long-term problems.* Workshop sponsored by Solutions Consultation and Training, Calgary, AB.

Carey, M., Walther, S., & Russell, S. (2009). The absent but implicit: A map to support therapeutic enquiry. *Family Process, 48*(3), 319–331. https://doi.org/10.1111/j.1545-5300.2009.01285.x

Carson, D. K., & Casado-Kehoe, M. (Eds.) (2011). *Case studies in couples therapy: Theory-based approaches.* Routledge.

Chang, J. (1998). Children's stories, children's solutions: Social constructionist therapy for children and their families. In M. F. Hoyt (Ed.), *Handbook of constructive therapies* (pp. 125–145). Jossey Bass.

Chang, J. (2021). Solution-focused brief therapy: A pragmatic approach. In L. Lorras, P.-E. Binder, & F. Thuen (Eds.), *Håndbok i individualterapi* (pp. 321–338). Fagbokforlaget.

Chang. J., & Nylund, D. K. (2013). Narrative and solution-focused therapies: A twenty-year retrospective. *Journal of Systemic Therapies, 32*, 72–88. https://doi.org/10.1521/jsyt.2013.32.2.72

Chang, J., & Phillips, M. (1993). Michael White and Steve de Shazer: New directions in family therapy. In S. Gilligan & R. Price (Eds.), *Therapeutic conversations* (pp. 95–111). Norton.

Dass-Brailsford, P. (Ed.) (2010). *Crisis and disaster counseling: Lessons learned from Hurricane Katrina and other disasters.* Sage.

Dattilio, F. M. (2010). *Cognitive-behavioral therapy with couples and families: A comprehensive guide for clinicians.* Guilford.

De Jong, P., & Berg, I. K. (2013). *Interviewing for solutions* (4th ed.). Brooks/Cole.

de Shazer, S. (1985). *Keys to solution in brief therapy.* W. W. Norton.

de Shazer, S. (1988). *Clues: Investigating solutions in brief therapy.* W. W. Norton.

Doherty, W. J., Harris, S. M., & Wilde, J. L. (2015). Discernment counseling for "mixed-agenda" couples. *Journal of Marital and Family Therapy, 42,* 246–255. https://doi.org/10.1111/jmft.12132

Escudero, V., & Friedlander, M. L. (2017). *Therapeutic alliances with families: Empowering clients in challenging cases.* Springer.

Fisch, R., Weakland, J. H., & Segal, L. (1991). *The tactics of change: Doing therapy briefly.* Wiley.

Harway, M. (Ed.) (2005). *Handbook of couples therapy.* Wiley.

Keeney, B., & Ray, W. A. (1993). *Resource focused therapy.* Routledge.

Kolski, T. D., & Jongsma, A. E. (2014). *The crisis counseling and traumatic events treatment planner,* with DSM-5 updates (2nd ed.). Wiley.

Korman, H., De Jong, P., & Jordan, S. S. (2020). Steve de Shazer's theory development. *Journal of Solution Focused Practices, 4*(2), Article 5. Retrieved March 12, 2022 from https://digitalscholarship.unlv.edu/journalsfp/vol4/iss2/5

Madigan, S. (2019). *Narrative therapy* (2nd ed.). American Psychological Association.

Miller, G. (2011). *Fundamentals of crisis counseling.* Wiley.

Morgan, A. (2000). *What is narrative therapy? An easy-to-read introduction.* Dulwich Centre Publications.

Nelson, T. (Ed.) (2020). *Integrative sex and couples therapy: A therapist's guide to new and innovative approaches.* PESI.

Peluso, P. R. (Ed.) (2007). *Infidelity: A practitioner's guide to working with couples in crisis.* Routledge.

Roberts, A. R., & Ottens, A. J. (2005). The seven-stage crisis intervention model: A road map to goal attainment, problem solving, and crisis resolution. *Brief Treatment and Crisis Intervention, 5,* 329–339. https:/doi.org/10.1093/brief-treatment/mhi030

Sandoval, J. (Ed.) (2013). *Crisis counseling, intervention and prevention in the schools* (3rd ed.). Routledge.

Shipway, L. (2004). *Domestic violence: A handbook for health care professionals.* Routledge.

Slive, A., & Bobele, M. (2011). *When one hour is all you have: Effective therapy for walk-in clients.* Zeig, Tucker, & Theisen.

Taibbi, R. (2018). *Brief therapy with couples and families in crisis.* Routledge.

Tomm, K., St. George, S., Wulff, D., & Strong, T. (Eds.) (2014). *Patterns in interpersonal interactions: Inviting relational understandings for therapeutic change.* Routledge.

Watzlawick, P., Weakland, J. H., & Fisch, R. (1976). *Change: Principles of problem formulation and problem resolution.* W. W. Norton.

Yeager, K. R., & Roberts, A. R. (2015). Bridging the past and present to the future of crisis intervention and crisis management. In K. R. Yeager & A. R. Roberts (Eds), *Crisis intervention handbook: Assessment, treatment, and research* (pp. 3–36). Oxford University Press.

13 A narrative approach to strengthening child and family relationships

Helen Nelson

Overview

This chapter outlines the narrative approach to counselling, with a focus on reducing the harm of relational aggression and bullying. Bullying occurs in a relationship of power imbalance. The narrative approach seeks to empower children or family members to identify and name a "problem" that is interfering with healthy relationships using their own language. This sets the issue as separate from the identity of the person. As the history of the narrative is traced, times when the problem was not powerful in achieving its goal are explored. Names are given to the characteristics that were behind these "unique outcomes." The practitioner listens deeply and enquires in a way that helps people explore as experts of their own experience, and to name the problem, unique outcomes, and a desired outcome or solution. Learning tasks are provided to help scaffold the distance between the presenting problem and desired outcome, supporting understanding and development. This is important to building personal agency, preparing children and families to deal with crisis and disaster. Consistent with the systems approach to school-based family counselling, scaffolding may be provided by family, peers, school staff, and community members. This chapter introduces the reader to the basic principles of the narrative approach and refers the reader to a wider range of resources.

Background

School-based family counselling is framed within an ecological systems perspective. This model centres each child surrounded by family, school, community, overarching policies, and history. Each child has their own story, shaped in the context of the many surrounding systems, or layers, of influence. Nurturing care provides a foundation for secure identity and a background through which children learn to approach new and different situations. The path of development is punctuated by critical periods in which outcomes can be enriched or hindered by children's experience in their own environment. For example, during recognised peaks of aggressive behaviour, children learn to regulate behaviour and develop resilience within supportive relationships

DOI: 10.4324/9781003201977-16

and structures of care (Runions, 2008). Through this, they also learn to give back to others in a positive way. In contrast, unresolved relational stress can become embedded into neurobiology, with associated internalising problems or externalising behaviours (Gunnar & Bowen, 2021). These, in turn, disrupt concentration, learning, and long-term health outcomes. There is plasticity to neurobiology, promoted as stress hormones subside when children find a safe base of care. For example, being truly heard without judgement by an adult or peer and feeling supported as the child explores how to overcome difficulties. This chapter will introduce the value of nurturing care through the narrative approach of deep listening, with a focus on relational aggression and bullying.

In early childhood, there is a normative peak in physical aggression, following which most children learn to regulate their behaviour in the context of nurturing relationships (Runions, 2008). As children develop cognitive and social skills, they gain greater capacity for self-reflection and compare themselves with peers, placing more and more importance on peer relationships (Pfeifer & Peake, 2012). From the ages of 8–11 years, they increasingly encounter relational aggression defined as "the manipulation of peer networks and relationships to cause harm" (Runions, 2008, p. 109). For example, the intentional spreading of gossip and lies about a peer with the purpose of gaining social status. This occurs most frequently among peers at school. At this time of increasing cognitive capacity, children's development is supported as they access support from family, school staff, or peers (Nelson et al., 2020). However, some aggression is cleverly hidden from adults and peers, resulting in social isolation and harm to those who are targeted (Runions, 2008).

Bullying is a type of aggression, differentiated by repetition, intensity, and goal orientation, in a power imbalanced relationship (Kaufman et al., 2020). Those who bully others choose a target who is unlikely to find help to defend themself, and those who are bullied feel unable to change the situation because of the experienced power imbalance (Kaufman et al., 2020). Children who bully others harness power through the peer group. The experience of being bullied has been described by children in school Grades 4–6 as leaving them feeling "lonely and insecure," "like there's nobody with them," or that "they don't belong anywhere" (Nelson et al., 2018). The resulting social exclusion of the bullied child poses a threat to mental and physical health through neurobiological embedding of a harmful and unresolved stress response (Nelson et al., 2020). Two overarching experiences of power imbalance have been found in recent studies, related to physical strength and popularity (Kaufman et al., 2020; Nelson et al., 2020). Most children who were bullied perceived that the goal of the one who bullied them was to achieve status. In relation to these findings, Kaufman et al. (2020) concluded that unique strategies must be found to tackle bullying, for example, teaching children to find support. However, many children experience an increase in social isolation after seeking support from an adult at school or home (Nelson et al., 2020).

The difficulty of finding support is heightened when socially clever aggressors intentionally hide aggression and bullying from those who might help. In the school environment, these aggressors may even make a favourable impression on adults and be regarded positively by staff (Nelson et al., 2020). This poses a question, what does it look like for children to find support when they experience relational aggression, or are bullied in a way that is cleverly hidden from adults? Children and school staff have reported that bullying can become worse when the teacher helps, related in part to punishment of those who bully others and of peers, or to a culture of blame (Nelson et al., 2020). Blame is attributed to cultural norms through which status is attributed and social power misused (Nelson et al., 2020). Children who are bullied perceive a powerlessness to overcome and may view this problem as part of their own identity, instead of seeing it as external to self, driven by cultural patterns and norms. Perceived power imbalance is minimised as family and school staff listen and support children as they problem solve, in an effort to understand how they might resolve the situation themselves.

SBFC practice using a narrative approach can provide a secure base through which children (or family) identify and name a problem using their own words, and identify a potential solution. Children identify the solution through narrative, as they recall a time when the problem was not powerful in achieving its goal (Morgan, 2000; White & Morgan, 2006). For example, a script recalled from a time of secure identity. The meanings that are given to each experience form the story or narrative. This strengths-based approach of empowering children fits within the systems model of school-based family counselling (Gerrard et al., 2019).

Procedure

Consistent with SBFC, narrative therapy is based on the concept that relational problems are a product of the social structure or culture that holds a problem in place. First introduced by White and Epston (1990), narrative practices aim to separate a named "problem" from the identity of the child and/or family, creating an opportunity for change (Morgan, 2000). The practitioner listens without judgement or blame, acknowledging people as the expert of their own experience. Meanings given to experiences are explored, as are times when the problem has had less influence over the child or family. These "unique outcomes" provide a path to explore a new story that is set apart from the problem (Morgan, 2000).

White and Morgan (2006) revisited the development of narrative practices and outlined three position maps to guide practitioners through narrative practice. The first map guides the narrative practice of inviting development of a rich story. The second map guides the practice of promoting the child and/or family's capacity to achieve their desired solution. Third guides conversations that scaffold the child and/or family as they learn to distance from the named problem and to problem solve toward a new story. These three maps are outlined with a focus on the child; this could equally read child and family (see White and Morgan, 2006 for a fuller description):

1   Development of a rich story founded on "unique outcomes" or "exceptions" (White & Morgan, 2006, p. 2). This moves back and forward between the following stages:

   a   Giving the child an opportunity to characterise their experience, for example, using language or by drawing. Inviting the child to define and name the problem. This places the child at the centre of the conversation. The SBFC practitioner listens to the narrative and engages with the child with respect, acknowledging the child as the expert of their experience (White & Morgan, 2006). The SBFC practitioner sees the child and the problem as different and does not decide what the problem is so as not to lead the child to a name.

   b   Having named the problem (thus externalising the problem, setting it apart from the identity of the child), the SBFC practitioner gives the child space to explore the agenda of the named problem and what that problem is up to. The "activities" of the problem (how it is affecting the child's daily life and relationships) and how the problem plans to affect the child's future (White & Morgan, 2006).

   c   Evaluate the consequences of the problem – how it is affecting the child's life.

   d   Give the child space to justify the evaluation, why they are unhappy about the agenda and consequences of the problem. Identify the child's wishes and longings for their own life (White & Morgan, 2006).

2   As the history of the story is traced, a time before the problem may be identified, supported through discovery of the beliefs and ideas that keep the problem powerful. As these beliefs and ideas are explored and named, the times when they haven't held power are explored as "unique outcomes." This challenges truths that have been constructed to hold the problem in place, helping the child separate from the problem (Morgan, 2000). White named the second position map the "statement of position" (White & Morgan, 2006, p. 1). The map guides the practitioner in drawing out the significance of the unique outcome or exception. The following steps may not occur in a linear way during the conversation.

   a   The child recalls a time when the problem did not succeed in its agenda and the child prevailed. The child identifies, names, and defines a characteristic that lead to the "unique outcome."

   b   The child identifies how their life might look when they draw on this characteristic that prompted the "unique outcome" or "solution."

   c   The SBFC practitioner evaluates how the child and their family might receive new developments as the child moves away from the problem and toward the new outcome.

   d   The child and family justify the evaluation, telling why they would receive the new outcome or solution in such a way.

From thin descriptions and thin conclusions to "rich and thick description"

Through deep listening, and asking questions of the expert – the child who is telling the story, the SBFC practitioner joins with the child to explore the meanings that have been given to events. Morgan describes this initial description of the problem as a thin description, often created and spoken over the child by others who have "power of definition" (Morgan, 2000, p. 13). This may lead to a "thin conclusion" about the identity of the child (Morgan, 2000, p. 13). For example, a Grade 6 girl spoke of the response of school staff when she sought help after being bullied, "They ignore me like it was my fault" (Nelson et al., 2018, p. 286). This perceived attribution of blame speaks into a thin story and deepens the power imbalance felt by the child. It is the opposite of deep listening or hearing children as the experts of their own experience. Thin descriptions and thin conclusions can spiral into a dominant story of problem (Morgan, 2000).

The narrative perspective uses externalising conversations to trace the history of the problem in the context of the child's life. This helps the child to see the problem as separate to their identity and "begins to disempower the effects of labelling" (Morgan, 2000, p. 31). The problem (for example, bullying) is viewed as separate from the child and "assumes people have many skills, competencies, beliefs, values, commitments and abilities that will assist them to reduce the influence of problems in their lives" (Morgan, 2000, p. 2).

Keeping the deeper context in mind

The SBFC practitioner listens for the names given to problems by the child and asks questions to determine what contributes to invisible power relations that hold a problem in place. In doing this, the SBFC practitioner must be aware that the problems named and unique outcomes identified by children may exist within the context of deeper harmful issues, including abuse. To simply focus on the named problem without addressing the deeper issue could "contribute to silencing the child's experience and reduce the likelihood of the abuse being addressed" (Morgan, 2000, p. 23). For this reason, the SBFC practitioner "must keep checking on the broader context" of the child's/family's life (Morgan, 2000, p. 23).

3. The third step named by White is that of "scaffolding conversations" (White & Morgan, 2006, p. 2). White (2006) comments that although a narrative practice was not informed by Vygotsky's sociocultural theory, his experience of narrative practice gave confirmation to Vygotsky's developmental theory (White & Morgan, 2006). Vygotsky theorised that children's cognitive development occurs in the context of their social relationships. This theory is also consistent with the developmental systems perspective that informs school-based family counselling (Gerrard et al., 2019). Vygotsky used the term "scaffolding" to represent the important role of others as children grow in personal agency. Social relationships provide a scaffold as children learn to distance from the named problem and to problem solve toward the unique outcome (White & Morgan, 2006).

   a. Children learn as other people make a social investment into their lives. The SBFC practitioner helps to scaffold the gap between the problem and unique outcome by the deep listening and enquiry that allows children to explore as the expert of their own experience. Based on this exploration, the SBFC practitioner provides learning tasks that the child can reach although it will require effort. Family members, school staff, and peers may contribute to the scaffolding.

   b. The learning tasks provide the child with an opportunity to move step by step toward the desired new outcome.

   c. In the process of moving from the old to the new, the child learns "chains of association" that support understanding and development (White & Morgan, 2006, p. 44).

   d. The child learns "personal agency" (White & Morgan, 2006). To act responsibly and contribute positively to outcomes associated with their personal well-being and relationships.

Deep listening

Deep listening is central to the narrative approach, allowing children to feel heard. This provides a safe base, a central component of secure development. The automatic stress response continually shapes brain pathways and the associated physiology of the body, in turn, shaping how children react to each new experience, make decisions, and learn (Gunnar & Bowen, 2021). For example, when children report bullying to an adult and their experience is dismissed, they experience the opposite of being heard and are left feeling alone. This elevates the neurobiological stress response, including a fight or flight reaction, and heightens the harm of being in a power imbalanced relationship (Nelson et al., 2018). Children may react to this perceived power imbalance with an inward focus of self-protection or fear, or through externalising behaviour. These hinder their capacity to learn. Vygotsky emphasised the important role of relationships to scaffolding as children move from what they know to what is possible (White & Morgan, 2006). Such scaffolding includes a secure base of emotional support for children who seek help to understand how they might resolve relational aggression or bullying. A secure base is supported in school systems that are structured to provide support to children, families, and school staff (Gerrard et al., 2019; Runions, 2008).

Multicultural considerations

The narrative approach aims to remove the power of a problem that has held over a child or family using a gradual scaffolded process. However, intergenerational trauma can make it very difficult for individuals and groups who have experienced ongoing harm to find a new story. For example, dangers and difficulties experienced by refugee children and families, or the history of abuse and exclusion known by many First Nations people. For these groups, school can provide either a safe base of support and belonging or it can be unsafe through the experience of racism and bullying.

Children construct knowledge from within as they respond to and reflect on their own experience, ask questions, and accommodate to their own environment. As children face physical or social threats or challenges, the stress system helps them maintain stability through change. It provides a buffer to the brain and body during the challenge and is automatically reduced when the stress subsides. The effects of ongoing trauma can damage brain plasticity through a persistently elevated stress system, inhibiting the capacity of a child to bounce back from hurt and heightening their unconscious fight or flight response. This is reflected in behaviour and may be seen by some as intentionally disruptive and wilful, rather than the result of ongoing biological embedding of adversity.

When using a narrative approach, the SBFC practitioner must be aware of issues that may be inappropriately minimised if they are overlooked, for example, when a named problem occurs in a social or political context of racism. Ignoring the context may contribute to harm experienced by the child and family. From a systems perspective, school-based family practitioners can help shape the context of how children and families who have experienced chronic adversity are understood and included in a welcoming school environment. For example, refugee children described a time when a friendship with a local child was established, or when they received social recognition, as a significant episode that supported their well-being and feeling of belonging at school (Fazel, 2015). This can inform part of the scaffolding process for

The narrative approach invites people to strength and hope as they access awareness of personal agency. The SBFC practitioner listens deeply with awareness that what is visible is often rooted in what has gone before, for example, the intergenerational trauma experienced by Australian Aboriginal people following colonisation. For Australian Aboriginal people, well-being is embedded in the health of the community, including a strong sense of identity, ceremony, storytelling or "yarning," and a deep connection to the land (known as Country) (Kingsley et al., 2013). The SBFC practitioner listens with respect and does not approach the conversation from the position of knowing an answer; doing so may perpetuate the intergenerational harm. Instead, using a systems approach, the SBFC recognises the unique capacity of the community to contribute to the scaffolding process. For example, Australian Aboriginal Elders teach children to use "deep listening" to learn about Country and to be "ready for the two worlds" that they walk in (https://www.napcan.org.au/product/national-child-protection-week-2021-poster-deep-listening/).

individual children and for groups. In addition, each culture has traditional knowledge, wisdom, and story that are passed through generations, as narrative, or through art, dance, and ceremonies or festivals. The SBFC practitioner advocates for social inclusion and recognition of the value and heritage of cultures and groups.

Challenges and solutions

This section discusses the challenges of a narrative perspective specific to relational aggression and bullying. Children who are able to overcome adversity are often described as resilient. Twum-Antwi et al. (2020, p.79) promote the concept of resilience as "the ability of one or more systems (e.g., a child, family, a school) to successfully withstand, overcome, and adapt to adversity." This focus removes the attribution of resilience to an individual and is consistent with the narrative approach and with the systems approach of school-based family counselling. Children learn to adapt and overcome adversity over time as they encounter increasingly complex interactions within social systems of care (White & Morgan, 2006). For example, when a child feels truly heard by an adult or peer, without dismissal or condemnation, they experience a safe base of support that allows the stress response to subside (Gunnar & Bowen, 2021; Twum-Antwi et al., 2020). This promotes brain plasticity, allowing children to explore how to overcome a difficult situation with a trusted person, to adapt, and to learn. The change is incremental. If the potential solution does not initially achieve a positive outcome, the child can return to the safe base and explore a way forward with a trusted person. This is similar to the security experienced by a toddler who leaves the caregiver to explore, and stumbles or falls, then returns to the caregiver for comfort before running off again to explore.

Children who are bullied do not always feel that they have access to a safe base of support. Children from Grade 6 have given examples of their experience after telling an adult carer of bullying. A girl said, "sometimes my dad just says to ignore them… cause he doesn't want to get involved" (Nelson et al., 2018, p. 286). A boy spoke of his reluctance to tell a teacher when it results in punishment of others. "Because they've been in trouble so they're gonna get you in trouble" (Nelson et al., 2018, p. 285). Another girl gave the following example in response to a discussion about relational harm, "I was involved in one of those things and the reason why I moved to (this school) is because it happened at my old school with my teacher and kids, I got bullied" (Nelson et al., 2018, p. 286). When a child feels dismissed or isolated, the heightened stress response is not turned off. This can be experienced as a feeling of being overwhelmed, a sense of fight or flight, loneliness, blame, fear, or anxiety. This, in turn, impedes the ability of the child to feel safe at school, to focus, and learn.

In contrast to being told or disciplined, non-punitive relational support using a narrative approach will shift responsibility for resilience from the child, to a system in which the child is centred within a relational network of support (Gerrard et al., 2019). Over time, the child will learn to directly or indirectly support others, becoming a resource within the family, school, and community (Twum-Antwi et al., 2020). Using a whole school approach, it may be helpful to explore beliefs around bullying. For example, is relational aggression acknowledged in the school or do staff and parents acknowledge physical bullying only? Does the school culture promote social, academic, or sporting status in a way that contributes to hidden aggression and bullying? Does the community celebrate diversity and different cultural heritages? Is the community committed to deconstructing cultural norms that result in social isolation?

Conclusions

The narrative approach places the child or family member at the centre, giving them the opportunity to characterise their own experience. The SBFC practitioner uses non-judgemental listening to ensure that children are heard, inviting them to name the problem, setting it apart from their own identity. Then to think of a time when this problem did not achieve its goal of harm, and to name the characteristic that minimised the power of the problem. In doing so, children have the opportunity to connect their identity to a positive script, scaffolded by supportive relationships. Through deep listening and recognising children as the expert of their own experience, the narrative approach provides a safe base of support for children as they seek to overcome relational aggression by peers. Using a systems approach, narrative therapy can promote school and family resilience, strengthening the ability of children and families to cope successfully with crisis and disaster.

Resources

The first two resources are comprehensive introductions to narrative therapy. The third is an article describing the application of narrative practice in a school, and is specific to bullying. These resources, and many more including videos and online courses, are available through the Dulwich Centre: https://dulwichcentre.com.au

Morgan, A. (2000). *What is narrative therapy? An easy-to-read introduction.* Dulwich Centre Publications.

Alice Morgan explains the principles of narrative therapy, and gives easy to read examples of narrative practice. The book is very easy to read and accessible, a great introduction to narrative therapy.

White, M., & Morgan, A. (2006). *Narrative therapy with children and their families.* Adelaide, S. Australia.

In chapter 1 of this book, Michael White reviews developments of his work in narrative practice over 20 years, with a focus on working with young children and families. He provides examples of his work with three children and their families to illustrate three position maps of narrative practice.

Williams, M. (2010). Undercover teams: Redefining reputations and transforming bullying relationships in the school community. *Explorations: An E-Journal of Narrative Practice,* 4–13.

Narrative therapy has been used in schools with children who are bullied and with children who bully others. This article demonstrates the use of narrative to co-author a new story for a child who was being bullied. The authors view the source of bullying in a relationship narrative, and describe how narrative therapy was used to transform bullying identity as a group of children were selected to co-author the new story together.

References

Fazel, M. (2015). A moment of change: Facilitating refugee children's mental health in UK schools. *International Journal of Educational Development, 41,* 255–261. https://doi.org/10.1016/j.ijedudev.2014.12.006

Gerrard, B. A., Carter, M. J., & Ribera, D. (Eds.). (2019). *School-based family counseling: An interdisciplinary practitioner's guide.* Routledge.

Gunnar, M. R., & Bowen, M. (2021). What was learned from studying the effects of early institutional deprivation. *Pharmacology Biochemistry and Behavior, 210,* 173272. https://doi.org/10.1016/j.pbb.2021.173272

Kaufman, T. M. L., Huitsing, G., & Veenstra, R. (2020). Refining victims' self-reports on bullying: Assessing frequency, intensity, power imbalance, and goal-directedness. *Social Development, 29*(2), 375–390. https://doi.org/10.1111/sode.12441

Kingsley, J., Townsend, M., Henderson-Wilson, C., & Bolam, B. (2013). Developing an exploratory framework linking Australian Aboriginal peoples' connection to country and concepts of wellbeing. *International Journal of Environmental Research and Public Health, 10*(2), 678–698. https://doi.org/10.3390/ijerph10020678

Morgan, A. (2000). *What is narrative therapy? An easy-to-read introduction.* Dulwich Centre Publications.

Nelson, H. J., Burns, S. K., Kendall, G. E., & Schonert-Reichl, K. A. (2018). The factors that influence and protect against power imbalance in covert aggression and bullying among preadolescent children: A thematic analysis. *Journal of School Nursing, 34*(4), 281–291. https://doi.org/10.1177/1059840517748417

Nelson, H. J., Kendall, G. E., & Burns, S. K. (2020). How covert aggression contributes to the power imbalance experienced by children who are bullied. In N. Kaplan Torin (Ed.), *Proceedings of the 2020 Oxford Symposium in school-based family counseling* (pp. 166–189). Institute for School Based Family Counseling.

Pfeifer, J. H., & Peake, S. J. (2012). Self-development: Integrating cognitive, socio-emotional, and neuroimaging perspectives. *Developmental Cognitive Neuroscience, 2*(1), 55–69. https://doi.org/10.1016/j.dcn.2011.07.012

Runions, K. (2008). A multi-systematic school-based approach for addressing childhood aggression. *Australian Journal of Guidance and Counselling, 18*(2), 106–127. https://doi.org/doi.org.dbgw.lis.curtin.edu.au/10.1375/ajgc.18.2.106

Twum-Antwi, A., Jefferies, P., & Ungar, M. (2020). Promoting child and youth resilience by strengthening home and school environments: A literature review. *International Journal of School & Educational Psychology, 8*(2), 78–89. https://doi.org/10.1080/21683603.2019.1660284

White, M., & Epston, D. (1990). *Narrative means to therapeutic ends.* Norton.

White, M., & Morgan, A. (2006). *Narrative therapy with children and their families.* Adelaide, S. Australia.

14 Family-based interventions for children in crisis

Anjali Gireesan and Sibnath Deb

Overview

This chapter will look at different phases of crises that a family may undergo with the help of an example. This is followed by a detailed elaboration of three systemic approaches to counseling, which describes the parameters on which families may be assessed. The stages of counseling have been explained in which the points to be deliberated are brought to attention. The multicultural considerations, which are imperative in practicing school-based family counseling, and the challenges encountered in the process have also been elaborated upon.

Background

Children are surrounded by a dynamic environment. Both school and family form an active part of this environment. According to school-based family counseling (SBFC) metamodel, school and family both play an important role in prevention of crisis situations as well as intervention in the crisis situation. Systemic interventions have proved to be effective for children who have undergone crisis, such as child abuse and neglect, as well as chronic mental and physical illnesses (Carr, 2019). In this chapter, the endeavor has been to understand effective ways to intervene into the family and mold it into a strong resource for the children.

Crisis unfolds itself in multiple stages (US Department of Health and Human Services, 1994). Families that possess adequate resources to cope with stressors in the environment can manage the crisis of an individual member or the whole family. Certain families realize that there is a dearth of resources and they seek outside help. But there are families which neither understand their limited capabilities to deal with a stressor nor approach the environment for help. The tragic case we describe here happened in Burari district, New Delhi, India. The family consisted of eleven members in which there were seven adults and four children (House of secrets, 2021).

Step 1: Precipitating Event: *In this example, the death of the eldest member of the family, Mr. Bhopal Singh, was perceived as a very traumatic event. The family abided by his rules and obeyed his decisions. Suddenly, there was a lot of uncertainty in the lives of all members.*

DOI: 10.4324/9781003201977-17

Step 2: Perception of the Event: *Mr. Bhopal Singh was the head of the family. Everything happened on his instructions. He was the strongest financial contributor of the family as he had sold all his land in the village, to come to an urban locality, where there were better opportunities for his son. Though all the members were equally affected, his youngest son, Lalit Singh was the most affected, as he was very attached to his father.*

Step 3: Disorganized Behavior: *Things had started to look gloomy within the family. The financial condition was deteriorating. At this point in time, Lalit started claiming that his dead father visited him in his dreams and has given solutions to their problems.*

Step 4: Seeking New and Unusual Resources: *The family started believing in the dreams of Lalit. They started following his instructions for day to day activities, educational advice, as well as business-related activities. They got validation from the positive results of the advice and the instructions being followed. Lalit took the place of the head of the family and directed all family members as his father used to do.*

Step 5: Series or Chain of Events: *Though Lalit's instructions were helping the family to become financially stable, his own mental health was deteriorating every day. His psychosis of being visited and "possessed" by his father was becoming stronger. The family members started experiencing "shared psychosis". The children maintained diaries for all the family members in which all ritualistic instructions were penned down systematically. There used to be a schedule of séances with Mr Bhopal, which were documented.*

Step 6: Previous Crisis Links Current Crisis: *Lalit had a history of encountering traumatic events, like a bike accident in adolescence, in which he had injured his head and also had been attacked by his co-workers. In both these incidents, he experienced a loss of control, which led to experiences of acute anxiety. The loss of his father and the unstable economic condition of the family, had unlocked his anxiety associated with his previous experiences. This affected the severity of the crisis that the whole family experienced.*

Step 7: Mobilization of New Resources and Adaptation: *The Bhatia family embraced the instructions being provided by Bhopal Singh through Lalit. They adapted to it for 11 years. They never realized that they were experiencing a crisis situation. When the eldest granddaughter of the family got engaged, Lalit again experienced a loss of control. On the pretense that the members had done something wrong, a strange ritual was instructed to be conducted. All members were supposed to hang themselves from the ceiling in a particular pattern, with their eyes blindfolded and hands tied. Bhopal Singh was supposed to rescue them at the end of the penance. As a consequence of this delusion, the whole family died.*

The family was perceived to be a very happy one, where children were very well behaved and had a lot of respect for their elders. All children were doing well academically. Nobody thought that family would be undergoing a crisis of this magnitude. An effective intervention at the right time could have prevented this massive tragedy. SBFC practitioners can act as active resources for identification and management of such families, especially of a child, who has experienced some kind of crisis.

Procedure

In the following section, an attempt has been made to understand the process of family assessment and then administering family counseling for children in crisis (Gladding and Batra, 2007).

Step 1: Identification of a systemic approach to counseling

There are many ways in which maladaptive practices may be identified and hence regulated. In this section, three such approaches have been elaborated on (A) circumplex model of marital and family systems, (B) Bowen's family system and (C) structural family counseling. Each of them has a different way of looking at the family as a system and the possible source of the problem in it.

Circumplex model of marital and family systems

The circumplex model of marital and family systems is a comprehensive model that explains the dynamics of family interaction (Olson, Waldvogel, & Schlieff, 2019; Wilde, 2018). The three main dimensions on which the model operates are (1) family cohesion, (2) flexibility and (3) communication. Family cohesion and flexibility have a curvilinear relationship, whereas communication acts as a mediating factor in this model.

Family cohesion

Family cohesion directly points at the degree of bonding that is shared among the different units of the family. Here, interpersonal boundaries, the closeness between two or more family members, common interests, the support network available to the family and decision-making styles, are analyzed. The dimension varies from togetherness at one extreme and separateness and the other extreme. The levels are as follows:

1 **Disengaged**: Togetherness is very low at this level. Family members often experience loneliness and have very limited social support systems in the form of family. There is individualistic predisposition. Group dynamics get negatively affected as the family seldom has group goals to contemplate and work upon.
2 **Somewhat connected to connected**: At these levels, there is a low to moderate level of togetherness. There is shared participation in achieving some familial goals but "me-time" is equally important.
3 **Very connected**: At this level, togetherness ranges from moderate to high. Here, the concept of loyalty is evident and friends are common to more than two family members. More shared interests are prominent, which makes the time spent together enjoyable as well as voluntary in nature.

4 **Enmeshed**: At this level, there is very high fusion between the family members. Independent opinions are discouraged. Conformity and obedience are high within the family. Here, loyalty is demanded rather than voluntarily accorded by the family members.

Balanced levels of cohesion are somewhat connected, connected and very connected, whereas unbalanced levels of cohesion are disengaged and enmeshed. Maintaining a balance between the two extremes is important.

Family flexibility

Family flexibility indicates the degree of acceptance of change that is welcomed by the family. Three aspects in which this change is viewed are, the type of leadership prevalent in the family, roles addressed by different family members and the nature of relationships maintained between the family members. It is important for a family to be a system that is functional under different circumstances and crisis, and thus return back to stability as soon as possible. This promotes positive mental health development within the family. There are four levels to this model:

1 **Rigid:** At this level, there is one fixed leader of the family, who controls all the other family members. This level is characterized by an autocratic leadership style. Rules cannot have deviations. Each member has a role that needs to be addressed by them exclusively. For example, men of the family will be employed outside the house, whereas women of the family will take care of the household chores.
2 **Somewhat flexible and flexible**: At these levels, a Democratic leadership is followed. Most of the power still remains with one leader but opinions are encouraged from other family members, resulting in participative decision making. Some roles are fixed, whereas other roles are flexible. Rules are strict and are to be followed.
3 **Very flexible**: Leadership still exists but there is no fixed leader. Roles keep changing according to the need of the hour. For example, when the father of the family is sick, the son takes over temporarily to enforce and channelize family decisions. Roles are also shared and are more fluid.
4 **Chaotic**: At this level, lack of proper leadership is prominent. The members are left to fend for themselves and roles are quite unclear. There is prevalence of diffused responsibility, which leads to many confusions. Members cannot rely on each other to get the family tasks done.

  Each of these levels balances change and stability in different ways. Somewhat flexible, flexible and very flexible levels are more adept at understanding change and coexisting, as compared to rigid and chaotic levels.

Family communication

Family communication is considered to be an important bridge between family cohesion and family flexibility dimension. The levels discussed earlier benefit a lot from an effective communication paradigm. Observation parameters included in this model are:

1 **Listening skills:** Listening skills are very important as it helps to receive the messages in an adequate manner. In an enmeshed family, where rigidity is prevalent, the emotions of the family members may be ignored and attention is paid only to the instructions of the leader. In a separate structured family, decision making is more participative, as some amount of empathy is expressed and attention is paid to more than one family member.

2 **Speaking skills:** A boundary needs to be maintained to refrain from taking over the expression of opinions from others. In a connected flexible family, emotions are given importance and everyone gets an equal chance to put forward their opinions. This facilitates a very healthy and productive discussion.

3 **Self-disclosure:** This relates to the ease with which members of a family can share their experiences with each other. The environment needs to be conducive to provide the probability of having such experiences and a platform to share it. In a disengaged chaotic family, these experiences may be so varied that the members might not be interested in each other's experiences.

4 **Tracking:** There is a need to focus on the direction in which the communication is progressing. This is possible only when family members share emotional bonding, have common goals and interests, and have a positive outlook toward each other.

5 **Respect and regard:** These are the tools to assure if there is healthy communication between the family members. The higher the degree of respect and regard for the family members, the better is the communication between them.

Based on the circumplex model, various inventories are available to assess the family on dimensions of cohesion and flexibility. Some of them are Family Inventory Package (self-report method to assess perception of each member of the family system), Family Adaptability and Cohesion Evaluation Scales (FACES IV) and Clinical Rating Scale (evaluation of the counselor or clinician to the family in session). Figure 14.1 shows the different types of families that are possible, depending upon their levels of cohesion and adaptability.

Bowen's system theory

Stress management is an essential part of any family life. Often, the perspectives on various stressors and its associated coping strategies are passed on from one generation to the other. It is the transmission of chronic anxiety that

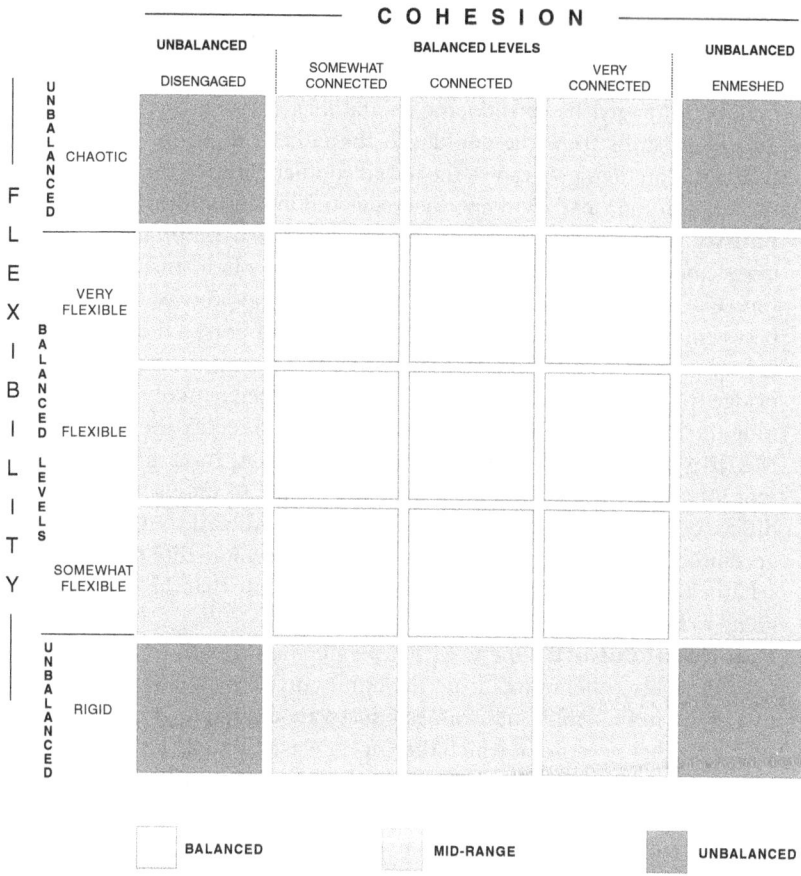

Figure 14.1 The circumplex model of marital and family systems

forms the major postulate of Murray Bowen's Family System Theory (Brown, 1999). The degree of this inherited chronic anxiety has direct emotional and physical consequences for an individual, as well as the whole family. As anxiety increases, it leads to systemic dysfunction in a family that mandates help and the subsequent change. Some of the important concepts of this theory are as follows:

1 **Differentiation of the self:** Family is an integration of multiple selves. Fusion, caused by emotional dependency, often leads to dilution of interpersonal boundaries, thus undermining the role that each family member is supposed to address to the best of their capabilities. The individual self needs to be emphasized.

2 **Emotional triangle:** One of the ways in which a family copes with arising anxiety is through the inclusion of a third party in the system. For example, the anxiety resulting from conflict between a mother and daughter, because of permission to stay out during the night for a party, may be managed by introducing the father's decision in the equation. The focus shifts from the conflict to the father's decision. This sort of triangulation does not resolve the initial conflict between the mother and the child. It may lead to temporary relief and more conflicts in future.

3 **Family projection process:** Projection is when we project our feelings, emotions and behaviors onto others. We often misinterpret the source of the emotion here. In the family projection process, this happens between a parent and a child. The perception of personal inadequacies is projected onto the child and there is a consequent action in order to bridge these onto the children. As a result, children actually start exhibiting the inadequacies and then, there is a need to rectify the problem.

4 **Multi-generational transmission process:** In a family where more than one child is present, the differentiation among the children differs because of the process of triangulation. All children may not be accommodated in the triangle of the parents. The more differentiated the self, the better is the prognosis for the further family that the individual is going to be a part of.

5 **Emotional cut-off:** One way that people manage anxiety in families is by detaching themselves from the family unit emotionally. This leads to a break in the emotional connectedness, though there is no resolution to the conflict because of which the cut-off was initiated. This unhealthy practice keeps making appearances in different relationships, present or revisited.

6 **Sibling position:** Individuals having similar sibling positions in their respective families are observed to have similar characteristics. For example, two individuals who hold the eldest sibling position in different families may share common characteristics, like assuming leadership roles and addressing responsible duties. If such individuals become a part of the same family, then there is a chance of conflict. This also depends on the degree of differentiation among these individuals.

7 **Societal emotional process:** A turmoil in the society will alter the flow of information in the family. Also, a harmonious society will facilitate this flow. Thus, it is necessary to understand the societal environment of the family to diagnose and treat their problems.

8 **Nuclear family emotional process:** There are certain relationship patterns that help in ascertaining where the problem lies in a family. These are (1) marital conflict, (2) dysfunction in spouse, (3) impairment of one or more children and (4) emotional distance.

These family patterns are frequently tracked using a diagram called the genogram which shows connections between family members (see Figure 14.2).

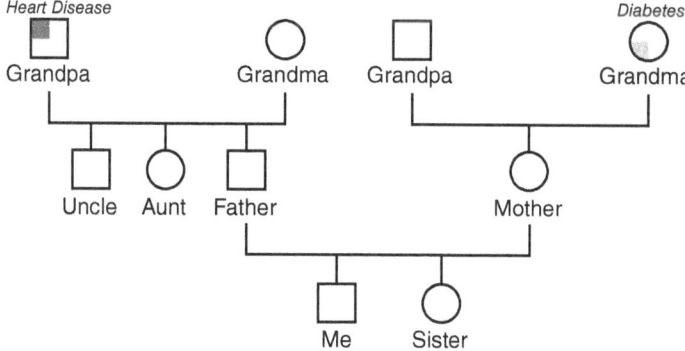

Figure 14.2 Example of a genogram

Structural family counseling

A systematic structure lays the foundation of a strong family. Absence of a structure to rely on results in chaos and increases the severity of the problem. Structure of a family is the focal point of this therapy. Another aspect that is paid much attention to is the creation of clear and precise interpersonal boundaries (Vetere, 2001). Some of the techniques employed in this therapy are:

1 **Family mapping:** This is a visual representation of the family and its dynamics. The activity propels the members to view themselves and their relationships in an objective manner. It gives them an efficient tool to analyze the behavioral patterns and the existing structure. The process also helps the counselor to identify the problematic areas and hence make appropriate treatment goals.
2 **Reframing:** This is a cognitive restructuring exercise where a particular problem is viewed from a relatively positive perspective. For example, a situation that was initially called "traumatic" may be relabeled as "painful". Reasons for the same are substantiated.
3 **Boundary making:** There are three types of boundaries that might exist among family members: (1) rigid, (2) clear and (3) diffuse. Rigid boundaries indicate unconnectedness, while diffuse boundaries indicate unhealthy unconnectedness among the family members. It is important to establish clear boundaries, which lead to healthy connectedness and thus improve family dynamics. For example, in enmeshed families, children do not have much opinion in decisions since the elders of the family perceive that they know what is best for their children. When a child is in crisis, the already dependent child expects the parents to voice their emotions and concerns. Parents may not fully comprehend the situation and dilute or exaggerate the severity of the situation. In boundary making

exercises, an activity is provided, which helps to observe if everyone participates equally. If the parent is cutting off the child at multiple places, then roles are emphasized and the environment provides for a more participative decision making.

Step 2: Pre-session planning

The counselor needs to understand the crisis that the child has undergone and hence plan the interaction with the family. The main objective here is to improve upon the family dynamics and interaction in such a way that the child gets a social support mesh to rely on and feel comfortable. In this phase, demographic information is collected from the primary counselor and family members and the basic idea and assumptions are drawn regarding the child and the family.

Step 3: First phase

The first phase of family counseling overlaps with principles of any other type of counseling. The difference lies in the number of people with whom the interaction needs to be taken place. Initial steps involve rapport formation with each unit of the family, individually, as well as a group. The basic foundation of the patterns of family interaction is understood. Some of the significant elements included are:

1 Empathetic understanding of the perceptions of each family member.
2 Physical environment in which the family has set itself. For example, the social distance between the different family members.
3 Verbal behavior among the different family units. For example, the tone and pitch that the parents use with children, difference of attitude between the siblings and the ways in which the extended family, if any, are made a part of discussions.
4 Body language of all members like exchange of smiles, maintenance of eye contact, use of hand gestures, etc.
5 Identification of coalitions (members who are closer to each other) and if there is scapegoating in the family (problem attribution to individual members of the family).
6 Leadership styles and parenting styles prevalent in the family.
7 Conclusions need to be drawn regarding the interpersonal boundaries that are maintained in the family as a whole.

The inclusion of different parameters depends on the therapy chosen to follow. For example, if following a Bowen's family system therapy, the SBFC practitioner may assess degree of differentiation of the self, fusions that may exist, various family projections and triangulations present, transmission process that has been inherited, the social environment in which the family is embedded in and the type of emotional process that is prevalent in the family.

Step 5: Second phase

After the initial identification of family dynamics, goals are formulated. In this phase, the counselor helps the family to achieve the goals by making appropriate changes within the family structure and their interaction patterns. The nature and focus of the change to be implemented vary with the therapy that is adopted.

In Bowen's family system, the focus is on the differentiated selves of each family member, reducing the occurrences of multiple triangles and family projections, prevention of emotional cutoffs and management of familial emotional processes. In the circumplex model of family systems, the focus is on establishing a balanced family system type and shifting quickly from the unbalanced family system, in order to make peace with the changing environment. One way to do this is by improving the communication skills. In structural family counseling, the focus is on restoring a healthy structure in the family, so that the family works as a whole unit, rather than individually. This leads to strengthening of the social resources available to the family.

The course of the change to be implemented is to be closely monitored by the SBFC practitioners. During this process, the resources that may help the family are identified both by the family and by the SBFC practitioners. For example, introduction of a crisis SBFC practitioner may help the family in understanding the stages of crisis and enhance pre-crisis preparation (safety and support considerations), in-crisis action (coming out with certain possible alternatives for handling the crisis situation, formulating action plans and ensuring that the plans are followed thoroughly) and post-crisis recovery (debriefing). The SBFC practitioners may also employ other counseling techniques, like self-disclosure and confrontation, to regulate the interaction patterns among the family members. Role plays, in which role reversal may be practiced, are often helpful. For example, in rigid families, where the controlling power is limited to one leader, the role play may involve power being vested upon different family members and obtaining consensus to agree on the instructions being imparted by all family members.

Changes have to be made, which surpass the superficial level. These are called first-order changes. For example, in the family where a child has experienced intra-family sexual abuse, it is true that the removal of the perpetrator from the family will be helpful but only making this change will not help the child. Here, a second-order change (change from one family system to another) is necessary, so that the child feels safe in the immediate environment. Psychoeducational assignments are helpful in sustaining changes and bringing about second-order changes. For example, a fairy tale about bravery can be prescribed for reading and the child might be led to perceive and identify with the hero of the tale, which will instill confidence to better face life situations. Here, it is important for the family members to actively listen and participate in the discussion, so that the child feels that everyone believes what the child is actually saying.

Step 6: Third phase

This constitutes the last phase of family counseling. It signifies that improvements have been made and are being acted upon more frequently in the family. The goals that were set down initially are achieved and the family functions well now, especially to provide support to the child in crisis.

- **Future considerations:** The SBFC practitioner appreciates the work of each member of the family unit and gives a brief overview of the entire process that all of them have undergone together. A plan is laid to continue the good work that the family has done. For example, a plan is laid out for helping the child in crisis, where it is specified which family member will facilitate the child. This is told to the child as well, who knows now the person to approach, when he/she is facing problems. It gives confidence to the child that he/she is not alone in his/her problem. Since a second-order change is more probable now, the improvements will be long-lasting and are not just at the surface level.
- **Preparation for tough times:** Stressful situations cannot be eliminated from the environment. However, the perceptions can be managed. Family counseling makes the family empowered to take on stressors in a healthier way.
- **Follow-ups:** In combination with promoting and encouraging independence, the family is assured of the SBFC practitioner's support and availability through the procedure of follow-ups. In these sessions, the improvements are monitored and small doubts that the family have in their new environment are deliberated on.

Multicultural considerations

Families are meshed in cultures intricately. The cultures define the principles, ideals and beliefs that a family follows. While practicing family counseling, the following points need to be kept in mind from a cultural perspective:

a   Understanding the culture of the family is important to identify the appropriate treatment model.
b   The SBFC practitioner should be aware of personal stereotypes and biases embedded in his or her own culture, so that there is minimal interference and cultural transference can be managed.
c   Identification of who is in charge within the family is important. Respect for this hierarchy in the treatment procedure facilitates rapport building and therapeutic alliance.

d   A special emphasis on understanding the religious affiliations of the family is needed, so that their sentiments are not hurt in the process and the spiritual journey can also become part of the therapeutic journey.

e   The SBFC practitioner should be familiar with the language of the family and conduct family counseling in the local language.

f   Family counseling services need to be offered with informed consent and confidentiality of information is to be maintained.

Challenges and solutions

When there is an attempt to standardize and arrive at a resource that may help children in crisis, it is not without its challenges. Table 14.1 outlines some of these and their possible solutions.

Table 14.1 Challenges and solutions for children in crisis

Challenges	Solutions
1 Acceptance of the presence and degree of the problem that a child is experiencing because of a crisis. The family's hiding tendency and fear of stigmatization may aggravate the degree of the crisis being experienced by the child.	It is important to educate about the universality and the commonness of the problem being experienced by the child during a crisis period, both outside and inside the therapeutic setup. This will facilitate openness among families, to accept the situation and come forward with help. The uniqueness of each problem needs to be validated.
2 Bringing the family together in a therapeutic setup. Time and infrastructural constraints may impede the process of family counseling.	Initial sessions, wherein the counselor is building a rapport and collecting basic information, may be conducted through various online platforms that are conducive to all family members. As the involvement and familiarity of family members increase, face to face sessions should be introduced in pre-decided school premises, as per everyone's convenience. Once the exercises introduced by the counselor have started showing results, follow ups can again be resumed through online platforms.
3 The SBFC practitioner may experience burnout in the process of managing both individual and family therapy cases simultaneously.	It is important to prescribe and establish the guidelines when it comes to taking up a number of counseling cases at a time by one SBFC practitioner. If the maximum number of caseload is reached, there should be a provision by the school management to take on an additional SBFC practitioner on a contract basis, till the time the workload is adjusted. This will increase the efficiency of the SBFC practitioner, facilitate a positive impression of the school management, as well as ensure best services to the children.

(Continued)

Challenges	Solutions
4 Emergencies like Pandemics and Epidemics may result in panic, where parents might not be able to understand, whether their child is facing a problem, because of some crisis.	Parents need to be actively educated regarding signs that a child is experiencing a mental or physical problem, because of a crisis. A small handbook may be published for all parents to read, in which the guidelines may be provided, as well as certain activities may be prescribed, which will help them understand their child better.
5 Limited awareness of school mental health practitioners with respect to family counseling.	Family counseling is a significant resource that a school can effectively capitalize upon. In case of limited awareness on the same, schools should invest in training their mental health practitioners in specific courses on systemic therapies, which will be beneficial in the long run

Conclusion

Family is an important resource which, if put in action efficiently, can prove to be a significant factor for management of children in crisis. The skilled SBFC practitioners, trained in the practice of family counseling, are a necessity these days, especially when we consider the present context of the COVID-19 pandemic. The role of SBFC practitioners is very important in arranging special trainings for mental health professionals, especially for school counselors, in order to deliver professional services to families who require it, for the safety of the children. It is also necessary to assess the situation objectively and capitalize on the strengths of this paradigm, rather than be discouraged by the challenges it presents. Let us all move in a positive direction and make this world a better place for the children to inhabit.

Resources

Harris, N. B. (n.d.). *How childhood trauma affects health across a lifetime.* TED: Ideas Worth Spreading. https://www.ted.com/talks/nadine_burke_harris_how_childhood_trauma_affects_health_across_a_lifetime?utm_source=-whatsapp&utm_medium=social&utm_campaign=tedspread
This TED gives insight as to how adverse childhood experiences have long term consequences for them.
Munakata, Y. (n.d.). *The science behind how parents affect child development.* TED: Ideas Worth Spreading. https://www.ted.com/talks/yuko_munakata_the_science_behind_how_parents_affect_child_development?utm_campaign=tedspread&utm_medium=referral&utm_source=tedcomshare
This video may enhance the SBFC practitioner's knowledge about parenting and how to convince parents about their importance in management of children in crisis.
Tseng, W. S., & Hsu, J. (2018). *Culture and family: Problems and therapy.* Routledge.
This book is a comprehensive view on the cultural aspects to be kept in mind while practicing family counseling.

References

Brown, J. (1999). Bowen family systems theory and practice: Illustration and critique. *Australian and New Zealand Journal of Family Therapy*, 20(2), 94–103.

Carr, A. (2019). Family therapy and systemic interventions for child-focused problems: The current evidence base. *Journal of Family Therapy*, 41(2), 153–213.

Gladding, S. T., & Batra, P. (2007). *Counseling: A comprehensive profession*. Pearson Education India.

House of secrets: The Burari deaths [Video]. (2021). Netflix - Watch TV Shows Online, Watch Movies Online. https://www.netflix.com/title/81095095?trkid =13747225&s=a&t=wha&vlang=en&clip=81439423

Olson, D. H., Waldvogel, L., & Schlieff, M. (2019). Circumplex model of marital and family systems: An update. *Journal of Family Theory & Review*, 11(2), 199–211.

US Department of Health and Human Services. (1994). Crisis intervention in child abuse and neglect. *Administration for Children and Families*. Retrieved July, 2, 2012.

Vetere, A. (2001). Structural family therapy. *Child Psychology and Psychiatry Review*, 6(3), 133–139.

Wilde J. L. (2018). The circumplex model of marital and family systems. In: Lebow J., Chambers A., & Breunlin D. (eds) *Encyclopedia of couple and family therapy*. Springer, Cham. https://doi.org/10.1007/978-3-319-15877-8_413-1

Part IV

School prevention

15 Big Talks for Little People

Child Mental Health Module

Phillip T. Slee

Overview

The *"Big Talks for Little People: Child Mental Health Module"* is a primary school module which aims to help school students better understand their mental health and enhance their well-being. The digitally delivered module comprises six lessons incorporating six social and emotional learning (SEL) topics on mental health for young children. The focus on SEL topics, including relationship building, self-awareness, social awareness, self-management and responsible decision making, emphasises the preventative features of the intervention. In addition to the six lessons, there are eight teacher information sheets providing teachers with further information and links to resources on topics such as "trauma informed teaching", "anxiety", "bullying" and "proprioception". Teachers can use a digital platform to run the six-lesson module in their classrooms. The focus is on early intervention and prevention for all children in each class. The digital module is designed to be updated in response to new events, e.g. COVID-19 and bushfires. The six-lesson downloadable outlines are each accompanied by a digital animation depicting the topic for that lesson, e.g. conflict resolution intended to promote classroom discussion.

Background

The coping procedure focussed on in this school/classroom-based intervention involves assisting primary school-aged children to correctly identify and understand their emotions and feelings and strengthen their friendship network at school. That is, a focus of the module across the six lessons is on assisting primary school-aged children to correctly identify and appropriately express emotions as part of their school life and interactions with other students. Research (Saarni, 1999) suggests that emotional awareness is one of the most rudimentary skills required for competent emotional functioning. The same author has argued that emotion awareness and emotion expression contribute to developing in a child "a sense of subjective well-being and adaptive resilience in face of future stressful circumstances" (p. 10) consistent with hedonia. An overview of research typically demonstrates that young people

DOI: 10.4324/9781003201977-19

with high emotional ability show lower levels of anxiety and depression, fewer school problems and fewer externalising problems. The coping procedure fits with the SBFC model particularly in terms of its prevention and school focus.

Emphasis was given in the module to supporting students to identify and address anxiety. Anxiety is one of the most frequently reported issues for young children with Goodsell et al. (2017) reporting a national prevalence of 6.9% for anxiety disorders in young people. Peer relationships are central features of social anxiety (Chansky & Kendall, 1997). It often precedes the development of early onset major depression (Wittchen, Stein, & Kessler, 1999). A source of anxiety for pre-adolescent children is the anxiety of being negatively evaluated by peers which may be reflected in school bullying. Across the arts and literature, "friendship" occupies a special niche. The ancient Greeks set a great deal of store by the notion of friendship, e.g. as reflected in Homer's epic poem *"The Illiad"* in which the friendship of Achilles and Patroclus is the key element. The Greek philosopher Aristotle devoted a considerable portion of the *Nichomachean Ethics* to a careful examination of the concept of friendship. In the most recent developmental psychology literature, the interest in friendship has waxed and waned, but presently is the focus of a good deal of research. Friendships are a source of skill learning, e.g. listening, insight into one's behaviour and a source of support during stressful times. A formative period in developing these skills is early and middle childhood. The recognition, understanding and expression of emotions and feelings is a significant part of friendship "making and breaking" particularly in relation to issues such as bullying.

The basic underlying premise of the programme is focussed on early intervention particularly for those students impacted by trauma. In the module, trauma in the broadest sense is considered: e.g. environmental trauma, including bushfires, floods or earthquakes, and personal trauma: e.g. including school shootings or the death of a teacher or classmate. Complex trauma is caused by exposure to severe stressors that are repetitive or prolonged. These stressors may be related to abandonment or harm by a trusted adult or occur during developmentally vulnerable time periods such as early childhood or adolescence. Complex trauma has been linked to many negative outcomes for children.

"To a large extent, the basic tenets of SEL overlap with the principles of trauma-informed instruction. Where they have differed are on questions of intensity — both the intensity of the stress children are experiencing and the intensity of the instruction required to help them" (Pawlo, Lorenzo, Eichert, & Elias, 2019). For instance, children who've suffered traumatic experiences often benefit from highly predictable routines, which can be effective in promoting a sense of safety and reducing fear.

From a trauma-informed perspective, the emotional stability of the adults in the school takes on special importance. Many students affected by trauma will have had caregivers who were unavailable or unable to provide consistent caregiving, and for these students, supportive relationships with adults at school are especially salient.

In relation to attachment theory, it is noted that: "In particular, encouraging attachment-focused responses to student behaviour, rather than punitive reactions, may provide corrective relational experiences and encourage positive relationship-building among students, improving their attachment and socio-emotional well-being" (Crosby, Day, Baroni, & Somers, 2019). The four Rs of trauma-informed practice include:

Realisation (that trauma is widespread and multivariate).
Recognise (manifestations and symptoms or trauma).
Respond (practices informed by research).
Retraumatising (prevent doing this at all costs).

(Galguera & Bellone, 2020)

Procedure

The development of the module

The module was developed as a digitally delivered resource suitable for the classroom. A rapid literature review utilising systematic review methods was conducted focussed on the mental health of primary school-aged students. The findings informed the content of the module classroom lessons, teacher information sheets and digital animations.

Concurrently, a range of "experts" in child mental health were interviewed (e.g. psychiatrist and senior school counsellor) using a non-probability "snowball sampling" methodology helping further clarify the module content.

Simultaneously, an audit identified 200 well-being programmes available to Australian schools
(Dix et al., 2020). Some 56% had "low" quality evidence supporting their effectiveness.

The digital platform and the animations were developed by an animation company. The content of the platform was informed by data gathered in the preceding stages.

A unique element of the resource was a series of animations. In developing the short animations for the module, a number of considerations were taken into account. Audio content was kept to an absolute minimum to cater for students with special needs, e.g. hearing loss and for students for whom English was a second language. In terms of the visual content of the animations, it was important that they be relevant for multicultural groups, that is, they did not depict a mainstream cultural group. Animation was considered better than real actors – safer as it is a step removed from reality. The animations were developed so that they were genderless, colourless and ageless catering for a wide developmental range.

Overall, the animations were developed to be short (i.e. 30–60 seconds in length), targeted, simple, able to be shared with parents and based on clear concepts of social and emotional learning (SEL) concepts such as friendship skills. The intent was to create characters that were identifiable and so they

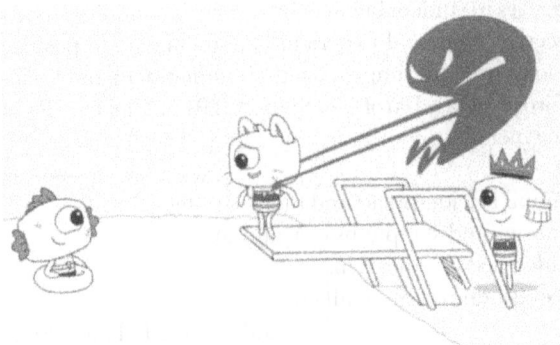

Figure 15.1 A "risk-taking" event involving three of the "peeps" ("Kit", "Sarge" and "Float")

were given names such as "Brim", the character wore a hat or "tek" where the character related to the world of technology. Each animation depicted a scenario, e.g. bullying or making friends designed to help development of empathy by creating scenarios without solutions and for promoting discussion. In Figure 15.1, the scenario depicts a "risk-taking" event involving three of the "peeps" ("Kit", "Sarge" and "Float"). The scene depicts "Kit" about to possibly engage in a "risky" event. The "feel" (emotion) is depicted as possibly restraining "Kit" from taking a risk.

As the animations developed and were trialled with small samples of primary school-aged students they evolved into two forms. The first form was the "peeps" (people) represented in a cartoon like fashion according to the criteria described earlier. There were nine characters in all represented individually by names such as "Tek", "Twig" and "Brim".

Evaluation of the pilot programme

In 2021, a pilot evaluation of a new Australian primary school six-lesson mental health programme, "Big Talks for Little People: a primary school mental health program", was undertaken. As described in this chapter, the digitally delivered module includes lesson content focussed on key SEL skills, e.g. relationships development including multi-media and practical teacher "information sheets". The research was conducted with approval from the Flinders University Human Research Ethics Committee with all participants and parents providing active consent. Five pilot schools were recruited from a sample of eight schools which had approached the researcher. In choosing the schools, maximum variation sampling was employed based on seven-point index of socio-economic dis-advantage (least to most) used in South Australian schools. All participating teachers received professional development.

Method: A mixed-method quasi-hybrid design methodology was utilised. An online survey was completed by students from five schools pre-test ($n = 173$) and three schools matched post-test ($n = 68$) with semi-structured interviews with teachers ($n = 4$) and a focus group of students ($n = 18$) conducted at the completion of the module. Student questionnaire data was gathered online, including the use of three standardised and internationally used measures of well-being.

Results: Students at post-test self-reported significant positive improvements in positive emotional state (PES), recognising and expressing emotions and reductions in anxiety and bullying. Teachers and students strongly endorsed the digitally delivered programme and its lesson content and animations, including the pre-programme teacher professional development.

In summary, preliminary evidence from this pilot study suggested that the six-week teacher delivered programme has some capacity to enhance student mental health and well-being. Further research is required to address the limitations of the research design of this initial pilot phase and prepare the module for upscaling.

In implementing this newly developed programme which was positively evaluated in classrooms in 2021 (the outcomes are described later in this chapter), the first step involves professional development for the teachers who will be actually teaching the programme. In a systematic review of the literature pertaining to well-being programmes, Dix et al. (2020) concluded that "Evidence suggests that well-being programs delivered by 'trained' classroom teachers (e.g., a program designed to build the capacity of the teacher first, supported by resources for students) were marginally more effective in impacting students' well-being outcomes than programs delivered by external professionals". This finding highlights the importance of teacher professional learning and their essential role and capacity to influence student well-being outcomes. No difference was found on academic outcomes due to the mode of delivery.

Schools are complex organisations that pose significant challenges for the delivery and evaluation of health promotion initiatives. In considering schools as sites for mental health promotion initiatives such as well-being, the matter of how an intervention developed outside of the school is taken up and enacted in the often "messy and typically busy" world of the classroom is significant. The question of how an intervention programme is conducted faithfully in the classroom is a vitally important issue because it reflects on the outcomes of the programme which brings us to the matter of the effectiveness of school-based interventions and factors that enhance and degrade effective implementation.

The gap between research and practice has been a longstanding concern. The increasing demand for evidence-based practice means an increasing need for more practice-based evidence. As Durlak and DuPre (2008) note:

> Social scientists recognise that developing effective interventions is only the first step toward improving the health and well-being of

populations. Transferring effective programs into real world settings and maintaining them there is a complicated, long-term process that requires dealing effectively with the successive, complex phases of program diffusion.

(Durlak and DuPre, 2008, p. 327)

Durlak et al. (2011) identified a number of key elements that should be incorporated in the implementation of any school-based programme to help ensure quality and maximise outcomes from the intervention. These are:

- *Adherence* (a.k.a. fidelity, compliance) is the degree to which the core components of a programme are delivered as intended.
- *Exposure* (a.k.a. dosage) refers to how much of the original programme has been delivered and the quantity of the programme to which participants have been exposed.
- *Participant responsiveness* is associated with the degree to which the programme stimulates the interest or holds the attention of participants and the extent to which participants engage with the programme.
- *Quality of delivery* relates to the instructors' programme delivery skills and how well different programme components have been conducted.
- *Programme differentiation* is the extent to which a programme's theory and practices can be distinguished from other programmes (i.e. programme uniqueness) so that there is no contamination from other programmes.

In addition to these five domains, Durlak and DuPre (2008) identified three other important aspects of implementation, which are particularly relevant to school-based programmes. Specifically, these are:

- *Adaptation*, which refers to the changes made in the original programme during implementation and the extent to which it is modified and adapted.
- *Control monitoring*, involving a comparison of differences to non-participating schools and their outcomes.
- *Programme reach*, which refers to the proportion of the target audience who have participated and is the rate of involvement and representativeness of programme participants.

Implementation quality is vitally important in the effective delivery of well-being programmes in schools and classrooms. A key element helping ensure implementation quality as noted by Dix et al. (2020) is that the teachers delivering the programme receive professional development. In this regard, all of the teachers who were involved in delivering the "Big Talks for Little People…" received professional development. A custom-designed PD programme (1–2 hours duration) was delivered by two experienced researchers for all teachers delivering the programme. The outline of the PD is as follows:

i   Introduction to the module and its framework
    Framework: Big Talks for Little People: A Framework for Prevention & Intervention
    - **P** – Prepare – and consider the issue of mental health
    - **E** – Educate – and develop an understanding of the issue
    - **A** – Action – develop an action plan for intervention and prevention
    - **C** – Coping – identify the strategies needed to cope
    - **E** – Evaluate – develop strategies for assessing the evidence-base
ii The explanation of the digital platform for the delivery of the Big Talks for Little People program
iii The nature of mental health problems amongst primary school students, e.g. anxiety and depression
iv Demonstration of the use of the six teacher information sheets on topics such as "trauma informed teaching"
v   Registration of teachers to enable access to the digital platform.

The second step focusses on familiarising teachers with the eight practical teacher information sheets on the topics of children's anxiety, the brain, SEL, trauma-informed teaching, proprioception, bullying, self-efficacy and teacher well-being. The support role of teachers starts with emotional coaching and teaching the students to acknowledge and validate their emotions, acknowledge emotions in others and know that it is okay, for example, to express anger. As a step towards this goal, teachers may need to be taught how to model some of these behaviours such as how to help others without rescuing, how to offer support without taking over and how to support in a conflict situation. Student supporters need support and training about how to be a friend and knowing how and when to ask for help. By connecting up neuroscience, we can explain to students "verbal pain and physical pain have the same effects in the brain" and lead into conversations about belonging and inclusion. Inclusiveness should be taught as not necessarily about "liking" someone but still making them feel included. In relation to teaching, the emphasis is on the group and community rather than individual, encouraging a sense of community and emphasising the importance of student to student connection. It is also suggested that teachers create hooks and paraphernalia to remind students of the programmes being used, revisit multiple times and include activities like journaling to embed the learning. Emphasis is given to having friendship ambassadors, peer mediators – where students lead conflict resolution, peer mentors and lunchtime clubs, while providing student support as required by teachers. Emphasis is given to making the lessons visible with posters, etc., around the classroom. Emphasis is given to explicitly teaching concepts like understanding that some fellow students around them might be suffering and not showing it. Simple precepts such as treating others as you would have them treat you, encouraging in students the confidence to stand up when you feel like someone is being mistreated, and understanding of group roles. It was emphasised in the lessons in the module that role playing these concepts out in class is vital to providing a "lived experience" for students.

The third step involves familiarising the teachers with the online questionnaires developed to collect student and teacher data. The online data for the students is collected during the first and sixth lessons providing the opportunity to analyse change over time. Qualtrics is a data programming company which provides the platform for this data collection. The data collected from the students is anonymous and confidential as the students use their school identity number and the data is sent directly to the primary investigator. Data is collected using a series of Likert scales and open-ended questions on topics such as:

- Positive peer relationships, e.g. how many friends they have at school.
- Happiness about personal skills, e.g. sports.
- Happiness about their progress in school work.
- Peer relationships, e.g. their experience of bullying.
- Self-concept, e.g. how students feel about themselves.
- Self-esteem, e.g. how much they like/care for themselves.

In relation to the standardised questionnaires completed by the students pre- and post-test, the following is noted:

The Stirling Well-being Scale for Children (StirCWB Scale) was designed for students aged 8–15 years. Previous research piloted with children demonstrated that the scale had good theoretical grounding and "was understood… and… perceived by children to be measuring well-being" (Liddle & Carter, p. 7). Comprising 12 items, the StirCWB Scale assesses emotional and psychological well-being and the level of a child's PES as well as Positive Outlook (POL).

The Emotion Expression Scale for Children (EESC) is a self-report scale for primary school-aged students designed to examine two aspects of deficient emotion expression, namely (i) lack of emotion awareness and (ii) lack of motivation to express negative emotion. Difficulties with recognising emotion and expressing emotion have been linked to poor mental health and well-being (Penza-Clyve & Zeman, 2002). According to Saarni (1999), emotion awareness and emotion expression are skills of emotional competence and contribute to develop "a sense of subjective well-being and adaptive resilience in face of future stressful circumstances" (p. 10). Emotion awareness is the ability of attending to and understanding one's own emotions which is thought to provide a foundation helping cope with emotion experience.

The Social Anxiety Scale for Children–Revised (SASC–R; La Greca, Silverman, & Wasserstein, 1998) is a 22-item empirically derived inventory designed to capture conceptual distinctions between subjective and behavioural aspects of social anxiety, and its development was guided by theory and work regarding the nature of social anxiety.

The fourth step involves clearly illustrating the six lessons comprising the module for the teachers as part of the professional development session. The six lessons include:

- *Lesson 1*: Introduction to the Module

  The purpose of the lesson is to support students to develop knowledge, understanding and skills to create opportunities and take action to enhance their own and others' health, well-being, safety and physical activity participation. Students develop skills to manage their emotions. Using a 60-second animation, students are introduced to the characters in the animations. As illustrated earlier, the students are introduced to the characters "Peeps" and the "Feels" associated with emotions or feelings arising out of school-based incidents such as bullying. Each of the lessons provides teachers with guidelines, e.g. questions to ask, activities to run and ideas for using the animations, e.g. pausing and asking students to suggest what is happening in the scenario and what the emotions or feelings might be. The online pre-test data will be collected during this lesson.

- *Lesson 2*: What is Mental Health and Well-being?

  The purpose of the lesson is to understand what mental health and well-being are, and the importance of looking after it. The animation here directly addresses the issue of dealing with disappointment.

- *Lesson 3*: How Do I Look after Myself and Others?

  Purpose: Understand the signs they need to look out for to help manage their mental health and well-being. Build up the skills on how to have a supportive mental health. The animation used here focusses on resilience in the face of adversity.

- *Lesson 4:* Bullying: Face to Face and Online

  The purpose of the lesson is to understand what bullying looks like, both face to face and online. Learn skills on how to raise concerns safely and how to stop it. The animation provides a scenario of bullying to promote discussion.

- *Lesson 5:* Showing Compassion for Others

  The purpose of the lesson is to understand, grow and develop the skills required to be compassionate individuals who are part of the team. Use the diving board animation (see Figure 15.1).

- *Lesson 6:* Summary

  This lesson will summarise new knowledge, skills and understanding students have developed. The students recognise the influence of emotions on behaviours and discuss factors that influence how people interact. Use new concluding animation. The online post-test data will be collected during this lesson.

The basic underlying premise of "Big Talks for Little People…" is early whole school universal intervention. Interventions may be categorised broadly according to whether their purpose is primarily to prevent something, e.g. bullying, from happening or alternatively to deal with cases if and when they occur. However, a rigid distinction cannot be made; for instance, disciplinary actions taken when, for example, a case of bullying is identified may impact not only upon the person being treated but may also make it less likely that others will bully; that is, it may also have a preventative function. Some interventions are not primarily directed towards changing the behaviour of individuals but are concerned rather with establishing an environment or ethos in which a behaviour is less likely, for instance, by developing in members of the school community (including both teachers and parents) a better understanding of the problem and promoting more pro-social attitudes and empathic feelings towards others; or alternatively by reducing the motivation to bully by involving students more deeply in a school-related study. These may be described as preventative measures. Many programmes include both preventative and interventive elements.

By adapting a model described by Haggerty and Mrazek (1994), interventions may be targeted (Figure 15.2):

a   universally at whole populations,
b   selectively at a population at risk and
c   indicatively at "high-risk" individuals.

(a) and (b) are usually identified in terms of "prevention", whereas (c) encompasses "early intervention".

i   Universal Programmes: are targeted to the general public or a whole population group that has not been identified on the basis of individual risk, e.g. childhood immunisation.
ii   Populations at Risk. Here, the interventions are directed towards individuals or sub-groups of a population known to be at risk of developing problems, e.g. literacy programmes directed towards children from economically depressed areas.
iii   "High Risk" Individuals. Programmes are directed specifically towards high-risk individuals who may already be presenting with signs or

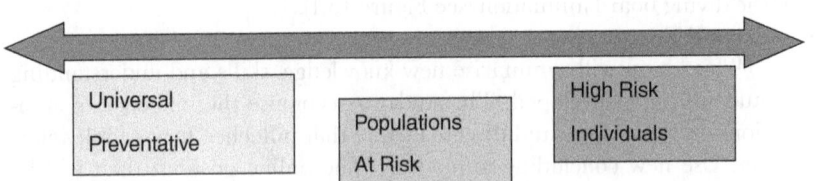

Figure 15.2 Three levels of intervention

symptoms, e.g. programmes to prevent depression in children who have one or both clinically depressed parents.

Generally as one moves across the continuum from universal preventative programmes to targeted programmes for high-risk individuals, the size of the population receiving the interventions decreases, while the degree of the psychological problems increases in severity.

Multicultural considerations

The "Big Talks for Little People: Child mental health module" has been developed with a number of very specific design features in mind in order to deliver the programme to all students in any classroom. One of the most defining trends in the last two decades has been globalisation and the increasing migration associated with it. Multiculturalism has become a defining feature in many of the world's economies with Canada, the United Kingdom, the United States and South Africa examples of nations that have embraced a strong immigrant-receiving tradition. In relation to Australia, as well as being home to the world's oldest continuous culture, Australians identify with more than 270 ancestries. For example in a primary school near the author in a class of 26 students, the first language of eighteen of the students is not English. As such, taking multiculturalism into account, the "Big Talks for Little people..." module has been developed accordingly. For example, the six lessons delivered by the teacher rely heavily on small group activities, student role plays and debates. A unique feature of the programme was a series of animations to be presented in each lesson. The animations were primarily visual to cater for multicultural groups. Animations were seen as is better than real actors – safer as they are a "step removed" from the situation being depicted. Designed for the 8–12 age group, they are genderless, with a neutral colour in skin, and ageless due to developmental range (see Figure 15.1).

Challenges and solutions

There are a number of challenges to be addressed if implementing the approach described in this chapter. The first of these involves the very practical issue of providing professional development. Factors limiting the uptake of professional development by teachers include the points that they are "time poor" and generally receive no "credit" for undertaking the professional development. Possible solutions to these challenges involve providing temporary relief to teachers to take classes, while the teachers undertake professional development. Another option that some education departments provide is professional development "certificates" that count towards some form of professional accreditation associated with salary advantages or possibilities for promotion. Another challenge concerns the issue that many teachers do not feel that their training has prepared them to address the social emotional learning of their students; for example, they may be trained maths, science or English teachers. The long-term solution here is to ensure that under-graduate teacher training does prepare them with appropriate courses or topics in areas such as child and adolescent development.

Conclusion

The *"Big Talks for Little People: Child Mental Health Module"* is a primary school module which aims to help school students better understand their mental health and enhance their well-being, particularly those impacted by trauma. The programme is consistent with important elements of the SBFC model particularly in terms of its prevention-based school focus. In summary, from a multi-informant perspective, the analysis of the qualitative data from the teacher interviews and student focus group proved significant in terms of providing insight into the end-users experience of utilising the module in the classroom and most importantly provided insight into the students' experiences of the module and the learning that accrued from it.

Resources

Askell-Williams, H., Lawson, M.J., Slee, P.T. (2009). Venturing into schools: Locating mental health initiatives in complex environments. *International Journal of Emotional Education, 1*(2), 7–14.

Clark, A., S., McQuail, S., & Moss, P. (2003). *Exploring the field of listening to and consulting with young children.* Research Report RR445. London: DfES.

Glasgow, R. E., Emmons K. M. (2007). How can we increase translation of research into practice? Types of evidence needed. *Annual Review Public Health, 28,* 413–433. doi: 10.1146/annurev.publhealth.28.021406.144145. PMID: 17150029.

Glazzard, J. (2019). A whole-school approach to supporting children's and young people's mental health. *Journal of Public mental Health, 18,* 265–265.

Liddle, I., & Carter, G. F. A. (2015). Emotional and psychological well-being in children: The development and validation of the Stirling children's well-being scale. *Educational Psychology in Practice, 31*(2), 174–185, doi: 10.1080/02667363.2015.1008409

March, J. S., Silva, S. G., & Comptom, S. (2005). The case for practical clinical trials in psychiatry. *American Journal of Psychiatry, 162,* 836–846. [PubMed] [Google Scholar]

National Action Plan for the Health of Children and Young People 2020–2030 (2020). Australian Government Department of Health. Canberra, Australian Capital Territory.

Wolfenden L., Williams, C. M., Wiggers, J., Nathan, N., & Yoong, S. L. (2016), Improving the translation of health promotion interventions using effectiveness–implementation hybrid designs in program evaluations. *Health Promotion Journal of Australia, 27,* 204–207.

The following links and references provide the interested reader with additional support including details for accessing the "Big Talks for Little People: Child Mental Health Module" as referred to in this chapter.

Website

Child Adolescent and Psychological Resources www.caper.com.au

Programs

Slee, P.T (2019). The PEACE Pack: *Coping with Bullying & Promoting Wellbeing.* Flinders University, Adelaide. South Australia

References

Chansky, T. E., & Kendall, P. C. (1997). Social expectancies and self-perceptions in anxiety disordered children. *Journal of Anxiety Disorders, 11,* 347–363

Crosby, S. D., Day, A., Baroni, B. A., & Somers, C. (2019). Examining trauma-informed teaching and the trauma symptomatology of court-involved girls. *The Urban Review, 51*(4), 582–598.

Dix, K., Kashfee, S.A., Carslake, T., Sniedze-Gregory, S., O'Grady, E., & Trevitt, J. (2020). *A systematic review of intervention research examining effective student well-being in schools and their academic outcomes.* Evidence for Learning: Melbourne.

Durlak, J. A., & DuPre, E. P. (2008). Implementation matters: A review of research on the influence of implementation on program outcomes and the factors affecting implementation. *American Journal of Community Psychology, 41*(3), 327–350.

Durlak, J. A., Weissberg, R. P., Dymnicki, A. B., Taylor, R. D., & Schellinger, K. B. (2011). The impact of enhancing students' social and emotional learning: A meta-analysis of school-based universal interventions. *Child Development, 82*(1), 405–432.

Galguera, T., & Bellone, M. (2020). Healing the Phoenix: Trauma-informed practice at the ground level. *Childhood Education, 96*(2), 6–13.

Goodsell, B., Lawrence, D., Ainley, J., Sawyer, M., Zubrick, S.R., Maratos, J. (2017). *Child and adolescent mental health and educational outcomes. An analysis of educational outcomes from Young Minds Matter: The second Australian Child and Adolescent Survey of Mental Health and Wellbeing.* Perth: Graduate School of Education, The University of Western Australia.

Haggerty, R. J., & Mrazek, P. J. (Eds.). (1994). *Reducing risks for mental disorders: Frontiers For preventive intervention research.*

La Greca, A. M., Silverman, W. K., & Wasserstein, S. B. (1998). Children's pre-disaster functioning as a predictor of posttraumatic stress following Hurricane Andrew. *Journal of Consulting and Clinical Psychology, 66*(6), 883.

Pawlo, E., Lorenzo, A., Eichert, B., & Elias, M. J. (2019). All SEL should be trauma-informed. *Phi Delta Kappan, 101*(3), 37–41.

Penza-Clyve, S., & Zeman, J. (2002). Initial validation of the emotion expression scale for children (EESC). *Journal of Clinical Child and Adolescent Psychology, 31*(4), 540–547.

Saarni, C. (1999). *The development of emotional competence.* Guilford press.

Wittchen, H. U., Stein, M. B., & Kessler, R. C. (1999). Social fears and social phobia in a community sample of adolescents and young adults: Prevalence, risk factors and comorbidity. *Psychological Medicine, 29,* 309–323.

16 Preventing school violence through student engagement

Emily J. Hernandez and Alia R. Elasmar

Overview

Violence prevention is an important component to violence intervention. It involves responding to crises or disasters that impact the school community which may occur at any time. Due to the unpredictable nature of crisis and disaster events, it is important to develop a model that is grounded in prevention to shift the system from a reactive mode of responding which then becomes cyclical, non-productive, and contributes to high levels of stress and burnout among the school staff and support structures. Reactive response models overwhelmingly tax the system and deteriorate a sense of safety and learning in the school. This chapter describes how focusing on the engagement of students to schools can serve as a form of violence prevention. While there are many aspects to student engagement, this chapter will focus on three important components that have been shown to be critical factors in student engagement: cultivating a positive school climate, establishing school organization and infrastructure, and fostering positive student interactions. School-Based Family Counseling (SBFC) practitioners working in school settings can work proactively within a prevention model focused on student engagement that dually serves as a component of the violence prevention efforts and plan for the school.

Background

As defined in Chapter 5 of this book, "Crisis Intervention with School Personnel", a school crisis is commonly defined as a sudden, uncontrollable, and extremely negative event that can potentially impact the entire school community (Brock et al., 2009). School crises can include natural disasters, death of a student or school personnel, harm to self or others, and acts of violence. In 2018 alone, there were 82 school shootings in the United States, the highest number since 1970 (CHDS, 2019). Death by suicide is currently the second leading cause of death among teenagers, next to car accidents (CDC, 2018). In 2017, two out of every 100 teenagers made suicide attempts serious enough to require medical treatment; seven out of 100 attempted suicide (CDC, 2018). This rate has increased during the COVID-19 pandemic.

DOI: 10.4324/9781003201977-20

These tragedies have various impacts on the school community that extend far beyond the events of the day.

Secondary trauma and grief affect students, families, and school staff in ways that may appear immediately following a school tragedy for weeks, months, or years later. Preventing violence in school is an integral part of violence intervention. Violence prevention strategies can establish systems and practices that help address root challenges that lead to crises. Violence prevention is important because these strategies help create a healthy structure for the school community in managing emotions, thoughts, and risky behaviors. Incidents of violence involve a crisis which places a school and school district in a difficult position to mobilize response. Therefore, schools naturally focus on reactive measures and procedures that follow when a crisis happens. The lack of a violence prevention approach can create a reactive cycle in which students and staff well-being are at risk and constantly must respond to tension instead of building connection. A violence prevention systems-based approach that includes the entire school community is an important approach to violence prevention. It is critical for SBFC practitioners to understand the role of student engagement as a key component in violence prevention.

Student engagement

Student engagement has been widely studied in educational research and is a term that is used to measure a student's relationship, or connection, to school. There are consistent themes that relate to student engagement: sense of belonging and being a part of a school; whether or not students like school; level of teacher supportiveness and caring; presence of good friends in school; engagement in current and future academic progress; fair and effective discipline; and participation in extracurricular activities (Libbey, 2004). Student engagement and the factors described above have been found to be highly associated with student outcomes and a robust predictor of achievement and behavior in schools (Appleton, Christenson, & Furlong, 2008; Shernoff & Schmidt, 2008). Christenson, Reschly, and Wylie (2012) refer to student engagement as the "glue, or mediator" that links the various important contexts (life, home, school peers, and community) to students which, in turn, has an effect on the outcome of interest and connection to school (p. 3).

Student engagement has become an important topic in the field of education. In general, there are widely known facts about student engagement that are important to understand as a foundational base for utilizing student engagement as a systemic prevention and intervention effort in a comprehensive school setting (Christenson et al., 2012). These commonly known facts are detailed in Box 16.1.

Studies show that student engagement is considered the main theoretical model in understanding student dropout (Christenson et al., 2008; Finn, 2006; Reschly & Christenson, 2006b). Hart et al. (2011) recommend that student engagement interventions be a part of the key to promoting school completion

---

Box 16.1 Known facts about student engagement (Christenson et al., 2012)

Student engagement is crucial to understanding student dropout

Engagement behavior is complex and much more than just attending school, or doing well academically.

Student engagement is associated positively with academic, social, and emotional learning outcomes.

Student engagement is a multi-dimensional construct that requires an awareness and understanding of affective connections within the academic environment and student behavior.

Context is important. Engagement is inextricably linked and influenced by the context of the student's life (school, peers, family, community). Focusing on the individual alone is not enough.

Student engagement and motivation must be a component of effective instruction for positive learning outcomes.

Measuring student engagement is a powerful tool to drive data driven decision making in schools.

There are evidenced based practices and interventions that are known to increase student engagement.

---

and academic outcomes and describe measures to be used as an assessment tool to target interventions for students who are at risk or used as prevention efforts at the school-wide level. The student engagement construct has been found to be a critical component in working with students who are struggling in their connection to school, with peers, and demonstrating risk behaviors. For these reasons, it is critical to include the student engagement construct in violence prevention and intervention programs because it can be a protective factor for preventing and intervening with crisis situations at schools.

Connection to SBFC model and framework

Student engagement can be viewed and applied through the lens of the SBFC model and framework. The SBFC model, as described by Gerrard and Soriano (2019), illustrates the primary focus of SBFC to be on the school and the family in the area of prevention and intervention. The model consists of four quadrants: school prevention, school intervention, family prevention, and family intervention. It provides a framework to help SBFC professionals stay focused on working systemically within a school structure which is at the heart of the SBFC approach (see Figure 1.1 in Chapter 1) (Gerrard & Soriano, 2019).

Student engagement falls largely in the area of the prevention quadrants if you are viewing the construct through the SBFC model and framework. In

Table 16.1 Findings: Three emerging themes and supporting strategies (Hernandez, 2014)

Theme	Supporting strategies		
Positive School Climate	Leadership	Whole-School Approach	
School Organization and Infrastructure	Student Safety and Learning	Campus Supervision	Student Groupings/ Cohort Model
Student Interactions	Cooperative Learning Model	Character Building and Social Skills	

order to increase student engagement within a school system, it is best to begin with a prevention-focused systems-oriented approach. A specific focus on prevention within a systems perspective reduces the need for intervention-related services. The focus on prevention shifts the balance from a reactive model to a more proactive one. The need for school and family interventions will always exist and is a definite need within school systems. The development of a school system that is heavily prevention-focused will allow for more time and use of deliberate and intentional interventions for youth and families by SBFC professionals (Hernandez, 2016).

The proposed procedure in this chapter is systemic in nature and also falls within the prevention quadrants of the SBFC model. The procedural steps are aligned with the findings of three critical elements for fostering student engagement in school systems: positive school climate, school organization and infrastructure, and student interactions (Hernandez, 2020). These three elements are core components to be addressed and developed in preventing school violence. There are supporting strategies found within each theme that are applied. The themes with their supporting strategies are depicted in Table 16.1.

A systemic approach focuses on the strength each individual has and builds a foundation that benefits all. The systemic SBFC approach to preventing school violence described in this chapter will include three themes and their supporting strategies: *positive school climate, school organization and infrastructure and student interactions.*

Procedure

This procedure was developed for SBFC practitioners that are working at a school site and steps include preventing and intervening with school violence through a lens of focusing on student engagement. Each step includes supporting strategies that are focused on preventing school violence from a systemic prevention-focused lens.

First step: Intentional focus on positive school climate

The first step in the procedure is to intentionally focus and address issues related to school climate. The SBFC practitioner needs to work collaboratively with the school site leadership to assess the climate of the campus and work toward establishing structures that are focused on a positive school climate. This step includes working with leadership and ensuring a whole-school approach is used. For these reasons, collaboration is key and the SBFC practitioner cannot accomplish this step of the procedure on their own.

School climate is a complex construct that has been identified as an important component for effective schools. Students learn better when they feel safe and connected to school. Connectedness, school engagement, and a sense of a safe classroom/school environment improve when norms and boundaries are in place, expectations are clearly outlined and enforced, and open conversations are held. SBFC practitioners must be active catalysts for change, collaborative partnerships, and leaders in reform efforts directed at promoting positive school climates.

Whole-school approaches are supported by research as being an effective practice in the overall violence prevention, and more specifically the prevention of bullying. Bullying is a common form of violence in schools. Effective practices in preventing bullying require more than a "one size fits all" approach. Sherer and Nickerson (2010) argue that strategies for the prevention of bullying need to take place across five categories; system-wide, school staff and parent involvement, educational approaches with students, student involvement, and interventions with bullies and victims. Casebeer (2012) asserted that school bullying is a complex issue in violence prevention that calls for a comprehensive approach based on the needs of each individual school culture. Thus, the most effective method for the reduction and prevention of bullying, and other forms of school violence, involves a whole-school approach unique for that school community. Klein, Cornell, and Konold (2012) emphasized the importance of school climate as a protective factor, and Sherer and Nickerson (2010) discussed the most effective, yet most under-utilized, approach to affect and change school climate as the use of system-level interventions. Based on research, the most effective practice in preventing school violence is to utilize a school-wide, whole-school, approach that aids in developing a positive school climate.

Improving positive school climate in schools through leadership utilizing a whole-school approach

SBFC practitioners collaborate with leadership at school sites and within districts to develop systems for violence prevention. The components below are important to take place when working on improving a positive school climate in a school system utilizing a whole-school approach.

School site leadership:

- Establishes belief systems that value and prioritize the emotional and physical safety of the school campus.
- Works on involving all stakeholders with the school vision, mission, and operations along with formulating partnerships with and involving parents in their child's education.
- Participates and facilitates professional development and training that encompasses inclusive practices of all members of the school community.
- Participates and facilitates professional development and training that educates staff about evidence-based practices for emotional and physical safety in the classroom.
- Practices transparency in their communication with the school community.
- Demonstrates value for effective and respectful communication by establishing norms around communication and modeling best practices.
- Must be a visible presence on the school campus to ensure school safety; the level of visibility should be prominent, consistent, and authentic.
- Engages caregivers and families by consistently communicating school events and expectations. This includes weekly newsletters, messages about school safety, values and expectations and how to model those expectations at home. This also includes holding workshops and meetings that are relevant to challenges families are facing with students (e.g. coffee with the principal, parent workshops, and skills for success).
- Partakes in actions that foster trust with staff such as collaborating and making decisions about school-wide practices together.
- Models school values and actively voices/labels school values as school community members are practicing it. For example, establishing acronyms for school values that are easy to remember and recall (R for respect; "thank you for respecting your friend/ teacher").
- Adopts systems that foster a positive school climate such as Positive Behavioral Interventions and Supports (PBIS) and a Multi-Tiered System of Supports. This enables a paradigm shift for providing support and setting higher expectations for all students through intentional design and redesign of integrated supports and services, instead of selecting a few components of intensive interventions.
- Ensures stakeholders (students, parents, teachers, staff, and community members) are treated as partners, welcomed, respected, and given the message that they are a necessary component to the school family.
- Ensures that there are clear visual images and displays around the school further communicating a welcoming message to all stakeholders and setting a positive tone with high expectations for all.
- Allows SBFC practitioners to work within a "whole-school approach" focusing on effective communication, developing capacity, community building, and ensuring engagement with multiple stakeholders. Stakeholders should include students, parents, community, and school staff.

- Ensures that teachers at the school are highly regarded, celebrated, respected, and seen as major change agents. Teachers are to be provided training and guidance toward the mission and vision of the school and work together with administrators as partners, a team, in collaboration toward the same goal.

Second step: Develop school organization and infrastructure for student engagement

The second step in the procedure is focused on the school organization and infrastructure. The SBFC practitioner works collaboratively on school issues directly related to safety and learning, effective supervision of the campus, and addressing infrastructure related to how students work together in courses.

Prioritize student safety and learning

In their research, Kutsyuruba, Klinger, and Hussain (2015) emphasize "School safety and well-being of students are important antecedents of academic achievement". Their research indicates that students have different perceptions and experiences with safety (Kutsyuruba et al., 2015). Later in this chapter, we will discuss multicultural considerations to provide insight on how to ensure a safe learning environment that is inclusive of all students' perceptions and experiences. Building a learning environment that is emotionally and physically safe requires the following foundational practices:

- Form a crisis response team on campus and establish roles and forms of communication between roles within the crisis team. Typical members of a crisis team include administrators, counselors, school psychologists, and other mental health professionals on campus.
- Crisis team will construct a crisis protocol that aligns with the district crisis protocol. Crisis protocol will include step-by-step process, risk assessments, interventions following risk assessments, safety plans, and re-entry plans.
- Implement school assemblies that reinforce school expectations established in PBIS system.
- Implement a school-wide social-emotional curriculum that is accessible and ready to use in all classrooms at a tier-1 level of support (i.e. Second Step, Responsive Classroom, and Inner Explorer).
- Adopt restorative justice practices and/or conflict resolution opportunities to provide a learning opportunity for students to practice regulating emotions and working through relational challenges.
- Engage in and facilitate trauma-informed care professional development to learn effective and equitable practices to address challenging behavior.

Effective campus supervision

Campus supervision is a simplified concept that all schools utilize in some form. An effective campus supervision plan and team is a critical component to ensuring safety and learning contributing to a positive school climate. The campus supervision team plays an important role in the prevention and early intervention of violence on campus. The manner in which campus supervision takes place on campus can also contribute to a positive school climate. Team members have a great opportunity to increase student engagement while ensuring that the campus supervision protocol is one that is positive and engaging focused on connecting with students, rather than punitive in nature. The SBFC practitioner may be a part of the campus supervision team or may collaborate regularly with the team if not available. The following guidelines have been developed to ensure effective campus supervision at a school site that fosters student engagement, thus serving in preventing school violence (Hernandez, 2014).

Campus supervision:

- Should be an organized, structured, goal-directed active form of supervision, and members of the team are trained and held accountable to quality supervision of students.
- Should be systematized and is a major consistent daily function of the school staff, including the administrators. Establish a core campus supervision team that meets regularly to discuss issues related to campus supervision and for constant improvement to the system based on feedback and observation.
- Requires the development of a campus supervision protocol to ensure that all members of the team are "on the same page" and expectations are clearly understood. The guidelines operationalize what the campus supervision should look like and focus on the main key points that they would like staff members to keep consistent. Training on these guidelines provides for a consistency in how campus supervision is performed.
- Team should embrace ownership over the role with a shared understanding that "This is our school, our students, our job". Everyone works together for the safety and structure of the whole.
- Should be "active" in nature. This "active" form of supervision requires staff to regularly be visible and provides consistency and ample opportunities for interactions with students.
- Can be extended as voluntary to the rest of the school staff. For example, an effective campus supervision program can be embedded into the school culture so that teachers may voluntarily supervise their hallways during transition periods without being asked because they want to do their part. Monitoring the hallways becomes an integral part of being visible and interacting with students.

Student groupings/cohort model

Schools can design the infrastructure of their school day so that students are grouped together in some form of a student grouping or cohorting model. Developing a grouping system, or cohort model, keeps students and teachers together in contiguous space areas. This grouping system allows for a large school to feel like a relatively small school for a student, as they become a part of a smaller community within their group. This sense of "smallness" creates increased opportunities for increased socialization and safety. This can create a safe and positive climate in the hallways. It also allows for teachers to have closer relationships with students and have a better sense of student needs. Further, all teacher teams for the entire grade should follow the same curriculum and implementing advisory periods can serve as a "school family" and teachers take "ownership" of those students by taking responsibility for their academic and social/emotional well-being. This advisory period allows time for students and teachers to develop relationships together and focus on non-academic content such as life skills, character development, and growing together as a class community. This time is also used to provide guidance as needed when they are struggling with academic or home issues. Implementing a grouping system at a school creates a sense of safety, community, equity, and access for all students. SBFC practitioners can be a part of the school system that helps in developing and implementing this model as well as a service provider working collaboratively with the students and staff within the infrastructure. The advisory period allows for more sustainable opportunities to provide prevention and intervention through the SBFC model while increasing student engagement because of the continuity of services and relationships.

Examples of how to implement a student grouping/cohort system may include:

- Student cohorts are developed based on student data with a balance of high and low performing students, inclusive of all students: English Language Learners, English Only, Gifted, and Students with Disabilities. The classes are equally balanced so that each class has students who represent all areas.
- Student groups are matched with a group, or team, of teachers that all work together with the same students. The classrooms for these teams are set up next to each other, so teachers are logistically close to each other to be able to communicate frequently. In addition, this physical arrangement allows students to not have to travel much between their classes, thus preventing absences and tardiness.
- The teacher teams work together to develop their curriculum uniformly and deliver the same content to all students.
- Implementation of a daily advisory that meets with students every morning to cover a multitude of topics, such as SEL curriculum, and focus on developing relationships and engaging with students.

- The advisory teacher stays with the same group of students for the duration of their stay at the school, allowing multiple years of a consistent, stable relationship with students and families. The advisory teacher also serves as a case manager of sorts, reviewing their students' grades, attendance, behavior, and works with the teacher team in communicating regarding students.
- The SBFC practitioner team can also adopt a grouping model and travel with their students in the same way. They remain with their students until they leave the school and transition to the next school. This allows them to develop strong bonds with their students and have enough time to work with students and families, before the year is over and they need to get to know an entire new group of students.

Third step: Focus on student interactions

The third step in the procedure is focused on student interactions. This involves taking a good look into what infrastructure is in place to mold the level of interactions students have among each other and with teachers. The SBFC practitioner will focus on models for interaction within the classroom and curriculum that are school-wide and focused on the prevention of school violence.

Cooperative learning models

The use of a cooperative learning model in classroom instruction is a key contributor to student engagement which contributes to violence prevention . Cooperative learning structures, such as "Kagan", is a scientifically researched instructional model that focuses on student interactions and communication in the classroom. The central role of the model stems from a belief that "it's all about engagement" (Murie, 2004). Cooperative learning is a teaching method that refers to small, heterogeneous groups of students working together to achieve a common goal. The students work together to learn and are responsible for their teammates' learning as well as their own. Basic elements of cooperative learning include positive interdependence, individual accountability, equal participation, and simultaneous interaction between students (Murie, 2004). The various structures utilized in the cooperative learning model increase the interactions between students and teachers in the classroom which has an overall positive effect on academic and social outcomes because students learn and practice communicating with each other in a positive proactive manner (Murie, 2004). The cooperative learning structures require students to constantly be interacting and engaging with each other and the academic content. It allows for the modeling, practicing, and reinforcement of positive social skills daily. This student interaction is structured and guided by the teacher but allows for flexibility and creativity. The cooperative learning model engages students academically because it uses student interaction as the main component for learning. In effect, students become not only academically engaged but also socially engaged with their peers and the class as a whole. In addition, the process of teaching students to work, discuss, challenge, and articulate their thoughts about something together stimulates learning and fosters positive social relationships. School leaders may consider incorporating the cooperative learning model to increase student engagement and focus on student interactions within their schools. This consistency, coupled with the relationships fostered between students and teachers, creates a sense of safety for students. School safety outside of the classroom is an important component that cannot be overlooked.

Guidelines for implementing cooperative learning structures:

- Collective decision making around cooperative learning structures to implement.
- Establish a shared belief system around the commitment to student engagement and fostering student interactions in the classroom.
- Develop a benchmark, or goal, for student interaction that can be understood by all, such as "50% of the student talk in the classroom should be that of students".
- Leadership to identify funding streams for implementing cooperative learning structures to include initial and ongoing professional development for all staff.
- Schedule professional development during the summer when students are not in session. Funding should be identified for compensation of staff for training.
- Cooperative learning structures to be implemented similarly in all classrooms.
- Prioritize the expectation for cooperative learning in the classroom and provide ongoing support, coaching and mentoring so that it becomes a norm at the school.
- Identify cooperative learning "champions" to serve as leaders and mentors for other staff that may be struggling with implementation. Celebrate success regularly.

Fostering student connections

If asked, many people can recall an important memory or relationship they had on campus while attending school. In fact, most people, if not able to recall a specific person or memory, can at least share the experience of how they *felt* at school. This demonstrates just how monumental student connections are to their learning experience. Fostering student connections is at times, misinterpreted as being a one-way connection from adult to student. However, fostering a true sense of student connection on campus comes from multiple directions. Student-to-student connections are some of the first forms of trust outside of family that students learn about and experience. Effectively fostering student connections includes modeling connection practices with all members of a school campus, providing spaces, time, and education for students to have space to connect in a healthy manner. This can seem overwhelming at first; nonetheless, below are some practices schools can begin to implement to impact student connections on campus in a practical manner as they continue to build more authentic school culture and connections:

- Establish community practices such as morning meetings or community circles in classrooms to increase sense of belonging and togetherness. This will also help students foster positive relationships and trust with peers and adults on campus.
- Practice reviewing community norms whenever a group of school community members are meeting. Community norms can be created and reviewed at staff meetings, parent meetings, board meetings, and classrooms.
- Facilitate homogenous and heterogenous focus groups as needed (tier-2 system of support) for students with specific goals/challenges. These groups can be counseling groups or academic groups.
- Promote empathy, understanding of differences, and perspective taking through curriculum, school-wide initiatives, and assemblies.
- Initiate leadership opportunities that all students have access to like little/big buddies and other mentorship opportunities.
- Normalize and model asking for help on campus from multiple adults/ leaders on campus, so students feel comfortable enough to use resources available to them.

Multicultural considerations

When carrying out school violence prevention procedures, a school must consider the demographics of its school community and use equitable practices to ensure safety and inclusivity of all. In order for school crisis leadership to be effective, it needs to be inclusive. It intentionally and consistently includes those in our decision making who may have differing views, identities, and experience. This provides the foundation of cooperation and transparency that will be needed during and after a crisis. Leading through inclusive leadership requires our awareness of who is and is not at the table, and what plans we do and do not consider. This includes the need for debriefing and reflecting on the unintentional infliction of stress and trauma for specific populations. A violence prevention procedure should include culturally responsive strategies and services. Culturally responsive strategies include asking clarifying questions when interviewing/assessing students and their families for crisis intervention or prevention. It means fostering trust with local community leaders that represent the diverse population that the school serves. Establishing trust with students and their families requires creating intentional spaces in schools that are welcoming and comfortable, as well as conversations that are calm, composed, and personable. Often when professionals speak with students and their families, we tend to hold more importance on being formal than on fostering a presence that fosters a positive relationship. It is highly unlikely that school leaders will know all student backgrounds and the implications when working with all cultures. However, using these strategies help create a space that allows students and their families to have the opportunity to teach us and take ownership of their academic journey. Inclusive strategies are equitable in the sense that they acknowledge a collaborative relationship in which all members of the school community are important and involved in serving the whole child in the best way possible.

Challenges and solutions

As with the implementation of any systems-based interventions, one of the greatest challenges is time. Perhaps, this is one of the reasons that these interventions can be difficult to implement and sustain. School systems, especially larger ones, have frequent turn-over of staff and leadership which can further exacerbate the difficulty of implementation. Systems-based interventions require time, committed staff, and are not a quick approach to change. A solution would be to train core leadership and staff to take the lead on implementing change and commit to a minimum of two to three years at one location for sustainability of implementation. Another challenge is the buy-in of district leadership and staff. This approach would be most successful with the support of larger district staff and resources to support the efforts at the school site. Further, this support should be accompanied by a commitment of funding for resources in order to allow the site to follow through with implementation and ensure sustainability.

Conclusion

In conclusion, this chapter aimed to provide strategies that SBFC practitioners could participate in with their schools and leadership teams to prevent school violence by engaging students holistically. Implemented effectively, preventing school violence is a multifaceted task. As defined in previous sections of this chapter, school violence includes emotional and environmental harm. Not only does preventing school violence require these foundational strategies highlighted in this chapter but it's also clear that the entire school community is involved and responsible in upholding a safe school. Students are key stakeholders and engaging students in taking ownership of their learning environment is an essential component to crisis intervention and prevention.

Resources

Websites

Kagan cooperative learning

Kagan Publishing and Professional Development. (n.d.) Retrieved May 16, 2022
Kagan Publishing and Professional Development Kagan Online: https://www.
kaganonline.com/

*Kagan cooperative learning is built on a single tenet that is student engagement. When students
are actively engaged, it positively impacts learning. In classrooms that utilize cooperative
learning structures such as Kagan, all students must be engaged and accountable.*

MTSS

Multi-Tiered System of Supports. (n.d.) Retrieved May 16, 2022 California
Department of Education: https://www.cde.ca.gov/ci/cr/ri/

*California's MTSS focuses on aligning initiatives and resources within an educational organi-
zation to address the needs of all students. It is an integrated, comprehensive framework for
local educational agencies (LEA) that aligns academic, behavioral, and social-emotional
learning in a fully integrated system of support for the benefit of all students. MTSS offers the
potential to create systematic change through intentional integration of services and supports
to quickly identify and meet the needs of all students.*

SEL and second step

Socioemotional Learning (SEL) Second Step Program. (n.d.) Retrieved May 16,
2022 Second Step: https://www.secondstep.org/

*Children need social-emotional skills to thrive both in the classroom and in life. Social-emotional
learning (SEL) curricula teach children techniques to: gain confidence, set goals, make better
decisions, collaborate with others in work and play, and navigate the world more effectively.*

Violence prevention

Center for the Study and Prevention of Violence. (n.d.) Retrieved May 16, 2022
Center for the Study and Prevention of Violence: https://www.secondstep.org/

*The CSPV have studied and implemented programs on violence prevention in schools and com-
munities across Colorado, the United States, and abroad. We know from this work that there
are tools and knowledge for preventing violence. We also have the ability to assess, intervene,
and support people who have been swept up in the current of violence. The CSPV bridges the
gap between research and practice.*

Books

Student engagement

Christenson, S., Reschly, A. L., & Wylie, C. (2012). *Handbook of research on student
engagement* (Vol. 840). New York: Springer.
Guides readers through the field's rich history, sorts out the component constructs, and identifies knowledge gaps to be filled by future research. It serves

as a valuable resource for researchers, scientist-practitioners, and graduate students in such varied fields as clinical child and school psychology, educational psychology, public health, teaching and teacher education, social work, and educational policy.

References

Appleton, J. J., Christenson, S. L., & Furlong, M. J. (2008). Student engagement with school: Critical conceptual and methodological issues of the construct. *Psychology in the Schools*, 45(5), 369–386.

Brock, S. E., Nickerson, A. B., Reeves, M. A., Jimerson, S. R., Lieberman, R. A., & Feinberg, T. A. (2009). *School crisis prevention and intervention: The PREPaRE model*. National Association of School Psychologists.

Casebeer, C. M. (2012). School bullying: Why quick fixes do not prevent school failure. *Preventing School Failure: Alternative Education for Children and Youth*, 56(3), 165–171.

Centers for Disease Control and Prevention (CDC). (2018). Suicide rising across the US. Retrieved from https://www.cdc.gov/vitalsigns/suicide/

Center for Homeland Defense & Security (CHDS). (2019). Incidents by year. Retrieved from https://www.chds.us/ssdb/incidentsby-year/

Christenson, S. L., Reschly, A. L., Appleton, J.J., Berman, S., Spanjers, D., & Varro, P. (2008). Best practices in fostering student engagement. In A. Thomas, & J. Grimes (Eds.), *Best practices in school psychology* (5th ed.). Bethesda, MD: National Association of School Psychologists.

Christenson, S., Reschly, A. L., & Wylie, C. (2012). *Handbook of research on student engagement* (Vol. 840). Springer.

Finn, J. D., & Owings, J. (2006). *The Adult Lives of At-Risk Students: The Roles of Attainment and Engagement in High School. Statistical Analysis Report.* NCES 2006-328. National Center for Education Statistics.

Gerrard, B. & Soriano, M. (2019). School-based family counseling: The revolutionary paradigm. In B. Gerrard, M. Carter & D. Ribera (Eds.), *School-based family counseling: An interdisciplinary practitioner's guide* (pp. 1–15). Routledge.

Hart, S. R., Stewart, K., & Jimerson, S. R. (2011). The Student Engagement in Schools Questionnaire (SESQ) and the Teacher Engagement Report Form-New (TERF-N): Examining the Preliminary Evidence. *Contemporary School Psychology*, 15, 67–79.

Hernandez, E. J. (2016). Reducing bullying and preventing dropout through student engagement: a prevention-focused lens for school-based family counselors. *International Journal for School- Based Family Counseling*, 7, 1–13.

Hernandez, E. (2020). Chapter 9. School prevention: How to increase student engagement. In B. Gerrard, M. Carter, & D. Ribera (Ed.), *School-based family counseling: A practitioner's guide* (pp. 258–282). Routledge.

Klein, J., Cornell, D., & Konold, T. (2012). Relationships between bullying, school climate, and student risk behaviors. *School Psychology Quarterly*, 27(3), 154.

Kutsyuruba, B., Klinger, D. A., & Hussain, A. (2015). Relationships among school climate, school safety, and student achievement and well-being: a review of the literature. *Review of Education*, 3, 103–135. https://doi.org/10.1002/rev3.3043

Libbey, H. P. (2004). Measuring student relationships to school: Attachment, bonding, connectedness, and engagement. *Journal of School Health, 74*(7), 274–283.

Murie, C. (2004). *Effects of communication on student learning.* Kagan Publishing.

Reschly, A. L., Appleton, J. J., & Christenson, S. L. (2007). Student engagement at school and with learning: Theory and interventions. *Communiqué, 35,* 18–20.

Reschly, A. L., & Christenson, S. L. (2006). Prediction of dropout among students with mild disabilities: A case for the inclusion of student engagement variables. *Remedial and Special Education, 27*(5), 276–292.

Sherer, Y. C., & Nickerson, A. B. (2010). Anti-bullying practices in American schools: Perspectives of school psychologists. *Psychology in the Schools, 47*(3), 217–229.

Shernoff, D. J., & Schmidt, J. A. (2008). Further evidence of an engagement–achievement paradox among US high school students. *Journal of Youth and Adolescence, 37*(5), 564–580.

17 Adverse and positive childhood experiences

The role of Buddhism and resilience

Nidup Dorji and Sibnath Deb

Overview

Children and youths are undeniable determiners of peace and stability and assets of any nation. They are future leaders and cornerstones to societal transformation. For a better tomorrow, it is imperative to recognize and nurture the talents of the children and youths, and also identify their challenges and counter them. The number of youth is steadily increasing in every part of the globe and a lot must be invested in youths to secure promising returns. Adverse childhood experiences (ACEs), though differ, range from 33% to 88% across countries, impacting all dimensions of life, including health and well-being across lifespans. The prevention of ACEs and promotion of positive childhood experiences (PCEs) and resilience could improve health and well-being and better citizens. The broad objective of this chapter is to provide a broad guideline for organizing trainings for school teachers on promotion of Buddhist philosophy, mindfulness, and life skill education among school students, to enhance their coping skills (resilience) and deal with adversities in life such as crises and disaster. Mindful practice is one of the core values of the psychological well-being of children and youth. Everyday school activities based on guided meditation sessions in the morning assemblies, classrooms, and other gatherings are found to be very beneficial to improve the attention span, skills for conflict resolution, empathy, and calmness among children. An example on the blend of scientific and Buddhist approaches to adversities applied in the schools of Bhutan is provided. Understanding interdependence over independence, impermanence, and exercises of value and life skill-based education, SBFC practitioners using mindfulness practices could potentially facilitate children to grow and become productive and responsible individuals who are resilient in situations of crisis and disaster.

Background

Children and youth are the centre of growth and development in any society. The role of children and youth in national development is vital for the overall development of the nation. Investments in children and youths are akin to preparing the next set of world leaders. Youth socialization with surrounding people

DOI: 10.4324/9781003201977-21

affects human development. Parental and peer pressure can be beneficial but can also become toxic for the youths. 'Listening to young people and hearing their voice' is a way of engaging with the future. It also means educating youth in policy processes and recognizing them as a political force.

Evidence-based support

Adverse childhood experiences (ACEs)

ACEs are potentially stressful and traumatic events that occur within the first 18 years of life. Globally, the prevalence of ACEs stands at 57%, ranging from 33% to 88% across countries (Massetti, Hughes, Bellis, & Mercy, 2020). ACEs include many types of abuse (physical, emotional, sexual) and neglect (physical and psychological), exposure to violence in family and community, peer conflict, household dysfunction, parent issues, growing up with mentally ill or incarcerated household members. ACEs have a tremendous negative impact upon future violence affecting the lifelong health and opportunities of both victims and perpetrators. The adage *'It takes a village to raise a child'* continues to be relevant to this day and age.

ACEs, physical and mental health, and risk behaviours

Landmark studies on ACEs have clearly demonstrated strong relationships between ACEs and physical illnesses, such as respiratory, heart and liver diseases, cancer, stroke, diabetes, neurological symptoms and chronic pain, and autoimmune diseases (Anda, Felitti, & Corwin, 2014; Crandall et al., 2019; Dunne & Askari, 2012). Increasing ACEs are also linked to psychosocial and behavioural problems, including substance abuse, self-destructive behaviours, mental health symptoms (dissociation, sleep problems, sexual promiscuity, panic, uncontrolled anger), lower levels of gratitude, heightened insecure attachment in relationships, poor family cohesion, and lower perceived psychological well-being (Anda et al., 2014; Crandall et al., 2019; Ramiro, Madrid, & Brown, 2010). Health-risk behaviours are demonstrated mostly in the form of smoking, alcohol use, risky sexual behaviour (Ramiro et al., 2010) and sexually transmitted diseases (Anda et al., 2014), fuelling the global burden of diseases (Hughes et al., 2017).

ACEs and its co-occurrence, economic loss, and healthcare use

ACEs are associated with low educational attainment and poor interpersonal skills, which, in turn, limit the socio-economic advancement for the individuals and their families (Dunne & Askari, 2012). Individuals with higher ACEs are more likely to report not completing high school, being unemployed and living in households below the poverty line (Metzler, Merrick, Klevens, Ports, & Ford, 2017). They are also associated with increased healthcare utilization, thus financially burdening the healthcare system of countries that deliver free healthcare services (Kalmakis & Chandler, 2015; Metzler et al., 2017). A study on ACEs in Bhutan also showed that the experience of physical and emotional abuse, violent treatment of household members, bullying, and alcohol/drug use co-occurred with other forms of ACEs (Dorji, Dunne, & Deb, 2020).

ACEs prevention is better than curing ACEs

The emphasis on prevention is never enough. As ACEs impact human development across the lifespan, they are major determinants of future health. The key to prevention of ACEs and all its sequels is the disruption in the intergenerational transmission of ACEs (Anda et al., 2014). ACEs are now recognized as a serious international health and social problem. The pervasive influence of ACEs across lifespan requires a shift in the focus to include its prevention strategies, resilience building, and informed service provisions (Anda et al., 2014; Hughes et al., 2017). The Sustainable Development Goals (SDGs) placed focus on childhood development, to secure lifelong health. Nurturing the care within the family through interactions, being attentive to children's efforts to learn and connect with their world, is crucial (Daelmans et al., 2017). Fostering protective factors, such as self-value, self-regulation, hope and goal setting, supportive belief structure in the family, friends, communities, supportive academic functioning, coupled with knowledge and application of thinking, social, and emotional skills could assist in reducing ACEs prevalence (Thompson & Klika, 2015). The presence of supportive parents and teachers in childhood is believed to nurture healthy growth and development of the individual. A successful ACE prevention programme requires an integrated and ecological system of care at all levels. In schools, the role of teachers and counsellors can be vital in helping a child feel safe and secure.

Positive childhood experiences

Positive childhood experiences (PCEs) are experiences of building a sense of belongingness and connection in childhood. Although less is known about how PCEs provide protection and counter negative impacts of ACEs, research has demonstrated that exposure to PCEs can improve future social experiences, build healthy relationships, and predict better productivity and responsibility in adulthood (Narayan, Rivera, Bernstein, Harris, & Lieberman, 2018). This is because exposure to PCEs and supportive relationships helps children build resilience to withstand adverse experiences and mitigate its negative consequences (Sege et al., 2017). Furthermore, countering ACEs helps buffer their negative effects on health, protect against stress, depression, and sleep difficulties (Crandall et al., 2019). Some studies have indicated that PCE predicts positive outcomes, including current and future health conditions, positive functioning during adulthood, success in school, and less substance use (Kosterman et al., 2011). Academic institutions and public health programmes seek to promote PCEs, which may improve lifelong health and overall well-being. The importance of PCE in predicting positive functioning in early adulthood merits the attention of parents, teachers, and friends, who potentially have greater influence in actively providing prosocial opportunities to the children (Kosterman et al., 2011), which, in turn, would help buffer the negative effects of ACEs.

Adversities and resilience

Resilience is a positive adaptation or the ability to maintain or regain mental health in the face of adversity (Wald, Taylor, Asmundson, Jang, & Stapleton, 2006). Positive psychology explains that resilience can be perceived as a human capacity to face, overcome, or benefit from the challenges of life. While resilience is dependent upon the degree and the impact of adversities, lifespan research reveals that many people are able to move forward in life, recuperate, and achieve good functional status amidst adverse experiences. Evidence suggests that exposure to moderate levels of adversity can predict better mental health and well-being since exposure to stress provides an opportunity to develop toughness and allow the individual to appraise situations more positively, by tapping in their inner resources and perceive them as manageable (Seery, Holman, & Silver, 2010). However, resilience does not occur in isolation, as it is supported by a series of complex protective factors, including caring relationships. Protective factors are positive qualities found within environmental, social, familial, and friendship contexts.

Potential benefits of Buddhist philosophy in enhancing resilience among children and youth in crisis

Buddhism, the world's fourth-largest religious faith, with over 520 million followers, originated in India about 2,600 years ago. Buddhism is a way of life not merely a religion. Therefore, anyone can adhere to the principles of Buddhism to lead daily life with happiness and contentment.

Buddhist principles seek to ingrain certain ethical ideologies in the youth. These include **Sila** – which encompasses virtues, good conduct, and morality; **Samadhi** – that includes concentration, meditation, and mental development, which strengthens and controls the human mind, besides helping individuals to maintain good conduct; and finally, **Prajna** – that embraces discernment, insight, wisdom, and enlightenment, which are imperative to maintaining a pure and a calm mind. The Buddhist traditions teach not to harm others (like ahimsa), leading a contented and decent life, abstaining from being unkind to others, and refraining from abusive practices. Exercising these principles will not only assist in cultivating morality in youth but will also infuse a sense of conviction to lead a purposeful life with high resilience.

Buddhist ethics are concerned with views and practices that help individuals act in ways that help than harm. Faith/confidence, virtue, knowledge, generosity, and wisdom are the five qualities that Buddha considered as the hallmark of Buddhist philosophy.

Rather than speaking of actions being right or wrong, Buddhism speaks of being skilful (kusala) or unskilful (akusala). Buddhist philosophies are the ideal foundation for world peace, the equitable use of natural resources, and harmonize living with nature. This faith stresses on inner satisfaction and a peaceful state of mind, which are central towards developing divine values of kindness, generosity, honesty, optimism, tolerance, contentment, happiness, and psychological capital.

Advocating to inculcate the invaluable virtues of Buddhist mindfulness practices, optimism, and concentration will enhance the resilience capacity of children and youth to deal with any crisis situation.

Studies have indicated that higher levels of religious faith and spirituality are associated with more optimistic life orientation, greater perceived social support, higher resilience, lower levels of anxiety, helping individuals interpret life events, giving them the opportunity to discover meaning and purpose in life, and maybe also helping in the psychological integration of traumatic experiences (Koenig, 2006).

Buddhism is all about self-reflection and transformation. However, the challenge here is how the contemporary generation is willing to look within, when the outside world is filled with attractions and distractions. Buddhism discusses the significance of cause-condition-effect (karma), interdependence, and impermanence. There is nothing religious about these laws. Science supports the idea that health and well-being are not randomly distributed in the population. Individuals are the makers of their own problems and suffering, as is their happiness and well-being. Imagine how the world would be today if human beings were taught to understand that they belong to the land not the vice versa. Most humans today believe that nature belongs to them. This has led to all the negative consequences as a result of nature's destruction. Activists like Greta Thunberg, who fight for the earth, are not enough. As is encouraged in Buddhism, the practice of a universal pious outlook can be the solution to problems and can strengthen harmonious relationships with nature. This would, in turn, promote the notion of interdependence of this cosmos and challenge the belief of independence from the natural world. While the cup and its beauty what most think important are not neglected in Buddhism, the tea is more important than the cup. We drink tea and it nurtures us. Some of the famous quotes of Gautam Buddha are:

> *Never regret being a good person to wrong people. Your behaviour says everything about you, and their behaviour says enough about them.*
> *Change is never painful. Only resistance to change is painful.*
> *If anything is worth doing, do it with all your heart.*
> *All that we are is the result of what we have thought.*

Mindfulness and life skill education

In Buddhism, mindful practices, such as the simple technique of noticing the breath, are widely accepted, which mainstream mental health experts now recommend as an important method of managing stress. Mindfulness practice enriches the mind with skilful methods and teaches it to deal with whatever situation life throws at us. The purpose of mindfulness is to help individuals perceive reality more clearly and enjoy a more fulfilling life (Weiss, 2004). Most of the problems that the world today faces are rooted in lack of mindfulness. The 'mindfulness education', which is recognized as an integral part of the Bhutanese education system, involves the training of one's mind to look within and become aware of one's actions of body, speech, and mind (Thinley, 2012). Mindfulness education encapsulates the essence of making one's mind productive. This is critical for today's children and youth, especially in developing countries like Bhutan, which constantly face the increasing impacts of globalization, urbanization, and economic modernization. Furthermore, the adoption of life skills in the mainstream Bhutanese education system, and its implementation, has significantly played greater roles in the prevention of violence among children, the reduction of substance use, and the promotion of learning. Life skills include strengthening thinking ability (critical, creative, decision making, and problem solving), social skills (interpersonal relationships, empathy, effective communication, self-awareness), and emotional growth (coping with emotions and stress), which facilitates children to grow into responsible adults (Birrcll et al., 1997; Gyeltshen & Longpradit, 2020). Continuing life skill education facilitates children facing everyday challenges (Royal Government of Bhutan, 2009).

In disseminating the essence of Buddhist philosophy, online or in-person school-based family counselling (SBFC) could play a significant role in crisis and disaster management and sensitize parents to deal with the emotions of children sensitively, in addition to providing life skill education to children and youth. Furthermore, this promotes teaching one's children about the right to speech – such as translating one's feelings into words, either through writing to oneself, or attending to the issues of children with love and care, rather than letting the child engage in activities that negate the importance of family.

Procedure

Teachers can be empowered with knowledge and skills in imparting value-based education to children for facing the adversities in life (such as crisis and disaster) with a positive outlook. Three-day training programmes can be organized by the SBFC practitioner for the school teachers, to train them on core values of Buddhist philosophy, mindfulness, and life skills education. The steps which can be followed for organizing the three-day training programme include (i) secondary research, (ii) needs assessment, (iii) recruitment, (iv) planning and implementation, and (v) evaluation.

Step 1: Secondary research

Secondary research is very useful to provide information about effectiveness of such training and/or orientation programmes. In general, value-based training programmes are conducted for the school teachers to impart values among children. The SBFC practitioner should attempt to gather information about a similar value-based training programme that might have been conducted, methodology followed for conducting the training, its effectiveness, and challenges faced in organizing it. In addition, the SBFC practitioner should identify experienced resource persons through personal acquaintances and the selected group of teachers should be invited from different schools with the help of local authorities.

The SBFC practitioner should read the available literature on the same subject, so that he/she can come out with a broad outline of the curriculum for the training programme.

Step 2: Needs assessment

Understanding the school teachers' perception of issues and challenges faced by the students is crucial for the SBFC practitioner. For the same, two to three focus group discussions (FGDs) can be conducted by inviting school teachers from 8 to 10 nearby schools. In every FGD, 8–10 teachers may be invited, with a combination of both male and female teachers. The duration of the FGD should not be more than 40–45 minutes. To gather views and opinions of school teachers about the concerns of school students, semi-structured questionnaires can be used to collect both qualitative and quantitative data. Need assessment of the teachers in terms of knowledge and understanding about Buddhist philosophy helps to encourage active participation of the teachers in the training programme.

Step 3: Recruitment

The recruitment of school teachers should be based on voluntary participation, and they should have experience in advising students and have a passion for guiding students with empathy. The head of nearby school authorities may be asked to nominate four to five teachers for the training programme, based on their experience and interest. Emotional stability, interpersonal relationships, and communication skills of a school teacher are to be considered by the school authorities while recommending a teacher for the training programme.

Step 4: Planning and implementation

Planning a three-day programme schedule for training of school teachers, for imparting value-based education to the students, is a very important activity for the SBFC practitioner. The draft programme schedule should be shared with the school administrators and the resource persons for their valuable feedback and accordingly, it should be finalized in consultation with two to three senior and experienced school teachers. The training programme schedule may be a little flexible. While planning for training like this, the SBFC practitioner should decide upon the total number of potential participants and a suitable location should be selected with audio-visual facilities. Prior consent should be obtained from all the participants for attending the programme. The resource persons to be invited should be selected based on their experience and expertise. It has to be decided whether it would be a one-time training or a series of programmes, for reinforcement of information and skills among teachers. In addition to providing training materials, a good working lunch and snacks must be arranged, along with an experience certificate, which will be motivating for the teachers to actively engage in the training programme.

A leaflet for the training programme should be developed professionally, providing the necessary background information, objectives, and expected outcomes of the training, along with potential benefits for the participants. It should be shared with the heads of different schools. Three to four volunteers may be engaged to take care of logistics and for the smooth functioning of the training programme.

Step 5: Evaluation

Any training programme is subjected to review or evaluation, either by the organizers or by external experts. Evaluation of the training programme by the participants helps the organizers to understand its effectiveness and shortcomings, if any, and facilitates taking corrective measures while organizing similar programmes in the future. In addition, the evaluation report of the training will provide insights for the professionals involved in the training programme. If the training is funded by any agency, the agency will also require a copy of the evaluation report. There are different ways to evaluate the effectiveness of any training programme. For example, it could be evaluated by using the same structured questionnaire. It can be done after the training, after collecting views and opinions of some of the participants or all the participants, following an informal interview method, or by using a semi-structured questionnaire or structured questionnaire. However, the training evaluation questionnaire should not be very lengthy as many of the participants may be tired at the end of the training programme.

Example of a teacher training programme on Buddhist philosophy

An example of a teacher training programme is provided below. Broadly, there are six steps involved in the process. They include (i) warm-up, (ii) introduction of background of the training programme and its objectives, (iii) rules of the training, (iv) lecture on Buddhist philosophy, (v) group exercise, (vi) summarizing the learning experience, and (vii) evaluation of the training.

Step 1: Warm-up: This session should start with a self-introduction, followed by sharing of personal experience in dealing with students' issues and challenges in general. Three to four teachers may be asked to come forward to share their experience in addressing students' issues, where they could see some positive transformation, based on their guidance and inputs. This exercise would help the SBFC practitioner to set the tone of the training programme and justify the teachers' involvement in it.

> **Facilitator:** Good morning! I welcome everyone to this training program. The broad objective of this training program is to exchange our knowledge and understanding about Buddhist philosophy and provide an in-depth understanding about it. Dear friends, we are going to start today's session with self-introductions. We would urge all of you to write about a special incident where you addressed issues and challenges of your students in the school. Five minutes are allocated for this small exercise.

(School teachers complete the exercise.)

> **Facilitator:** Thanks everyone for this. I hope you enjoyed the exercise and could recollect one incident. Now I would like to ask five teachers to share their experiences which they have noted down and have a little discussion on the same.

Step 2: Introduction of the Background of the Training Programme and Its Objectives: The objective of this session is to talk about the context for organizing the training programme for the school teachers, citing evidence, and clearly stating the objectives of the training and its long-term objectives.

> **Facilitator:** Now I am going to give all of you a brief introduction about the background for organizing this training program and its objectives which would help all of you to understand the intentions of the training program.

Step 3: Rules of the Training: Discussing the basic rules of the training at the beginning is very important for its smooth implementation.

> **Facilitator:** Dear colleagues, we need to follow some rules during the training program and they include asking questions one by one. During the lecture, there should not be any gossiping. It is important to respect the views of others and not make any comment which might hurt another participant. It is important to not mention outside the group the name of any participant or any personal sharing made during the training.

Finally, it is important to attend all the sessions, if there is no serious health issue. I hope the rules are clear. However, if any of you have any questions, please feel free to speak to me.

Step 4: Lecture on Buddhist Philosophy: Two special lectures will be delivered by two experts on Buddhist philosophy, clearly emphasizing upon the strengths of Buddhist philosophy in imparting values among school children and in dealing with crisis situations logically. The lectures will be followed by question and answer sessions.

> **Facilitator**: Dear colleagues, I am sure all of you enjoyed the lectures and clarified your doubts. I would urge some of you to share your views about the session, freely and frankly.
> Participant 1: It was an interesting and informative session.
> Participant 2: My first attendance at such an interesting session.
> *Participant 3*: Now I understand the value of Buddhist Philosophy.

Step 5: Group Exercise: A group exercise is very helpful to have a better understanding of the issue and for skill development. Now, we propose to have two group exercises dividing all the participants in two groups on the same issue. One case study related to adversities experienced by the children at times of crisis will be shared with the participants, for deliberation and discussion. Each group will select a participant as their group leader who will, in turn, share the outcome of the group exercise. Forty minutes of time can be given for discussion, to come out with possible solutions and see how Buddhist philosophy can help in this situation.

> ***Case Study***: Following the death of a much respected teacher the students are grieving.
> **Facilitator:** Discuss how Buddhist philosophy would be applied to deal with the hypothetical case.

Leader of Group 1: He/she might say, 'Our group would address this challenge with the students by reminding them of The Four Noble Truths, especially (*All aggregated things are impermanent and therefore all things have no inherent existence; All aggregated things attached to self are painful and therefore, Nirvana is beyond concepts*).'
Leader of Group 2: He/she might say, 'Our group would instead emphasize teaching the students the Eightfold Path with a particular emphasis on (*Right Understanding and Right Mindfulness*)'.

After the group exercise, one group leader, nominated by the group members, will present the outcome of the group exercise.

> **Facilitator**: How did you find the exercise? It seemed to me that all of you enjoyed the group exercise, exchanged your views and arrived at a

conclusion based on a unanimous opinion. Can two or three of you share your experiences of the exercise?

Participant 1: It was a good experience. Sometimes we had disagreements, but finally we agreed to some points after hearing the view of others.

Participant 2: It was a great learning experience for all of us.

Step 6: Summarize the Learning Experience: This session is very important to reflect upon what the participants learn after attending the three-day training programme. The following questions may be asked of the participants for reflection:

What did the participants learn or relearn?

How can they use the learning experience in helping school students to cope with stressful crisis situations?

What parts of the training program were most helpful?

What is the take home message for the participants?

Step 7: Evaluation of the Training: Evaluation of the training by the teachers helps to have a clear idea about its effectiveness and shortcomings. The views of the participants are helpful in effectively developing future training programmes. There are various methods to evaluate the training programme. It could be an end term evaluation or pre- and post-assessment methods. One can collect both qualitative and quantitative opinions from the participants, with respect to some parameter, for assessing the effectiveness of the training. Nevertheless, the SBFC practitioner can adopt any method to evaluate the effectiveness of the training and should share the outcome of the evaluation with the participants, the resource persons and with the funding agency, if funded by any organization.

Facilitator: Thanks for providing your valuable feedback about the training, which would help us to understand the effectiveness of the training and take corrective measures for organizing future similar training programs.

Multicultural counselling

Any training programme should take into consideration the socio-cultural background of the participants. The SBFC practitioner should ask the resource persons to deliver the lecture in the local language, if the participants are not comfortable with English. Logistic arrangements should be made based on multicultural consideration. Further, the participating teachers of the training should be sensitized to impart value-based education, based on Buddhist philosophy, after considering the cultural and social diversities of the students into account, in terms of race, ethnicity, religion, sex, and socio-economic class of the students.

Challenges and solutions

Organizing a training programme for the school teachers is a positive step, which is highly appreciated by some school authorities while some look at such training programmes as a waste of time. The latter group are often not willing to permit teachers to attend any training programmes, whether it is for personal knowledge of the teachers or for students' benefits. Sometimes, lack of teaching staff discourages school authorities from nominating and sending teachers for training. In those situations, the school authorities may be asked to nominate one teacher, instead of more, so that it does not affect their teaching-learning process. The preconceived notion of some teachers about any issue is another challenge. If any such notion is observed in any participant in the warm-up session, it can be addressed in the rules of the training.

Conclusion

Children and youth are assets to any society and greater investments in them would potentially reap an astounding return. Today, they are confronted with multiple challenges and issues, including ACEs. ACEs are avertable and counterable. Their negative influences can be mitigated. Value-based education based on Buddhist philosophy presented by the SBFC facilitator provides exposure to teachers about enhancing PCEs and minimizing negative experiences, so that, in turn, they can help the children who have ACEs. Mindfulness practices, life skill-based education, and SBFC strategies aid in enabling the realization of the causal-effect relationship (that an individual is the maker of their own problems and suffering, happiness, and well-being), promoting interdependence, and coping with impermanence. It could potentially improve the resilience of the children in facing a crisis or disaster by fostering healthier social relationships, enhancing learning, and promoting a sense of responsibility.

Resources

Chodron, T. (2001). *Buddhism for beginners*. Shambhala Publications.
This book provides a thorough tour of the Essentials of Buddhism, while remaining clear and accessible without veering into oversimplification.
Gunaratana, B., & Gunaratana, H. (2011). *Mindfulness in plain English: 20th anniversary edition*. Simon & Schuster.
The book offers a solid & convincing clarity of the purpose and rationale for building a mindfulness practice. It's a title you'll want to keep on your shelf for revisiting and refreshing your practice as it develops. Since Mindfulness in Plain English was first published in 1994, it has become one of the bestselling — and most influential — books in the field of mindfulness. It's easy to see why.
Hanh, T. N. (2015). *The heart of the Buddha's teaching: Transforming suffering into peace, joy, and liberation*. Harmony.
This book presents a number of core concepts of Buddhism. Each core concept is presented in a simple form for the interest of the readers.

Power, J. (1995). *Wisdom of Buddha: The Samdhinirmocana sutra.* Dharma Publishing.
A translation of the text which was a primary influence in the development of the Mahayana schools of Buddhism. An important text to practicing Buddhists, as well as students of philosophy and religion, but one which is best approached with some familiarity with Buddhist thought and history.

Rahula, W. (2007). *What the Buddha taught.* Open Road + Grove/Atlantic.
This book describes some of the essential parts of the Buddhist school of thought. Knowing them will make it easier to understand others.

Robinson, R. H., Johnson, W. L., Wawrytko, S. A., & Ṭhānissaro. (1996). *The Buddhist religion: A historical introduction.* Wadsworth.
This book provides a survey of Buddhism from a historical perspective.

The Dalai Lama & Cutler, H. C. (1999). *The art of happiness: A handbook for living.* Wheeler Publishing.
The Art of Happiness is a very readable collection of interviews, stories, and meditations which present Buddhist Philosophy with a twist of Modern Psychology.

References

Anda, R., Felitti, V. J., & Corwin, D. (2014). Adverse childhood experiences and long-term health. *ACEs: Informing best practice, AVA/NHCVA, section, 1.*

Birrell, R., Orley, J., Evans, V., Lee, J., Sprunger, B., & Pellaux, D. (1997). *Life skills education for children and adolescents in schools.* World Health Organization.

Crandall, A., Miller, J. R., Cheung, A., Novilla, L. K., Glade, R., Novilla, M. L. B., … Hanson, C. L. (2019). ACEs and counter-ACEs: How positive and negative childhood experiences influence adult health. *Child Abuse & Neglect, 96,* 104089. doi:10.1016/j.chiabu.2019.104089

Daelmans, B., Darmstadt, G. L., Lombardi, J., Black, M. M., Britto, P. R., Lye, S., … Richter, L. M. (2017). Early childhood development: The foundation of sustainable development. *The Lancet, 389*(10064), 9–11.

Dorji, N., Dunne, M., & Deb, S. (2020). Adverse childhood experiences: Association with physical and mental health conditions among older adults in Bhutan. *Public Health, 182,* 173–178. doi: https://doi.org/10.1016/j.puhe.2020.02.013

Dunne, M. P., & Askari, S. (2012). Adverse childhood experiences and chronic diseases among adults. *Journal of Medicine and Pharmacy, 2*(1), 22–27.

Gyeltshen, D., & Longpradit, P. (2020). *An evaluation of the life skill education program implementation for its enhancement in the schools in PemaGatshel district, eastern Bhutan.* Paper presented at the AU Virtual International Conference Entrepreneurship and Sustainability in the Digital Era.

Hughes, K., Bellis, M. A., Hardcastle, K. A., Sethi, D., Butchart, A., Mikton, C., … Dunne, M. P. (2017). The effect of multiple adverse childhood experiences on health: A systematic review and meta-analysis. *The Lancet Public Health, 2*(8), e356–e366.

Kalmakis, K. A., & Chandler, G. E. (2015). Health consequences of adverse childhood experiences: A systematic review. *Journal of the American Association of Nurse Practitioners, 27*(8), 457–465.

Koenig, H. G. (2006). *In the wake of disaster: Religious responses to terrorism and catastrophe*: Templeton Foundation Press.

Kosterman, R., Mason, W. A., Haggerty, K. P., Hawkins, J. D., Spoth, R., & Redmond, C. (2011). Positive childhood experiences and positive adult functioning: Prosocial continuity and the role of adolescent substance use. *Journal of Adolescent Health*, *49*(2), 180–186.

Massetti, G. M., Hughes, K., Bellis, M. A., & Mercy, J. (2020). Global perspective on ACEs. In G. J. G. Asmundson & T. O. Afifi (Eds.), *Adverse childhood experiences* (pp. 209–231). Academic Press.

Metzler, M., Merrick, M. T., Klevens, J., Ports, K. A., & Ford, D. C. (2017). Adverse childhood experiences and life opportunities: Shifting the narrative. *Children and Youth Services Review*, *72*, 141–149.

Narayan, A. J., Rivera, L. M., Bernstein, R. E., Harris, W. W., & Lieberman, A. F. (2018). Positive childhood experiences predict less psychopathology and stress in pregnant women with childhood adversity: A pilot study of the benevolent childhood experiences (BCEs) scale. *Child Abuse & Neglect*, *78*, 19–30. doi:10.1016/j.chiabu.2017.09.022

Ramiro, L. S., Madrid, B. J., & Brown, D. W. (2010). Adverse childhood experiences (ACE) and health-risk behaviors among adults in a developing country setting. *Child Abuse & Neglect*, *34*(11), 842–855. doi:https://doi.org/10.1016/j.chiabu.2010.02.012

Royal Government of Bhutan. (2009). *Guide Book for Teachers*: Comprehensive School Health Programme, Ministry of Health and Ministry of Education.

Seery, M. D., Holman, E. A., & Silver, R. C. (2010). Whatever does not kill us: Cumulative lifetime adversity, vulnerability, and resilience. *Journal of Personality and Social Psychology*, *99*(6), 1025.

Sege, R., Bethell, C., Linkenbach, J., Jones, J., Klika, B., & Pecora, P. (2017). Balancing adverse childhood experiences with HOPE: New insights into the role of positive experience on child and family development. Boston: The Medical Foundation.

Thinley, P. (2012). Mindfulness education in the Royal University of Bhutan: Context, present status and future possibilities. *Bhutan Journal of Research and Development*, *1*(1), 97–108.

Thompson, M. D. M., & Klika, B. (2015). Increasing resilience: Primary healthcare providers' opportunities to promote protective factors before and after childhood trauma. *Adverse Childhood Experiences: Informing Best Practices*, *6*, 12.

Wald, J., Taylor, S., Asmundson, G. J., Jang, K. L., & Stapleton, J. (2006). Literature review of concepts: Psychological resilience.

Weiss, A. (2004). *Beginning mindfulness: Learning the way of awareness*: New World Library.

18 Internet intimidation

Responding to cyberbullying of school children via the digital citizenship curriculum

Bishakha Majumdar

Overview

The ubiquitous presence of the internet in education, vocation, entertainment, and virtually all other dimensions of life makes it inevitable for the children of the digital generations to have an early and often unmonitored exposure to the world wide web. This exposure leaves the child vulnerable to the threats of cyberbullying. The proliferation of online education with the COVID-19 pandemic has further escalated such a threat. Families have a critical role to play in protecting their children from the threat of internet intimidation as well as in helping them develop resilience against potential attacks. This chapter lays out a plan for designing workshops or family education and counselling following the digital citizenship curriculum, such that the potential damaging influences of online exposure may be mitigated.

Background

The last decade has been remarkable for the proliferation of digital technology in almost all spheres of life – education, vocation, entertainment, healthcare, and other essential life services. From being a useful alternative, digitalization has often become the mainstay and the default mode for most of these experiences. Children growing up in this era are therefore called the digital natives – having early exposure to digital technology, regular access to technology at home, and using digital devices for the previous five years or more (International Telecommunication Union, 2017; Kesharwani, 2020).

Early digital access has multiple merits such as developing digital skills, and access to remote resources for education, vocational training, and entertainment. Children with a digital exposure and regular access are better prepared for the connected world of the future – as they are able to better negotiate the connected realities and better skilled at manipulating and innovating with digital technology. However, digital access also means an early and often unrestricted exposure to the adult world, leaving the child exposed to the dangers of cyber frauds and cyberbullying. Cyberbullying refers to concerted online attacks against one person or child, with an aim to discomfort, harass, or harm (Pham & Anderson, 2015). It is usually perpetuated by

DOI: 10.4324/9781003201977-22

a known peer group of the child or by strangers who ridicule or threaten the child for being different or for holding a contrarian opinion. Cyberbullying was identified as the foremost reason for harassment faced by the youth online (Anderson & Jiang, 2018). The risk further aggravated during the pandemic, with online classes. Eighty per cent of an Indian sample aged between 17 and 19 reported being cyberbullied during the pandemic (Jain, Gupta, Satam, & Panda, 2020). Closely related is the problem of cybersex and sexting that leave children vulnerable to online sexual predators (Adorjan & Ricciardelli, 2018). Children are easily manipulated into sharing personal information and photos, that are morphed to create pornographic content (Westerlund, 2019), for blackmailing the children or for executing financial frauds. Cyberbullying, online blackmailing, and cyberattacks have compelled children to self-harm and suicide (Chitre, 2019). Online games such as the Blue Whale have been suspected to use cyberbullying and blackmailing to drive children to suicides. Youth activism, political or otherwise, has been associated with cyberbullying, misogyny, and trolling (Marwick & Lewis, 2017).

A major influence in the online behaviour of children is the condition at home and involvement of parents. Lack of parental supervision, broken home, and low parental education has been associated with Problematic Internet Usage (PIU) among children (Chen et al., 2015). Again, Ying Ying et al. (2021) reported that monitoring of internet usage and role-modelling healthy internet behaviour by parents help children fight PIU and show responsible online behaviour (Hefner, Knop, Schmitt, & Vorderer, 2019). Li, Dang, Zhang, Zhang, and Guo (2014) too demonstrated the role of parental support in combating unhealthy addiction to the internet. It is therefore critical that parents are involved in protecting children from unhealthy internet usage and cyberbullying. Abreu and Kenny (2018) also recommended collaborative efforts among teachers, parents, lawmakers, and executives to decrease cyber victimization.

School-based family counselling

School-based family counselling (SBFC) refers to mental health interventions to help students overcome personal problems and excel in school performance (Gerrard & Soriano, 2013). The SBFC approach has its origins in the psychotherapeutic approach of Alfred Adler (Gerrard, 2008) and utilizes the linkages between the student, the school, and the family. The SBFC meta-model broadly classifies mental health interventions for school students along two parameters: focus on prevention or focus on remedial interventions, and (b) focus on school or on the family as the primary context for the intervention. Based on the two parameters, SBFC interventions may be classified as (1) school prevention, (2) school intervention, (3) family prevention, and (4) family intervention. While preventive measures focus on management, interventions as well as training and guidance, remedial interventions utilize counselling, crisis management, and support groups (Carter & Evans,

2008). SBFC approaches are powerful mental health interventions that bring together the school and family to solve problems faced by children. SBFC approaches guide families in finding mental health assistance in situations where professional help is either not accessible or not readily available, or situations that would benefit from family-based behavioural interventions.

A child's access to the internet beyond academic purposes usually happens at home, making family interventions particularly effective in teaching children safe online behaviour and protecting them from virtual threats. However, before they may guide the children, primary caregivers need extensive training on parental supervision and healthy online behaviour for children, as well as briefing about various technical resources for defending children online. SBFC interventions targeted at parents are increasingly emerging as a potent tool in the fight against online bullying of children. This chapter provides a detailed procedure for utilizing the SBFC framework to build awareness among primary stakeholders about the dangers of cyberbullying, the warning signs of online abuse of school children, and the process of providing the survivor of cyberbullying assistance without intimidating or alienating them.

Digital citizenship curriculum

Digital citizenship refers to the protocols of ideal behaviour on the internet that keeps the user and his or her ecosystem secure, healthy, and in compliance with national and international laws. The pervasive digitization of different aspects of life in the recent decades necessitates that the children growing up as digital natives are socialized early on in the digital do's and don'ts in the same way they learn about their rights and duties as a citizen. Dimensions of digital citizenship include digital literacy, digital access, digital health and wellness, and digital communication (Ribble, 2015).

Procedure

Family counselling by experts is an important way for imparting digital behaviour change communication. However, the efficacy of SBFC to school parents, caregivers, and children in digital citizenship behaviour depends on the extent to which the intervention is customized to the requirements of the target audience. To this end, the SBFC practitioner needs to take the following steps:

Step 1: Need assessment and categorization

Digital access and education have only recently emerged as one of the basic necessities of life, and that too in limited sections of the society across nations. SBFC practitioners may often come across parents and caregivers with vastly different states of readiness and knowledge when it comes to digital citizenship education. This will make holding a meaningful conversation in groups difficult, because what may be known for a group may not be familiar with the other. The first step to such an intervention needs to therefore relate to (1) need assessment of families in terms of how much their children are at risk of internet intimidation and (2) categorization in terms of their existing knowledge about the internet and their awareness of the problems of cyberbullying and possible solutions.

a. **Risk profile of children**: The SBFC practitioner should begin need assessment by assessing the extent to which children may be at risk due to their online behaviour. This may be assessed through anonymized surveys, or one-on-one interviews to know about the usage pattern of children. Important questions relate to (a) the number of hours children spend online, whether supervised or unsupervised, nature of device (personal/shared), (b) the types of activities conducted online – education, social networking, gaming, professional pursuits, etc., (c) websites visited, (d) nature of information shared – personal, financial, etc., (e) people interacted with – personally known, unfamiliar, (f) experiences of cyber threats – bullying, frauds, intimidation or blackmailing, hacking, (g) knowledge of resources to combat cyber threats – laws, institutional resources, etc., and (f) knowledge and skills of parents regarding cyber threats. Based on the above, children may be classified as being at low/moderate/high risks.

b. **Preparedness profile of parents and caregivers**: A similar exercise using anonymized surveys or interviews may be used for parents and caregivers to assess their preparedness for online threats for their children, their own online behaviour, and knowledge about resources. This may be useful to audit the information collected from students as well as to gain further insights into the digital affluence of the family and their risk profile when it comes to internet intimidation. Based on the above, families may be classified as being at low/moderate/high risks.

Once classification is done, the SBFC practitioner may classify families as belonging to low/moderate/advanced digital preparedness categories and plan separate sessions for each group. It may be interesting to note that digital knowledge and familiarity do not guarantee safety from internet intimidation. Often, a high level of knowledge, familiarity, and access will make families grow careless about cyber threats and provide children more unsupervised access than is suitable or desirable. Digitally trained families may also underestimate the cyber threats faced by their children due to an inflated sense of security. However, profiling and categorization may be important to customize knowledge interventions for the beneficiaries and to ensure that the specific threats to which a particular child is vulnerable are addressed immediately.

Step 2: Welcome and exposition

The SBFC practitioner needs to begin by establishing rapport with the counselling group of parents. As an icebreaker, the SBFC practitioner may ask the participants to list their main concerns with their children's online activities. The participants may be asked to list down the concerns in pairs, following which the responses may be discussed in small groups for further elaboration. This would help build an environment for discussion on cyberbullying as well as surface the main concerns in the minds of parents and caregivers regarding the online activities of their children.

SBFC practitioner: Welcome to today's discussion on safe internet behaviour and cyberbullying. The Internet is fast becoming an indispensable part of the lives of us and our children. Let us start off the discussion with some thoughts on what you feel are the concerns with your children's online activities? Please form a pair and list down at least five examples for the next twenty minutes.

(Parents work in teams and share feedback.)

SBFC practitioner: Excellent. Some issues that have arisen are concerns due to long hours spent online, lack of physical exercise, access to adult content, difficulty in monitoring, and risk of abuse. If you feel comfortable to share, what are some of the steps you have taken for redressal of these issues?

Once the key concerns have surfaced, the SBFC practitioner is likely to see common themes emerge, relevant to the topic of cyberbullying and other forms of cyber threats. At this point, the SBFC practitioner may summarize the first activity – by pointing out the commonality of issues faced by the children of today's generation. It is likely that parents with different levels of digital maturity will voice different concerns regarding cyber threats. Prior categorization based on digital maturity and access to resources would help in the emergence of common concerns.

Step 3: Exploration of the problem of cyberbullying

With the establishment of a common ground using the ice-breaking activity, the SBFC practitioner may enter the field of cyberbullying. The SBFC practitioner may begin by elaborating on the phenomenon of bullying and drawing parallels between bullying in real life and cyberbullying in the virtual world. It is important to draw attention to the fact that while the physical environment of a child is usually restricted to his or her home, school, and neighbourhood, the scope of the child's known environment expands tremendously in the virtual world. Thanks to social media, the child may be in contact with people who are of different age groups, in different regions of the world, and of different socio-cultural backgrounds. This often exposes the child to life experiences that are beyond his or her level of processing and maturity. Further, online interactions are likely to lead to polarization of thoughts, leading people to group with netizens with similar outlooks, and launch concerted attacks against those who happen to disagree. Children are often unsuspecting victims of such attacks, as they may draw flak for their opinions, photos, social backgrounds, or online activities. The SBFC practitioner may draw attention to the different forms of cyberbullying that can take place – driven by peers known to the child (e.g., school friends), peers personally unknown to the child (e.g., same-age netizens in online communities), or familiar/unfamiliar adults. The SBFC practitioner may also speak about the different forms of cyber-bullying – online shaming for divergent looks, characteristics, or opinions, trolling, making embarrassing photos/videos public, or morphing photos and videos with the intention of embarrassing the child.

One important aspect that needs to be highlighted at this stage is the potential of cyberbullying to escalate blackmailing the child into extortion, self-harm, or even suicide. The SBFC practitioner needs to establish the seriousness of the issue by sharing case studies and news events that show the debilitating impact of cyberbullying when undetected and unchecked. In addition, the SBFC practitioner needs to talk about the close relationship between cyber-bullying and cyber frauds – where children accidentally download malwares, causing their systems to be compromised into sharing intimate details and financial information of their parents.

Awareness about cyberbullying needs to be followed by debriefing and answering of the questions by the participants. It is possible that awareness about cyberbullying and its threats may lead to panic reactions in some parents, which needs to be addressed by focusing on the interventions and the legal measures available. However, some may downplay the risks involved. In these circumstances, the SBFC practitioner needs to provide a realistic appraisal of the situation – sharing statistics about the incidence of cyberbullying targeting children in the concerned geography, the hazards of cyberbullying, as well as the potential ways to counter them.

Step 4: Interventions

This is by far the most important stage of the group counselling intervention, where the SBFC practitioner needs to empower the parents and caregivers with tools to combat the threat of internet intimidation in children. To ensure that the participants feel involved and there is ownership towards the solutions generated, the SBFC practitioner may begin with a group exercise – asking the parents to generate preventive and curative interventions for cases of cyberbullying that involves active participation from parents and other family members. Encouragement needs to be provided. It is likely that several of the solutions generated would overlap with the best practices in this area. These need to be noted down and displayed prominently for future reference during the session.

Once the participants have discussed their potential solutions for the problem of cyberbullying, the SBFC practitioner may begin by highlighting the role of the parents, other caregivers, and other family members in teaching healthy online behaviour to children. The SBFC practitioner may at this point bring up the concept of digital citizenship and emphasize why it is critical to train children early in the concepts of ideal digital citizenship behaviour. Further, the role of the family in inculcating the right values and the best practice in the children needs to be emphasized.

Specifically, the following points need to be addressed by the SBFC practitioner.

1 Preventive Measures
  A *Building awareness*: The SBFC practitioner needs to highlight and speak about the role of the family in developing digital awareness in the child. While schools may provide early digital training to a child, for families with digital access, home is likely to be the first place where the child picks up digital training and online habits. Therefore, parents need to have age-appropriate conversations with children about the need to be watchful about their online presence and not share more than what is necessary. Children also need to be told about the threats of cyberbullying, cyber intimidation, their legal and ethical implications, such that they are both able to detect the early danger signals of cyberbullying as well as avoid displaying similar behaviour against others. The SBFC practitioner also needs to train the parents in the legal and community support measures available for survivors of cyberbullying, so that they may, in turn, train their children.
  B *Role-modelling ideal digital behaviour*: Research has shown a direct connection between parents' digital behaviour and PIU by children. Therefore, parents and other family members need to be told about role-modelling desirable online behaviour before children. This includes spending a rationed amount of time on social media daily, refraining from sharing personal details and photos in public, not posting controversial content online, and keeping one's financial details secure. Further, parents need to also exercise restraint in sharing photos of children on their social media handles without the latter's consent, such that their privacy remains protected.
  C *Monitoring and rationing digital access:* A critical aspect of preventing cyberbullying is to monitor the daily access of children to the online world. The SBFC practitioner may also introduce the parents to various child-friendly resources such as children's YouTube and restrict children's access to various OTT platforms. Parents need to be also updated about age limits for various social media sites and online resources, such that children do not have early access to them. The SBFC practitioner here may emphasize the need to keep digital devices in common areas of the house, where the child's online activities may easily be monitored. Parents need to also check the internet browsing histories of their homes periodically for any early signs of

concern. Another possible solution may be parents being present on the social media handles of children to watch out for signs of danger.

D   *Developing critical viewing skills*

The SBFC practitioner here needs to speak about training children into critical viewing and thinking, since extensive monitoring of a child's digital behaviour is neither possible nor desirable. The emphasis should be on making the child an ally in the fight against cyberbullying. The parents need to develop an open communication with the child such that they do not feel intruded upon by their family members but feel empowered to act as crusaders against cyberbullying.

The SBFC practitioner at this point may introduce the parents to small thought exercises and activities to play with the children to introduce them to the concepts of cyberbullying and potential danger signals in a simple, child-friendly way. Small case studies may be shared with the parents that could be shared with children to help them identify early alarms of internet intimidation, potential solutions, and places where they could seek help if in trouble.

SBFC practitioner: *In many households, the key challenge is that digital access is so ubiquitous that there are hardly any conversations between parents and children about the later online behaviour. In many other households, parents are not tech-savvy, so they tend to remain not participative in their children's digital behaviour. Both the approaches are likely to grow a distance between the child and his or her parents about the online world and the experiences that the child gains there. How do you feel one may combat this issue?*

(Parents share feedback. Responses may lead to further discussion)

SBFC practitioner: *In addition, if one is unfamiliar with the digital world, a useful way is to request children to teach one about internet browsing and social media. Donning the hat of an instructor would help the child feel empowered and responsible and would make him/her feel the need to practise and demonstrate ideal digital citizenship behaviour to his/her proteges. At the same time, it would normalize conversations about online activities at home, creating situations where the child can share any challenges without hesitation, and consider parents as allies in his/her online journey.*

2   Curative Measures

A   *Raising alert to concerned authorities – school, police, and community services*: Despite the best efforts, it is possible that cyberbullying may still infiltrate homes and schools to harm the children. Therefore, the SBFC practitioner needs to brief the parents about what danger signals to watch out for. These may include unusually long hours spent by the child on the internet, insistence on browsing in privacy, sudden and persistent negative mood especially after accessing the net, body image issues, and general loss of self-confidence. The SBFC practitioner needs to brief the parents about resources available to them online and in the community where they could seek police protection, legal resources, and mental health support for their children in case of cyberbullying. The SBFC practitioner may at the point provide easy reference materials such as IEC materials, posters, and flipcharts to the parents, so that they have the contacts of the resources readily available.

B   *Providing emotional support to the child*: Along with legal interventions, it is critical that children who are survivors of cyberbullying are provided emotional support by their parents and other family members. The SBFC practitioner may at this point speak about the importance of providing the child unconditional positive regard, rather than resorting to blame games, defending the child against future attacks, and rebuilding their confidence through monitored, safe digital encounters, and finding them professional mental health support wherever necessary. The SBFC practitioner at this point may bring in role plays to demonstrate how to hold a conversation with a child regarding cyberbullying, how to elicit information about potential threats, and how to rebuild their confidence in accessing online data.

   SBFC practitioner: *We have now been through the various interventions to combat cyberbullying. However, many of these are easier said than done. Let us practice some of the skills here. Imagine that you notice your child remains upset for a few days, especially after using the internet, but is not speaking out. (Designates one participant to play the role of the parent and another to play the role of the child.) How would you start the conversation as a parent?*

   After the role play…

   SBFC practitioner: *Excellent presentation. What challenges did you notice while executing the role play? Was it easy to help the child talk openly? What made him/her speak out about the issues? How would you close such a conversation?*

   (Parents share their feedback)

   SBFC practitioner: *One interesting way to start a conversation is to share one's own experiences with bullying. Stories where one has sought help, with successful results, is useful in demonstrating positive behaviour to children. In extreme cases, it may become essential to confront children with their digital history and offer help. However, one needs to be careful that the child does not feel alienated in the process. It is important to repeatedly assure that the child's well-being is the foremost concern in the minds of the parents and a safe environment alone will help the child gain more freedom of action in the virtual world.*

Step 5: Assessment

Once the interventions are discussed, the counselling session is nearing the end. At this point, the SBFC practitioner may launch an assessment of how far the training has been successful in training about a knowledge, skill, and attitude change in the parents and other caregivers of school children. This may be done either through a small, objective assessment testing recall of the information shared, or through spot quizzes, allowing participants to recall and reiterate important information in a fun way.

Second, the SBFC practitioner may check for acquisition of skills through role plays where the participants are given various situations related to digital safety of children at home – such as teaching a child about digital safety in a child-friendly way, monitoring a child's digital behaviour without being intrusive, negotiating with a child the potential signs of danger of cyber threat, counselling a child who has faced cyberbullying, etc. The SBFC practitioner may demonstrate some of the roles for the participants and then ask them to play out the rest. Role plays will allow the participants opportunities to practise the skills in a safe space and learn from each other the optimal ways of teaching children safe behaviour. Role plays will also help parents to appreciate the dynamics of digital citizenship curricula and the different questions and resistances that may come up while communicating the cyber-appropriate behaviour with children.

Another method of assessment that the SBFC practitioner may adopt is a pre-post assessment. If information has been gathered prior to the intervention about the knowledge, skill, and attitude of the participants, the assessment section may be used to reassess the participants and decide if there has been an improvement in their understanding and attitude post-intervention. Further, qualitative feedback on the intervention may be gathered, in terms of whether the training is perceived to be useful, if the participant would recommend the training and the resources shared to other parents, and whether the intervention has been successful in solving the specific problems encountered by the participants, if any.

The assessment section should also be used by the SBFC practitioner as an opportunity to solicit and answer questions and clarify doubts that may be lingering in the minds of the participants. The SBFC practitioner may use the opportunity to reiterate the important takeaways and share the important resources that the participants may use in case of any need.

Step 6: Conclusion and follow-up

Once the counselling session is over, all the session materials, including the information, education, and communication resources and the internet linkage information, need to be shared with the participants. Care needs to be taken that the material is provided in a language and form that is understood by the participants and could be stored and accessed readily by them.

Post-session, the SBFC practitioner needs to keep in mind that the information and skills shared may need to be reiterated periodically to facilitate retention and application. To this end, it is necessary to organize refresher training and counselling sessions where the information shared is rehearsed and new information and resources are updated. At the same time, these follow-up opportunities may be utilized by the SBFC practitioners to know the long-term impact of the interventions – in terms of if they have been able to address the problems of the children, if the participants have encountered any problems in implementing the recommendations, and if there are new insights that they have drawn from the process.

Multicultural considerations

The application of the digital citizenship curriculum, like other SBFC interventions, is subject to several cultural dynamics that need to be kept in mind while designing the interventions. Important concerns are the socio-economic status of the family, the nature of the family and the number of family members present to train and monitor the child, the national and the socio-religious culture of the target population, and the legal provisions for that geography.

Digital divide

The foremost concern while designing the interventions would be the digital divide. It is possible that the SBFC practitioner would encounter families with different levels of digital maturity and access. While it would be easy to facilitate the conversation with families having considerable digital access, in less-affluent households, parents may not be equipped to monitor the online behaviour of their children. In households that lack digital access, helping parents understand the cyber threats faced by their children may be a herculean task. Again, affluent households may be providing personal digital gadgets to even young children making monitoring difficult and leaving the children vulnerable to many potential threats. The SBFC practitioner therefore needs to segregate parents on their digital maturity, resources, and time, to customize training interventions.

Diversity

Cultural diversity may necessitate extensive customization of counselling content and even materials. For instance, in certain masculinity-oriented cultures of the world, it may be needed to place men and women in separate intervention groups for better understanding of the problem. The language of the materials also needs to be adopted according to the understanding and convenience of the participants.

Challenges and solutions

There may be several challenges that the SBFC practitioner may encounter while designing interventions. First, the success of a family-based counselling intervention will depend on the extent to which the solutions may be executed at home. However, the nature of the family may play a role here. While in a traditional family setup, it may be possible to monitor the child's internet usage regularly, in single-parent homes, or where both the parents are working, facilities for monitoring may not be available at all. In such situations, it is important for the parents to cultivate the child as an ally to the interventions, encouraging self-restraint and self-monitoring. In such cases, the SBFC practitioner may also emphasize technological tools for monitoring the online behaviour of the child. Firewalls, child locks, and close monitoring of browser history of children's devices for any problem will be useful in such situations.

Another potential problem is the attitude towards privacy. This could emerge as a concern with older children. While parental monitoring is often essential to maintain vigilance on the child's online activities, in many cultures emphasizing independence and autonomy, this monitoring may be perceived as intrusive by the children. Further, parents may be uncomfortable executing such vigilance. In these situations, again it is critical to obtain buy-in from the children along with the parents and make the former allies in the situation. This will help children feel empowered in the fight against cyberbullying and encourage them to take proactive steps to combat the menace, in the form of flagging harmful patterns of conversation, not engaging in harassing others, and in general maintaining decorum in online interactions.

One critical concern that the SBFC practitioner needs to talk about is the tendency to blame and penalize the survivor in case of any untoward incident online. Often, parents are unhappy with the long hours children spend on social media or at gaming. Therefore, any incident of cyberbullying or online harassment gets blamed on the child's online activities, with subsequent denial of access, suffocating vigilance, and repeated criticism. This further discourages the child from sharing their online challenges with parents, until things go out of their hands. IT is important not to resort to victim-blaming and criticizing the child when a problem surfaces. Rather, the child should be complimented for being brave and bringing the issue to the front, rather than hiding it. The SBFC practitioner may explain this to the parents through activities, where parents are asked to recount risk behaviours they undertake for pleasure, despite knowing its potential negative consequences – such as smoking, online buying and selling, blind dates, etc., and are made to develop empathy with the human tendency to underestimate risks and overestimate one's invulnerability.

Conclusion

Digital media is fast becoming ubiquitous in the modern world, bringing with it its own opportunities and challenges. To the children growing up as digital natives, digital access brings a wealth of opportunities inaccessible to the previous generations but also leaves them vulnerable to online crimes such as cyberbullying. Since digital access is becoming a constant in a child's life at both home and school, caregivers and schoolteachers therefore need to join hands to provide holistic protection and support to the child. The latter, mostly being digital non-natives presently, need specialized guidance and support in monitoring, preventing, and redressing the harm of cybercrimes against children. This chapter explored the concerns of digital bullying, the roles of schools and homes in protecting children from such crimes, and the SBFC processes by which the adult stakeholders may be trained in providing effective support to the school children. Effective adoption of SBFC intervention is likely to induct the future generations into a digital experience that is non-threatening, age-appropriate, and wholesome.

Resources

Bauman, S. (2014). *Cyberbullying: What counselors need to know.* John Wiley & Sons.
This book provides a comprehensive review of the phenomenon of cyberbullying, its antecedents and outcomes, and the role of the counsellors in preventing it.

Beale, A. V., & Hall, K. R. (2007). Cyberbullying: What school administrators (and parents) can do. *The Clearing House: A Journal of Educational Strategies, Issues and Ideas*, 81(1), 8–12.
This article provides recommendations for schoolteachers and parents to prevent and redress cyberbullying of schoolchildren.

Patchin, J. W., & Hinduja, S. (Eds.). (2012). *Cyberbullying prevention and response: Expert perspectives.* Routledge.
This book provides a lucid and comprehensive understanding of cyberbullying and the role of caregivers and schoolteachers in addressing the malaise.

Sabella, R. A., Patchin, J. W., & Hinduja, S. (2013). Cyberbullying myths and realities. *Computers in Human Behavior*, 29(6), 2703–2711.
The paper explores cyberbullying as a phenomenon, its similarities with traditional bullying, and its triggers.

Su, Y. W., Doty, J., Polley, B. R., Cakmakci, H., Swank, J., & Sickels, A. (2021). Collaborating with families to address cyberbullying: Exploring school counselors' lived experiences. *Professional School Counseling*, 25(1), 2156759X211053825.
This data-driven research presents the experiences of school counsellors in dealing with cyberbullying and offers practical tips in school-home collaboration.

References

Abreu, R. L., & Kenny, M. C. (2018). Cyberbullying and LGBTQ youth: A systematic literature review and recommendations for prevention and intervention. *Journal of Child & Adolescent Trauma*, 11(1), 81–97. https://doi.org/10.1007/s40653-017-0175-7

Adorjan, M. C., & Ricciardelli, R. (2018). *Cyber-risk and youth: Digital citizenship, privacy and surveillance.* London: Routledge. https://doi.org/10.4324/9781315158686

Anderson, M., & Jiang, J. (2018, May 31). Teens, social media, and technology 2018. *Pew Research Center Internet and Technology.* Retrieved July 1, 2021 from https://www.pewresearch.org/internet/2018/05/31/teens-social-media-technology-2018/

Carter, M. J., & Evans, W. P. (2008). Implementing school-based family counseling: Strategies, activities, and process considerations. *International Journal for School-Based Family Counseling*, 1(1), 1–21.

Chen, Y. L., Chen, S. H., & Gau, S. F. S. (2015). ADHD and autistic traits, family function, parenting style, and social adjustment for Internet addiction among children and adolescents in Taiwan: A longitudinal study. *Research in Developmental Disabilities*, 39, 20–31. https://doi.org/10.1016/j.ridd.2014.12.025

Chitre, M. (2019, October 6). UP: Rape victim commits suicide, writes names of the accused on hand. RepublicWorld.com. Retrieved July 1, 2021 from https://www.republicworld.com/india-news/general-news/muzaffarnagar-gang-rape-victim-commits-suicide-writes-names-on-hand.html

Gerrard, B. (2008). School-based family counseling: Overview, trends, and recommendations for future research. *International Journal for School-Based Family Counseling*, 1(1), 1–30.

Gerrard, B., & Soriano, M. (Eds.) (2013). *School-based family counseling: Transforming family-school relationships*. Createspace.

Hefner, D., Knop, K., Schmitt, S., & Vorderer, P. (2019). Rules? Role model? Relationship? The impact of parents on their children's problematic mobile phone involvement. *Media Psychology*, 22(1), 82–108. https://doi.org/10.1080/15213269.2018.1433544

International Telecommunication Union (2017). Measuring the Information Society Report Volume 1. Retrieved July 1, 2021 from https://www.itu.int/en/ITU-D/Statistics/Documents/publications/misr2017/MISR2017_Volume1.pdf

Jain, O., Gupta, M., Satam, S., & Panda, S. (2020). Has the COVID-19 pandemic affected the susceptibility to cyberbullying in India?. *Computers in Human Behavior Reports*, 2, 100029.

Kesharwani, A. (2020). Do (how) digital natives adopt a new technology differently than digital immigrants? A longitudinal study. *Information & Management*, 57(2), 103170. https://doi.org/10.1016/j.im.2019.103170

Li, C., Dang, J., Zhang, X., Zhang, Q., & Guo, J. (2014). Internet addiction among Chinese adolescents: The effect of parental behavior and self-control. *Computers in Human Behavior*, 41, 1–7. https://doi.org/10.1016/j.chb.2014.09.001

Marwick, A., & Lewis, R. (2017). Media manipulation and disinformation online. Data & Society Research Institute. Retrieved July 1, 2021 from http://www.chinhnghia.com/DataAndSociety_MediaManipulationAndDisinformation-Online.pdf

Pham, T., & Adesman, A. (2015). Teen victimization: Prevalence and consequences of traditional and cyberbullying. *Current Opinion in Pediatrics*, 27(6), 748–756. https://doi.org/10.1097/MOP.0000000000000290

Ribble, M. (2015). *Digital citizenship in schools: Nine elements all students should know.* International Society for Technology in Education.

Soriano, M., & Gerrard, B. (2013). School-based family counseling: An overview. In B. Gerrard & M. Soriano (Eds), *School-based family counseling: Transforming family-school relationships*, pp. 2–15, Createspace.

Westerlund, M. (2019). The emergence of deepfake technology: A review. *Technology Innovation Management Review*, 9(11), 40–53. http://doi.org/10.22215/timreview/1282

Ying Ying, C., Awaluddin, S. M., Kuang Kuay, L., Siew Man, C., Baharudin, A., Miaw Yn, L., … & Ibrahim, N. (2021). Association of internet addiction with adolescents' lifestyle: A national school-based survey. *International Journal of Environmental Research and Public Health*, 18(1), 168. https://doi.org/10.3390/ijerph18010168

19 An ACES approach to developing trauma-sensitive schools

Toni Nemia

Overview

This chapter is directed toward SBFC practitioners, classroom teachers, administrators, and all those who are interested in how Adverse Childhood Experiences (ACES) impair a student's ability to access the curriculum toward academic progress. It also introduces the concept of trauma-informed learning as an institutional foundation for creating safe environments, a space more conducive to learning. Most importantly, this chapter is written with an emphasis on educational practices in the United States of America and offers its contents to those who are facile at making multicultural adjustments.

Background

Adverse Childhood Experiences (ACES)

How did the concept of ACES come to the fore of public health, law, and education? In 1997, Drs. Vincent Felitti of Kaiser Permanente of San Diego, CA, and Robert Anda of the Centers for Disease Control, in Atlanta, GA, completed a study of 17,500 middle-class adults who were on a medically supported weight loss program, many already diagnosed with diabetes. These physicians were shocked to learn that although the success rate was high for shedding pounds, the return to weight gain was swift once the participants were re-interviewed after they were no longer part of the study. Dr. Felitti's "aha" moment came when he realized that as researchers he and Dr. Anda were not asking the participants the right questions in conjunction with the weight loss protocol. This crystallization resulted in the discovery that questions of psychosocial and family history were pivotal in researching issues of physical health. No longer could mental health be ignored as part of a complete wellness assessment (Felitti et al., 2019).

The original ACES questionnaire focusing on the importance of collecting data of family history was introduced. Ten questions on the following issues were asked and respondents were to score a "1" for every "YES" answer.

DOI: 10.4324/9781003201977-23

Before your 18th birthday, did you experience:

- Physical abuse
- Sexual abuse
- Verbal abuse
- Physical neglect
- Emotional neglect
- A family member who is depressed or diagnosed with other mental illness
- A family member who is addicted to alcohol or another substance
- A family member who is in prison
- Witnessing a mother being abused
- Losing a parent to separation, divorce, or death

The list of stressors has now been expanded to include issues of race, ethnicity, color, nationality, class, gender identity, sexual orientation, community violence, economic hardship, real life and cyber bullying, sexual coercion among cross age minors. Unfortunately, there are infinite possibilities.

Original ACES findings

The overall conclusions of the original ACES study indicated that the higher number of ACES one has endured, the more likely such an individual is at an increased risk for physical and mental illness in measurable ways. Many of the heart, brain, and endocrine illnesses have their roots in stress, to say nothing of the implications for mental health afflictions, alcohol and substance abuse, harm to self and others.

The connections among ACES, trauma, and key concepts

Concepts such as toxic stress, trauma, and epigenetics have emerged from the original study leading us to understand the impact which body, mind, and soul can be harmed through all kinds of adversity. For example, routine stress or anxiety is a part of daily living and can also help us to achieve successful accomplishments and complete tasks effectively. Toxic stress, however, is chronic and prolonged and can become disabling as it kicks the endocrine system into over drive. Adrenaline and cortisol are released into the system resulting in a hormonal flood of toxins. This experience contributes to the fight, flight, or freeze behaviors which result in reactive and impulsive actions rather than responsive and considerate behaviors.

Epigenetics, literally translated as "along, over, outside, or around," the gene structure speaks to the realities of trauma through the generations. International examples of Holocausts, genocides, and racial and ethnic cleansing devastation, for example, do not just impact the survivors of these atrocities but also live on in the descendants as well. If ever there were a convergence of nature and nurture, epigenetics has become emblematic of this age-old debate. Many trauma experts in a variety of professions hold the notion that the "body, mind, and soul" remembers in astonishing ways.

The contribution of Nadine Burke Harris, MD

Dr. Nadine Burke Harris – a pediatrician, the former Surgeon General for the State of California, internationally known public health advocate, author of *The Deepest Well*, and the founder of the Center for Youth Wellness in San Francisco, California – is a pivotal contributor to the implications of trauma and toxic stress in learning. (She resigned this position on Thursday, February 4, 2022, during the writing of this chapter, citing her own need for self and family care and naming the disparities in national health care between the affluent and the under-resourced.)

In many of her lectures, she describes the multitude of students who were referred to her clinic with a diagnosis of Attention Deficit Hyperactivity Disorder by San Francisco teachers and administrators (Harris, 2015). Her challenging and questioning of this pervasive diagnosis prompted her and her medical staff to interview children and families more deeply for psychosocial information. Just as Drs. Felitti and Anda concluded that they needed to understand the lives of their patients, their historical family contexts, Dr. Burke Harris shifted her inquiry with children and their families to a recognition and inclusion that social emotional factors and family dynamics must be included in initial physical health assessments. She concluded that, although there were some cases of correctly diagnosed Attention Deficit Hyperactivity Disorder, the majority of these referrals included children who had experienced trauma at an already tender age and were suffering from toxic stress (Harris, 2018).

Mitigating trauma and toxic stress

The factors which can mitigate trauma are built around the concepts of coping, flexibility, and resilience. Healthy eating, regular exercise, good sleep hygiene, a sound social structure of positive relationships, an attitude of faith or hope – these are just a few of the practices which strengthen one's resolve in the face of adversity.

Resilience and its hallmarks

Resilience involves the ability to recover and rebound from adversity and setbacks.

Examples of resilience characteristics include:

• the ability to know one's strengths and challenges and how to apply that knowledge in a crisis

- holding the attitude that life will present problems
- the capacity to maintain a sound social support network
- looking toward one's own locus of control and exercising good judgment rather than succumbing to the overall panic
- recognizing compassion for self and others

Building a resilient foundation is in fact one of main antidotes to lessening trauma.

Connecting the ACES findings with trauma-informed learning and schools which create safe havens

A trauma-informed school is one in which there is recognition and sensitivity to the fact that learning is adversely impacted, not only by what students bring to the front door of the building and don't leave at the threshold of the classroom, but also by what happens within the school climate (Overstreet & Chafouleas, 2016). The family concept is exhibited in both the nuclear family and the kin within a school.

Sandra Bloom, MD, a psychiatrist at Drexel University in Philadelphia, Pennsylvania, talks of the importance of institutions – government, law, physical and mental health, education – kindergarten to 12th grade and beyond through higher learning – as safe havens. Without the implementation and preservation of these entities as sanctuaries, there is a risk of losing a response to human needs and maintaining reactions which in fact run counter to these essentials (Bloom, 2013). Historically within the United States of America, there has been the creation of compassionate, mindful, and empathic schools. Contrary to popular belief, these schools do not forego academic performance. Rather, they foster all of the healthy, social emotional interactions among everyone – students, families, teachers, administrators, and support staff with the belief that learning will take place in safe and secure environments. With this ethic, such schools are not program- but process-oriented just as learning is. The most significant messengers are the adults who know how to be in addition to knowing how to do.

More mythology surrounds trauma-informed schools. There is a false belief that these schools lack discipline and compromise academic achievement for a laissez-faire environment. However, such is not the case. What is valued is an approach to behavior which includes discipline and consequences, not punishment, shaming, or retraumatization (Walkley & Cox, 2013).

A trauma-informed, responsive, and sensitive school incorporates the following:

- an awareness that climate and culture impact its community
- training and supporting staff in the impact of trauma on learning
- identifying vulnerable students
- establishing flexible accommodations for diverse learners

- developing disciplinary practices which are compassionate and appropriate to the infraction
- nurturing a collective consciousness of cultural, racial, national, ethnic, and gender differences
- creating a climate of cultural humility.

A little more needs to be said about discipline in confronting misbehavior, a fundamental piece in an educational community in which safety lessens chaos. The purpose of discipline is to foster emotional health, educate with healthy alternative and prosocial behaviors, and mitigate harm done in recognition of both the individual and the community. The overarching premise is that effective curriculum access can only take place in a harmonious environment.

The emergence of Social Emotional Learning (SEL)

The Collaborative for Academic, Social Emotional Learning (CASEL) is a major commercial and evidence-based curriculum which is marketed to a kindergarten through high school population and staff (Axelrod, 2010). According to CASEL, "the benefits of social and emotional learning (SEL) are well-researched, with evidence demonstrating that an education that promotes SEL yields positive results for students, adults, and school communities." Given the increased use of social emotional activities in schools, cautions have been raised. Are the accepted and recommended standards of prosocial behavior too narrowly defined by white, middle-class culture to the exclusion of diverse and other culturally valued ethics? Many teachers feel confined by a prescribed and costly curriculum and would rather use the global offerings of ephemeral materials provided by the real world. Such concerns need further exploration.

Relationship to the SBFC metamodel

The development of trauma-sensitive schools fits into the school prevention quadrant of the SBFC metamodel. When a disaster has already occurred, it is not the best time to initiate a trauma-sensitive school. However, if the school personnel have already developed trauma-sensitive procedures in their school, then when a school crisis (such as death of a student or teacher) or disaster (such as a flood or pandemic) occurs, the school community is more likely to display resilience in the face of serious emotional stress. In the case of school crises and community disasters, the old saying "prevention is worth a pound of cure" applies.

Procedure

Attitude and philosophy

How do trauma-informed teachers establish a context for learning in a trauma-sensitive way? The starting point is within one's self and the intention to become trauma-informed and responsive. Building an arsenal of coping strategies, maintaining a flexibility when change is necessary, adjusting rigid thinking, incorporating self-care and lifestyle activities which promote physical health and emotional well-being – these practices are at the foundation for building one's own resilience. Your resilience is critical to how you role model for others.

The application of these elements allows the SBFC practitioner to demonstrate the following attitudinal shifts around education and learning:

- accept that learning takes place in a community of support in which you are the role model
- maintain a consistent approach to disruption which does not enhance this energy
- remind oneself that building a community within the classroom and school takes time
- understand learning is not lost, but rather enhanced, by developing a trauma-informed approach
- believe that learning does not take place with one intervention, command, or lesson
- creative repetition and reinforcement are necessary to the process of learning.

How the move toward trauma-informed learning is presented to staff is no small task. Without the collective buy-in and collective advocacy from teachers building, this community will be difficult. Parental acceptance and support are also critical to developing and maintaining trauma-informed schools. Just as teachers hold the mandate of academic achievement in high regard, families also have an expectation that learning cannot be compromised for what might be perceived as non-academic activities. Initial and ongoing professional development for staff is complemented by educating families.

Steps to take

Essentials for the school principal, the teaching staff, and the SBFC practitioner in building the foundation of trauma-informed schools include the following.

1 Professional development at the administrative and faculty levels in trauma-informed school is critical to forming these safe environments. Provide brief readings, videos, evidence-based literature, experiential-based activities, or live testimonials on the inherent value to improving academics through meeting student psychosocial and emotional needs.
2 Who should take the lead? In a traditional top-down administrative model, the principal can take the lead by providing professional development and seeking buy-in. In a more collateral and collaborative model,

the encouragement can be initiated by anyone. In either case, professional development activities and dialogues, as stated in #1, are helpful. Include families at this information sharing phase.

3   Regardless of who leads with this idea, take steps to model prosocial behavior and discourse among the entire school staff. The adults in the building enact trauma-informed ways of being by listening well, maintaining an interested presence, reflecting back an understanding of what the speaker is saying, and responding with possible next steps.

4   Allow for discussions on current school climate so that everyone has the opportunity to air concerns and specific areas for improvement. Establish some agreed upon countable number of core statements for what your trauma-informed school will adopt and bring to life.

5   Develop a disciplinary policy of "do no harm" and "hold regard for the harmed." Provide constructive alternatives for those who do harm to make amends. Eliminate shame from the discipline.
   •   Ask the harmed individual what is needed for reparation to take place.
   •   Ask the individual who does the harm what might be needed for reparation to take place. Provide coaching and prompts if this individual has difficulty forming ideas.
        Offer to bare witness reparative conversations.
   •   Respect each individual's right not to participate.
   •   Offer the individual who has harmed a couple of alternative actions.

6   Restorative Practices: Establishing a restorative and reparative approach is in keeping with trauma-informed consequences for positive discipline (McCluskey et al., 2008). Consider how the following six core questions will shift the conversations.
   a   What happened? Model empathy and respect. Help the student to feel heard and understood.
   b   How were you feeling and what were you needing? Identifying and understanding underlying feelings which fosters insight.
   c   What were you thinking? This perspective focuses on thoughts. It allows the listener to model empathy with the intention of fostering the student's empathy with others.
   d   Who else has been affected? What do you think they might be feeling? This encourages a deepening of an empathetic perspective.
   e   What have you learned and what will you do differently next time? This question addresses the goal of Restorative Practices as it leads everyone a step closer to healing, understanding others, and developing a strong awareness of the human condition.
   f   How can harm be repaired? Rather than offering a punitive consequence, Restorative Practices offer concrete steps to making amends. It allows the student who has done harm to take responsibility for an action rather than receive a consequence in isolation.

Building community, specific activities for the classroom

Designate specific times for regular, interactive classroom conversation. Arrange seating in a circle. Consider offering any warm ups which allow for self-reflection, expressions of thoughts and feelings, all in an effort to foster relationship building. Give permission to students to "pass" or not speak on any topic.

Sample prompts:

- Describe/draw your dream home in detail. Where is the location?
- What are my three wishes for now or the future?
- What is something about me you wouldn't know by looking at me?
- If I weren't in school today, I would be _____ (fill in the blank)
- Tell the story of how you got your name.

Offer regular brain breaks

Brain breaks allow for a brief refocusing of mental exertion through some type of physical movement, mindfulness exercises, or sensory activities. Teachers act as role models for inspiration and participate actively with their students.

Sample ideas:

- Offer fidgets – hand toys, objects which allow students to discharge energy
- Encourage standing and stretching in place
- Create a specific dance move
- Offer a musical interlude
- Toss a bean bag or small stuffed animal around the room with students acting as pitchers
- Blow bubbles

Mindfulness and anxiety reduction

Sample ideas:

- Journal writing with a prompt, or free writing
- Teacher led guided imagery to create a safe, internal place for students

Sample verbal instructions:

Ask for 30 seconds of quiet time (eyes open or closed depending on comfort level of the student)
Imagine a blank artist's canvas ready for a painting:
Are you imagining yourself being inside or outside the painting you will make?

What color is the background?
What objects would you like to include? Where are these placed?
What people would you like to include? How would you arrange them?
Think about how this place you are painting gives you comfort, makes you
   feel safe?

Multicultural considerations

The advent of ACES and the expansion of what constitutes adversity in a child's life currently embraces a culture of social justice, acceptance of all peoples, respect for differences with an interest in understanding how unique different cultures can be. How multiculturalism translates into a trauma-informed environment, one which builds resilience, is emphasized in this chapter. Simultaneously, this writer acknowledges what have to be embedded and unconscious biases from an Amero-centric lens and a Western World psychological view.

Challenges and solutions

Were a trauma-sensitive environment to be a foundation and an institutionalized philosophy in schools, there would be a far less need to create such a milieu in the midst of catastrophes, crises, and disasters. The expressions "out of the ashes, rises the Phoenix" or "Crisis equals opportunity" are common reframes for how positive experiences can be cultivated as an outgrowth with difficult times. Yet, it must be acknowledged that the creation of safe havens is very important when adversity strikes. Perhaps the best approach is to start small and start now.

How the move toward trauma-informed learning is presented to staff is no small task. Without the collective buy-in and collective advocacy from teachers, building a trauma-informed school community will be difficult. Parental acceptance and support are also critical to developing and maintaining trauma-informed schools. Just as teachers hold the mandate of academic achievement in high regard, families also have an expectation that learning cannot be compromised for what might be perceived as non-academic activities. Initial and ongoing professional development for staff is complemented by educating families as well.

Conclusion

What a magnificent change it would be if schools became symbols of academic achievement in concert with social emotional interactions which reflect the best which humans can offer one to the other! Trauma-informed schools still remain in the minority within the United States of America. However, the growing research on the impact of ACES, along with the knowledge that students who have a peaceful mind allow for more sound learning, holds hope for the future. Although the focus of this book emphasizes ways of coping with disasters, it is important to remember that not all disasters are natural. War, climate change, and the ways in which people can exert power over others – all of these conditions are disastrous to humanity. What better setting to create a milieu where the emphasis is being smart in mind and smart in spirit than in a school setting!

Resources

The following websites offer information and activities on ACES and trauma informed schools. https://acestoohigh.com

This is an online news site that reports on research about positive and adverse childhood experiences, including developments in epidemiology, neurobiology, and the biomedical and epigenetic consequences of toxic stress. https://casel.org

This website is the Collaborative for Academic, Social, and Emotional Learning dedicated to the advancement of these practices for children and adults. https://childmind.org/healthyminds

This website is dedicated to children's mental health through a compassionate approach for the science of the developing mind. https://www.greatergood.berkeley.edu

This website provides an online compendium on topics for the psychological well being of children and adults. https://hearts.ucsf.edu

This site describes a collaborative project founded by the University of California, San Francisco Medical Center with partnerships in schools which are interested in becoming trauma informed communities. https://www.heysigmund.com

This is an online Australian resource dealing with anxiety, children and parents, the human mind and the way we work, love, play, behave, relate, and feel. It focuses on what it means to be human and how to master this art. https://www.pacesconnection.com

This website was formerly ACES Connections and it focuses on preventing adverse childhood experiences, healing trauma, and building resilience. https://en.wikipedia.org/wiki/Nadine_Burke_Harris

This is a Wikipedia description of Dr. Nadine Burke Harris, ACES information advocate.

References

Axelrod, J. (2010). Collaborative for academic, social and emotional learning (CASEL). *Encyclopedia of Cross-Cultural School Psychology*, 232–233. https://doi.org/10.1007/978-0-387-71799-9_77

Bloom, S. L. (2013). *Creating sanctuary: Toward the evolution of sane societies*. Routledge.

Felitti, V. J., Anda, R. F., Nordenberg, D., Williamson, D. F., Spitz, A. M., Edwards, V., Koss, M. P., & Marks, J. S. (2019). Reprint OF: Relationship of childhood abuse and household dysfunction to many of the leading causes of death in adults: The adverse childhood experiences (ACE) study. *American Journal of Preventive Medicine*, 56(6), 774–786. https://doi.org/10.1016/j.amepre.2019.04.001

Harris, N. B. (2015). How childhood trauma affects health across a lifetime [Video]. TED: Ideas worth spreading. https://www.ted.com/talks/nadine_burke_harris_how_childhood_trauma_affects_health_across_a_lifetime?language=en

Harris, N. B. (2018). *The deepest well: Healing the long-term effects of childhood adversity*. Houghton Mifflin Harcourt.

McCluskey, G., Lloyd, G., Kane, J., Riddell, S., Stead, J., & Weedon, E. (2008). Can restorative practices in schools make a difference? *Educational Review*, 60(4), 405–417. https://doi.org/10.1080/00131910802393456

Overstreet, S., & Chafouleas, S. M. (2016). Trauma-informed schools: Introduction to the special issue. *School Mental Health*, 8(1), 1–6. https://doi.org/10.1007/s12310-016-9184-1

Walkley, M., & Cox, T. L. (2013). Building trauma-informed schools and communities. *Children & Schools*, 35(2), 123–126. https://doi.org/10.1093/cs/cdt007

Part V
Family prevention

20 An internal family systems approach to building disaster resilience

Ralph S. Cohen

Overview

In the wake of increasing traumatic and stressful events that have been unfolding over the past several years, the educational environment has become severely impacted by such occurrences, affecting the adults and students alike. School shootings, gang violence, substance abuse, natural disasters, the breakdown of family structure, school shut-downs and the "pivot" to home-based learning due to the COVID-19 pandemic, and the loss of loved ones from COVID-19 are just some examples of the types of traumatizing and devaluing experiences faced in the current educational climate. Such occurrences constitute overwhelming challenges to all involved in the educational process, producing detrimental impacts on mental health, well-being, and resilience.

School-based family counseling (SBFC) professionals are called upon to intercede in such unprecedented situations, often with little guidance or support and without adequate preparation and training in their various disciplines to handle the depth and severity of the trauma that they encounter and experience personally. Such experiences take their toll on individual well-being, relationships, and organizations as well as how these experiences impact the teaching and learning processes necessary for fostering healthy development and effective responses to traumatizing situations.

In this chapter, the internal family systems (IFS) model, developed by Dr. Richard Schwartz (Breunlin, Schwartz & MacKune-Karrer, 1992; Schwartz, 1994; Schwartz & Sweeney, 2021), will be described as a new psychology for understanding both intrapsychic and interpersonal dynamics based on family systems principles. The IFS model provides a roadmap for understanding how we respond to trauma and how we can foster resilience in the wake of traumatizing events. We will briefly describe the basic concepts behind the IFS model and will focus in on specific ways that the model can provide SBFC professionals with tools to build their own resilience – to "put their masks on themselves first" so that they will be able to help others. An exercise will be offered to help the SBFC professional to use IFS principles to become grounded in the wake of overwhelming stress and to be able to separate from their own extreme responses to hold more "presence" in their roles as facilitators of resilience in others.

DOI: 10.4324/9781003201977-25

Background

The internal family systems (IFS) model was developed by Schwartz in the mid-1980s (Schwartz, 1994) and is now recognized as a leading methodology for healing trauma (Van Der Kolk, 2014). The IFS model has been recognized by the US Substance Abuse and Mental Health Services Administration (SAMHSA) as an "evidence-based model", which provides credence to the model's effectiveness in helping people cope with various social and emotional difficulties. The model was principally developed for mental health practice, but is also being employed outside of mental health applications, such as coaching (Liu, 2020), divorce mediation (Kroll, 2016), education (Goddard 2019a, 2019b; Hawkes & Hawkes, 2018), and medicine (Livingstone & Gaffney, 2016; Shadick et al., 2013).

The IFS model works with the idea that the human mind operates internally much like interpersonal systems do, which comprised two general components: "Self" and "Parts". The Self is seen in the IFS model as the core personality of each person, which provides organization and leadership within the internal system. The Self can be thought of as akin to being in the state of "mindfulness" that one achieves via meditation (Schwartz, 1994), but is ever-present and running in the background – it is the "seat of consciousness". Parts (as people generally refer to their inner components) consist of a large set of autonomous sub-personalities that interact and form relationships with each other and the Self. Our parts are myriad and diverse, each carrying talents, skills, beliefs, and experiences that contribute to the overall well-being of our inner systems. Like "external" systems (families, organizations, work groups, etc.), the internal system needs to have good leadership so that our parts can maximize their talents, feel valued and contributing, and have access to the system's resources. Schwartz (1994) has named the state of the Self's role in a leadership position vis-à-vis the system of parts as "Self Leadership".

The IFS model promotes **Self leadership**. A good leader provides balance, harmony, and direction to the system. Examples of such leaders are effective parents, teachers, administrators, orchestra conductors, etc. The Self serves as a good leader to our internal system, with its universal qualities that serve as resources for our parts: calm, curiosity, compassion, confidence, courage, clarity, connectedness, and creativity (Schwartz, 1994; Schwartz & Sweeney, 2021). At its best, a Self-led system allows us to experience these eight "C" qualities within a feeling of existing as a unified and grounded whole.

In the absence of connection to good leadership, the system breaks down, members of the system become polarized and self-protective, and wounding and trauma are likely to occur (Schwartz, 1994; Schwartz & Sweezy, 2021). This happens when the system is overwhelmed by traumatizing or devaluing experiences, very often during childhood, but also when we encounter such experiences as adults. When the system is overwhelmed, our parts lose trust in the Self's ability to provide leadership and some of them take on extreme, protective roles to mitigate harm that has occurred or to prevent exposure to harmful events moving forward. Other parts in our internal system directly absorb the extreme feelings, beliefs, sensations, and schemas of traumatic or devaluating experiences and seek relief or redemption from holding such painful burdens. Parts that hold these burdens are commonly referred to as "Exiles", since other parts of us try to protect us from feeling the pain of the burdens they carry or keep us from absorbing new burdens. Besides the impact of traumatic or devaluing events, parts can also internalize burdens from parents and previous generational traumas in the form of "legacy burdens", cultural burdens (such as from wartime or difficult immigration experiences), and racial burdens.

Extreme, protective parts fall into two categories: "Managers" and "Firefighters". Managers use a variety of tactics to push down exiled parts or to avoid situations that may trigger the surfacing of our exiled parts. Such tactics are pre-emptive and manifest as parts of us that try to control situations and other people through criticism of self and others, placating, avoiding, being pessimistic, being overly helpful or nurturant, and other tactics to soothe us or avoid triggering situations. Firefighters are parts of us that respond impulsively and try to "put out the fire" of extreme emotions once our exiles have been exposed and their burdens brought into conscious awareness. Firefighters, due to their impulsive natures, often create more problems for the system and further add to the burdens they are trying to mitigate. Parts that have taken on Manager and Firefighter share similar characteristics: anxiety, fear, and hypervigilance (Schwartz, 1994; Schwartz & Sweeney, 2021).

Schwartz (1994) explains that given that the extreme tactics of our protector parts often attract the very problems they fear, these protective systems become locked into repeating cycles of dysfunction and polarization, with various parts vying for power and control. This leads to a degradation of the system over time, due to the lack of leadership and trust within the system.

The antidote to this dysfunctional system is the re-installation of good leadership (e.g., the "Self" in the internal system or an effective principal in a school system or teacher in the classroom) to restore balance and harmony, and to promote the release of burdens that are picked up by its members as a result of extreme polarizations and trauma (Schwartz, 1994, Schwartz & Sweeney, 2021). The release of burdens can take place when our protectors are convinced that the Self can be trusted to handle the burdens of exiles without being overwhelmed and can bear witness to the stories of how burdens are absorbed. Once the story is told and lessons are learned from experiences, parts are able to release the extreme feelings beliefs of the trauma and can revert to their non-extreme, positive qualities and the entire system can return to a state of balance and harmony through Self leadership. The more a person's Self is able to "unblend" from burdened parts in their extreme, protective roles and release the troubling burdens of Exiles, the more the person is able to foster and manifest resilience and adaptive responses to traumatizing circumstances. This process has been shown to have profound and long-lasting effects on healing trauma (Van der Kolk, 2014) and even reducing the severity of symptoms of autoimmune responses of the body (Shadick et al., 2013).

IFS and the school-based family counseling metamodel

In recent years, there has been a growing movement in bringing IFS principles to schools to improve learning and foster resilience in students, teachers, administrators, parents and other stakeholders in the educational system (i.e., the Self Leadership Collaborative – see *Resources*). These efforts are beyond the scope of this chapter; many of those involved in this emerging field believe that foundation of creating a Self-led educational system begins with the adults' ability to be more Self-led on a personal level, which results in greater self-regulation, compassion, and effectiveness in building leadership, balance, and harmony in a school context.

The application of IFS to the SBFC metamodel is relevant to all four quadrants of the grid. (see Figure 20.1): it can be applied as a **school prevention** model in bringing self-leadership and understanding of parts into the school culture; It can be utilized in **school intervention** though teaching and modeling self-regulation (i.e., "unblending" Self from parts); it can be employed as a **family prevention** tool through introducing Self leadership to parents through psycho-education and workshops; and as a **family intervention** paradigm in the provision of IFS-oriented direct services to students, families, and couples.

IFS as an evidence-based practice

IFS was listed in 2015 on the US SAMHSA's National Registry for Evidence-Based Programs and Practices (NREPP) database as a promising treatment for a number of important mental and physical health conditions such as general functioning and well-being, anxiety, and depression. Because of this, it is now recognized nationally as an effective or promising evidence-based practice for these commonly treated conditions, and the research showing its effectiveness is continuing in order to improve the evidence base.

According to the description of IFS on the NREPP site:

> Internal Family Systems (IFS) Therapy is a psychotherapeutic modality developed in the mid-1980s, based on the observation that clients sometimes experience subpersonalities that come into internal conflict when dealing with challenges.
>
> The IFS model likens these subpersonalities to an 'internal family.'
>
> The IFS model uses mindfulness-based and other strategies to help people resolve internal conflicts in a satisfactory way. During sessions, therapists actively encourage participants to practice self-compassion toward subpersonalities and an internal dialogue. Participants attend individual sessions or group meetings with trained IFS therapists.

Procedure

IFS exercise: building resilience through differentiation of self and parts ("unblending")

The exercise presented here is designed to provide the reader with some basic tools for identifying and working with extreme parts in the service of building greater internal trust and connection with one's own Self.

Purpose

The purpose of this exercise is to help you to become familiar with working with your own "parts". Through this exercise, you can experience identifying your own inner parts, including polarizations of several parts, learning about what motivates them to do what they do. As you go through the exercise, you may feel yourself shifting from being reactive to parts that come up for you to holding more compassion, curiosity, and courage (i.e., qualities of Self leadership). The goal is to be able to sit with and explore a chosen part through inner dialog while manifesting these qualities.

This exercise will also give you a "felt sense" of unblending from parts of you that interfere with your ability to stay grounded in Self leadership and provides a roadmap for helping others to unblend from their parts.

For this exercise, you are asked to choose a "target" part to get to know better. It is recommended that you choose one of your "protectors" (e.g., an "angry" part, a "controlling" part, an "inner critic" part, a "caretaker" part, or any other part that tends to take you over in certain situations). By definition, any of these parts do not trust the Self's ability to lead the system; the desired outcome of this process is to "unblend" from protective part so that you can develop a "Self-to-part" relationship with your chosen target part. It is recommended that you avoid setting an "Exile" part as your target part for the purposes of this exercise; you may experience a backlash of protectors that would want you to get away from burdens that may be revealed by these parts. Examples of Exiled parts might be parts that carry feelings of abandonment, terror, loneliness, grief, neediness, betrayal, or any other deeply felt hurt or unresolved issues.

You may wish to work with a partner to do this exercise.

Figure 20.1 provides a visual flow diagram of the exercise.

Steps

1 Get comfortable; take a few deep breaths.
2 See if you can find different parts of you – focus on a thought, emotion, or sensation in your body, and pay attention to it.
3 As you focus on it, notice how you feel *toward* it. For example, do you cherish it, do you hate it, do you feel compassion for it, do you feel neutral toward it, etc.

4   If you feel anything besides curiosity, compassion or acceptance, then find other parts that are keeping you from getting to know it – see if they will be willing to separate from you so that you can get to know this part.

5   If you sense that there are other parts trying to distract you; if you find yourself in an internal dialog that is closing you down or critiquing this experience or process, or in other ways preventing you from participating fully, just ask the part or parts to step back and allow you the opportunity to experience something new. If you have a sense of fear about getting close to a part, just reassure the part that is fearful that you won't allow the part to overwhelm you or harm you.

6   You may find that these parts won't step back and that's okay – spend time finding out what they are afraid will happen if they let you approach this part/feeling.

7   If they are, then it's safe to approach it and get to know it better.

8   Updating – sometimes, parts become frozen in the past when they took on their protective roles and don't recognize you as your adult Self. When parts do not allow you to focus on the target part (i.e., to "step back"), it's good to update the part.

   Ask:

   Do you know who I am? (if it doesn't know, tell it)

   How old do you think I am? (Make sure it knows your real age)

   If the part doesn't know or sees you as younger or older than you really are, proceed with updating the part through inner dialog or showing it visual scenes of your being older, wiser, more experienced, more competent, etc. than when you were younger and lacking important resources. Show it how you better manage your life than when the part took on its protective role.

   The goal is to show it that you can be trusted more now and that it's safe for it to relax with your presence and allow you to focus on the target part.

9   Take a few minutes to get to know this part.

10 Ask it to not overwhelm you as you get closer to it. You can ask it a variety of questions: for example:

   a   How did it get that way?

   b   What's its role?

   c   What does it need from you?

   d   What other parts is it protecting or protecting you from?

   (Note: this question will sometimes elicit an Exile – this is an OPTIONAL question if you don't feel you know the answer in advance or feel resistance from other parts).

11 When you are ready, prepare yourself to return to the room. Make sure that you show appreciation for any parts that permitted you access to them.

Unblending

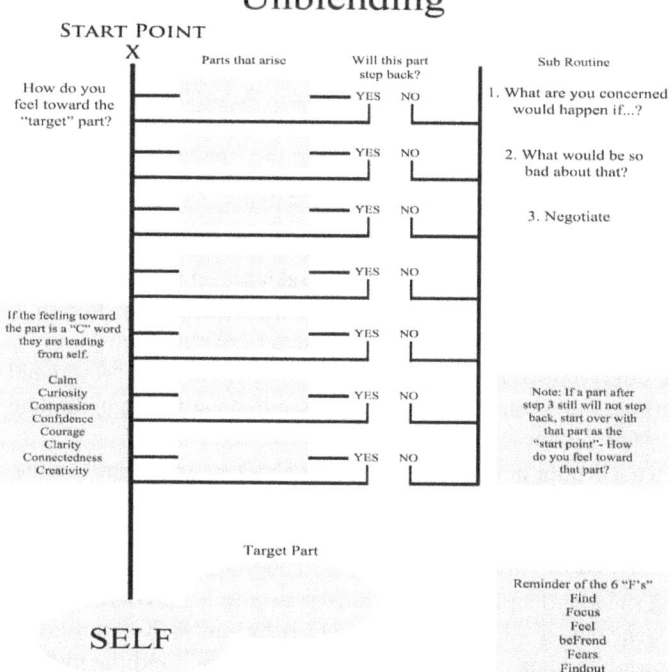

Figure 20.1 IFS unblending exercise

Note: For people who didn't "see" parts – don't feel bad if you didn't have pictures or scenes – many people don't.

Post-exercise reflections

1 How did you experience your parts? Visual? Inner dialog? Body sensation? Emotional? Evocation of memories/scenes in your mind?

2 As you focused on your chosen target part, did you notice other parts being reactive to your attention to it?

3 As you asked parts to "step back", did you notice any changes in how your felt toward or viewed your target part?

4 Did you have to update any parts? If so, how did they react to you after you gave it new information?

5 As you completed the process of becoming familiar with your target part, did you notice any shifts in attitudes of the parts that you asked to step back? Toward you? Toward the target part?

6 In what circumstances did your target part tend to take over? After this process, were you better able to relate to people or situations differently? Did you notice any changes in your current relationships?

Some people experience profound changes as a result of this exercise. If you feel that you need to do further work or would like to take more of a "deep dive" into what the model has to offer you in regard to personal growth or resolution of issues you have been carrying, it is recommended that you seek out the services of a trained IFS therapist to serve as a guide through your "inner journey."

Case example

Lisa, age 32, has been a third-grade teacher in a suburban elementary school for ten years. As a student teacher, she did her student teaching placement in a school near Sandy Hook Elementary School at the time of the shootings. Her ways of coping then were to try to push images of the event "into an imaginary box" and to distract herself from her feelings through "emotional eating". Over time, and with the help of a counselor, she felt that she had "gotten over it".

Recently, after learning about another school shooting in a nearby state, Lisa began experiencing feelings of dread and panic when she entered the school building to teach her class.

At first, she used coping skills learned in her counseling sessions to try to self-regulate but she found it progressively harder to curb her anxiety. During her lunch break one day, she decided to seek out Kathy, the SBFC practitioner in the building who had been trained in the IFS model and used the method to help Lisa to identify and separate from parts of her that were overwhelmed and interfering with her being able to function effectively at her job.

Kathy saw that Lisa was in distress and asked her if she needed help to regulate her emotions. Kathy explained to Lisa that she could help her to get to know the part of her that has taken over her with such high anxiety and to learn about why it was doing that to her. Thus, she could gain some distance from it and help it to express its fears in a safe way that would not overwhelm her. Lisa said that she would be willing to try.

Kathy walked Lisa through the steps of the above exercise and Lisa was able to identify the part of her that was so highly reactive and anxious about being in the school building and was able to feel separate from the part. As she continued, she encountered other parts that wanted to "get rid of" the anxious part or "hated it". As she asked these parts to trust that she could handle hearing from the anxious part, she developed more compassion for it and did not fear it anymore.

At that point, the anxious part began to show her scenes of the day of her internship when she became terrified of dying, including graphic images of the shootings. She asked this part to "take it slowly and to not overwhelm her", and it seemed to understand that she was fully present and willing to listen. This part expressed relief that it was being tended to and began to feel lighter in Lisa's body. This traumatized part was taken through steps to unload the burdens of the images and feelings of terror it carried, and Lisa reported that "it no longer was fearful and just wanted to rest". The parts of her that worked hard to prevent or stop her from feeling anxious were also updated about this release and saw that the "Anxious Part" was no longer a threat. Lisa reported that her internal experience was that these parts all wanted to "hang out together". By the end of the session, Lisa stated that her anxiety level was down to a "one or two" on a scale from 0 to 10 (10 being "Extremely Anxious").

Lisa visited Kathy two weeks later for a follow-up. She reported that she no longer felt anxious or panicked in the building. She was happy that she was able to focus on her students and her teaching again.

Multicultural considerations

The IFS model has been taught worldwide and with a wide range of diverse populations. The model seems to have tapped into some universal human principles that are very relatable on numerous dimensions across cultural boundaries.

In addition, the model has been used in non-clinical applications to address polarizations among various groups. One example is a project that was conducted on the Israeli-Palestinian border in which female kindergarten teachers from both sides of the border came together for training in IFS principles and were able to work on cultural and legacy burdens together, using IFS as a common "Language" (see *Resources*).

Challenges and solutions

The general theme of this chapter pertains to bringing the concept of Self leadership from the IFS model into the educational system – not as a "program" but as a new paradigm for understanding trauma and resilience in the educational context. We have introduced the idea that the leaders in the schools need to hold to and model Self leadership in their own internal psychology before they would be capable of providing the type of leadership in their spheres of influence that lead to resilience.

In introducing such a new paradigm, there are many challenges attached to such efforts. A few will be listed with some suggestions for possible solutions.

1 **Resistance of administrators to add another program to an already-taxed teaching staff**. Even if administrators recognize the need to support the emotional health and well-being of their staff, there is a great deal of pressure to prioritize achievement outcomes; thus, many of the programs that schools buy into are geared toward increasing compliance and controlling behaviors. While many of these programs are attractive and are touted as "evidence-based" or "best practices", ultimately it requires teachers to take time out of their already over-taxed schedules and duties to attend trainings to deliver these programs in

the classroom with little "return on investment" for the teachers. Many principals and superintendents are aware of the impact of asking teachers to take on yet another program that takes them out of the classroom.

2 **Changing social and emotional climate in the school to promote Self leadership vs. punitive or controlling discipline practices.** Given all of the pressures faced by teachers, staff, special services personnel, and school administrators, there is often a "bunker" mentality where the adults feel that they are constantly having to be reactive to emergent situations. The IFS model holds that when situations are being managed with a sense of reactivity, then we would expect to see an increase in reactiveness, polarizations, and self-fulfilling prophesies occurring in the day-to-day interchange in the school. In many of our schools, social control and providing "discipline" are the tools *de rigeur* to maintain structure and stability. This becomes a challenge to those who recognize the self-defeating dilemmas that such an approach creates and perpetuates. Even when well-meaning programs are introduced into a school or district, very often, the execution and sustainability of such programs get lost due to the dynamics outlined above in Challenge #2.

3 **Fears of protective parts to potentially open emotional wounds.** Teachers and administrators, like students, have relationships, roles and challenging circumstances beyond the school walls that carry emotional weight into the school building. As an "institution of learning", there often is an expectation (and a desire) to use the time in school to separate from outside issues and to focus on tasks and routines that seem more circumscribed, despite the day-to-day challenges faced in the school. By focusing on teaching or dealing with educational or behavioral challenges, staff can feel a sense of competence and control beyond what they experience when they go home; they can compartmentalize their stress and emotional challenges while they are at work. The stress and traumas that individuals carry are thus avoided or pushed away in their school roles only to re-emerge once they leave for the day (or sometimes manifest as "outbursts" or "breakdowns" or even somatically by way of illnesses in the school). Thus, the introduction of anything that can create a sense of vulnerability (such as discussing their "parts") can feel threatening and lead to further reinforcement of their inner and outer protective systems. The very protective nature of these strategies and tactics to avoid feeling overwhelmed can reinforce the very issues they are trying to mitigate.

Solutions

Many of the programs alluded to above rely on the adults to provide "content" and "skills" to students as ways of controlling disruptive behavior or to motivate students to function better in the learning environment of the school. Such programs as teaching "mindfulness" or "coping skills", running "restorative justice" groups, or "social emotional learning" skills all have in common the teaching of a curriculum to the students by adults. This requires that teachers and other staff take time to attend trainings, do outside reading and adjust their lesson plans to incorporate new learning structures or content, taking time away from what they see as their primary responsibility of imparting knowledge to their students. This creates a cycle of resentment and ultimately "burnout" for these front-line workers.

The IFS model, in introducing the idea of Self leadership, provides an antidote to the expectations that teachers and administrators in the school building will be able to teach yet another set of skills to their students with minimal training or promise of positive impact. Rather than providing new teaching mandates or giving workbooks or manuals to teach unpracticed skills to disinterested students, the IFS approach focuses on working with the adults to provide them with the tools and strategies that will help them to be better teachers and leaders in their interactions with their own inner worlds and their relationships with others – including their families and primary relationships, students, fellow educators, and the families of their students. IFS and the concept of Self leadership remove the stigma of extreme emotional and behavioral responses that are commonly defined as "mental health symptoms" and reframe them as "attempts at adapting to perceived and experienced stress".

The goal is to bring Self leadership into the school's ecology as a new language and a new way of "being" in support of creating balance and harmony among all involved. This will require the introduction of the IFS paradigm as a different approach than other social programs (e.g., Restorative Justice [Wachtel, 2012] and Social Emotional Learning [Weissberg, Durlak, Domitrovich, & Gullotta, 2015]) that directly and quickly impacts real-time outcomes in the day-to-day interactions in the schools. This is a new frontier in education and there is an international group of IFS-trained educational professionals who have been meeting regularly to discuss strategies for a successful and sustainable launching of this paradigm into our educational system. If the reader is interested in learning more, please go to the "Self Leadership Collaborative" website, listed below.

Resources

Additional information on the inclusion of IFS in NREPP can be found here: http://www.foundationifs.org/news-articles/79-ifs-an-evidence-based-practice
A listing of IFS-trained therapists in your area can be found on the IFS Institute website's provider directory at the following link: IFS Directory | IFS Institute (ifs-institute.com).
For CBFC professionals who would like to pursue formal training in the use of the IFS model, please visit Trainings | IFS Institute (ifs-institute.com) for a list of trainings. Many are on-line but several are in an in-person format.
IFS Video: Israeli-Palestinian intervention in which female kindergarten teachers from both sides of the border came together for training in IFS

principles and were able to work on cultural and legacy burdens together, using IFS as a common "Language". Link: (2015 Internal Family Systems Conference - ME | IFS Institute (ifs-institute.com)

The Self-Leadership Collaborative: An Innovative, Systemic and Sustainable Approach to Nurture Well-being for Students, Educators and Whole School Culture Inspired by the Transformative Paradigm of Internal Family Systems (IFS). URL: www.SelfLeadershipCollaborative.com

References

Breunlin, Douglas C., Schwartz, Richard C. & Kune-Karrer, Mac (1997). *Metaframeworks: Transcending the Models of Family Therapy.* Jossey-Bass.

Goddard, Rodger (2019a). *The IFS Teacher Manual: A Training Handbook for Using Internal Family Systems to Improve Teacher Effectiveness and Student Success.* Success Skills.

Goddard, Rodger (2019b). *The IFS Parent Manual: Using Internal Family Systems to Build Your Child's School and Life Success.* Success Skills.

Hawkes, Neil & Hawkes, Jane (2018). *The Inner Curriculum: How to Nourish Wellbeing, Resilience and Self-Leadership.* John Cott Educational.

Kroll, Linda (2016). *Compassionate Mediation (For Relationships at a Crossroad).* CreateSpace.com (Amazon Publisher).

Liu, Emily (2020). *Climax: Why Great Leaders Need Love Affairs: An Enlightening Leadership Fable.* New Chapter Press.

Livingstone, John B. & Gaffney, Joanne (2016). *Relationship Power in Health Care: Science of Behavior Change, Decision Making, and Clinician Self-Care.* CRC Press.

Schwartz, Richard C. (1994). *Internal Family Systems Therapy.* Guilford Press.

Schwartz, Richard C. & Sweezy, Martha (2021). *Internal Family Systems Therapy, Second Edition.* Guilford Press.

Shadick, Nancy A., Sowell, Nancy F., Frits, Michelle L., Hoffman, Suzanne M., Hartz, Shelley A., Booth, Fran D., Sweezy, Martha, Rogers, Patricia R., Dubin, Rina L., Atkinson, Amy L., Augusto, Rernando, Iannaccone, Christine K., Fossel, Anne H., Quinn, Jing Cui, Losina, Elena, & Schwartz, Richard C. (2013). A Randomized Controlled Trial of an Internal Family Systems-based Psychotherapeutic Intervention on Outcomes in Rheumatoid Arthritis: A Proof-of-Concept Study. *The Journal of Rheumatology.* August 2013, jrheum.121465; https://doi.org/10.3899/jrheum.121465

Van Der Kolk, Bessel (2014). *The Body Keeps The Score: Mind, Brain And Body In Transformation Of Trauma.* Penguin Books.

Wachtel, Ted. "Defining Restorative". International Institute for Restorative Practices. Retrieved 11 July 2012. What Is Restorative Practices? | Restorative Practices (iirp.edu)

Weissberg, Roger P., Durlak, Joseph A., Domitrovich, Celene E. & Gullotta, Thomas P. (Eds.) (2015). Social and Emotional Learning: Past, Present, and Future. In *Handbook on Social and Emotional Learning: Research and Practice* (pp. 3–19). Guilford Press.

21 Teacher development

Promoting teacher-family engagement to support crisis preparedness

Karen S. Buchanan and Thomas D. Buchanan

Overview

This chapter prepares SBFC professionals and school personnel to implement a three-stage professional development plan designed to support teacher and family collaborative relationships. Teachers build knowledge and skill around research-informed family engagement principles that are foundational to the support of diverse communities in a time of crisis.

Background

Teachers, as trusted individuals, are uniquely positioned to serve children and families in the event of a crisis. However, there is evidence that most teachers feel unprepared for this work (NAFSCE, 2022). Supporting the development of teachers who have the knowledge and skill to collaborate with families and connect them to resources will, among other important outcomes, encourage the relational foundation needed to assist parents/caregivers following an adverse event.

In *School-Based Family Counseling: Transforming Family-School Relationships*, Gerrard and Soriano (2013) write, "...family systems theory recognizes the interdependence of various systems in our society--be they the school, the family, or the community context--as well as the vulnerability of the child depending on these systems for his/her development" (p. 9). This provides a deeply rooted basis for partnerships designed to support the healthy development of children. With this interdependence in mind, and in alignment with the "School Prevention" quadrant of the SBFC metamodel, this chapter presents teacher development that can proactively support teacher knowledge and skills needed to support families in the event of a crisis or disaster.

Evidence-based support

The verbs "collaborate" and "connect" represent two research-informed family engagement principles addressed in the teacher professional development described below. These principles have strong support (NAFSCE, 2022).

DOI: 10.4324/9781003201977-26

Collaborate: Through collaborative conversations with parents and caregivers, teachers can grow in an understanding of families. This includes insight into the unique needs and concerns of diverse communities (Buchanan & Buchanan, 2020; Clark-Louque & Sullivan, 2020) and an increase in the teacher's knowledge of the learner, such as experiential funds of knowledge (Darling-Hammond & Oakes, 2019). Teachers who seek, respect, and honor the expertise held by parents/caregivers are able to apply this knowledge to classroom practice (Buchanan & Buchanan, 2020; NAFSCE, 2022).

Foundational to effective collaboration is the knowledge and understanding of those with which you are collaborating (Amatea, 2009). Teacher professional development can support the creation of collaborative relationships and effective communication with families (Darling-Hammond & Oakes, 2019; Leibforth & Clark, 2009).

Connect: Teachers connect when they build reciprocal relationships with families and when they foster interprofessional partnerships. Epstein writes:

> It is imperative for new teachers to understand family diversities, community resources, student experiences in and out of school, and how to use all available resources to maximize student learning and success. This knowledge and these skills are measures of teachers' professional skills and standing.
>
> (2018, p. 401)

Teachers should view themselves as a member of a collaborative, interprofessional team.

When a crisis or disaster occurs, teachers are positioned to provide needed support for students (Le Brocque et al., 2017) and for families (Mutch, 2020). Students and their families may be distressed by a loss of community. Teachers may be sought out as someone who will "know what to do" (Mutch, 2020, p. 4). Teachers can be key in helping students to build a strong support system by providing connections to school and community resources. Teachers who meet the complex demands of today's classroom envision and position themselves as part of a team of professionals and non-professionals who work collaboratively on behalf of the well-being and academic success of learners (Buchanan & Buchanan, 2020; Epstein, 2018). Strengthening the skills needed for reciprocal relationships with families and also for interdisciplinary work with SBFC professionals are areas of need worthy of well-crafted professional learning (Darling-Hammond et al., 2017). In addition to crisis preparedness, relational interprofessional efforts can strengthen family-school engagement and produce improved student outcomes (Epstein, 2018; Mutch, 2020). Relationships matter. Meaningful relationships with students, families, and colleagues are integral to vital aspects of teaching (Constantino, 2021; Darling-Hammond & Oakes, 2019).

Procedure

The following teacher professional development plan makes use of professional learning features, drawn from research, that positively impact teacher practice (Darling-Hammond et al., 2017). The plan follows a three-stage approach: ***Engage***, ***Apply***, and ***Reflect***. We suggest that the three-stage sequence occur over the course of four weeks. Revisiting this content over time will result in more powerful learning. As indicated in *Box 21.1, the* ***Engage*** and ***Reflect*** sessions are both designed for face-to-face or synchronous, virtual sessions. Sessions can be offered during a faculty meeting or as part of a designated professional development day. If delivered virtually, facilitators will adapt the small group work using features of the electronic meeting system being used; for example, when using zoom, facilitators can use the chat and zoom room features for small group engagement. The ***Apply*** activity falls between the ***Engage*** and ***Reflect*** sessions and is designed to be completed by individual teachers during their preparation time.

Box 21.1 Engage, Apply, Reflect

Stage 1: Engage session; face-to-face or virtual

This plan begins with a 30-to-40-minute session focused on engaging teachers in content designed to enhance collaboration with families through relationships and reciprocal communication. This session ends by asking teachers to "Give-It-a-Go" as they independently complete Stage 2.

Stage 2: Apply activity; "Give-It-a-Go; Family Conversations," completed independently

At a time of their choosing, teachers are asked to apply concepts from the ***Engage session*** in the "Family Conversations" activity. Facilitators send electronic messages to teachers encouraging them to complete the activity in preparation for the coming ***Reflect session***.

Stage 3: Reflect session; face-to-face or virtual

The final stage is a 30-to-40-minute session designed around collegial sharing. First teachers reflect on what they have learned about students and their families during the "Family Conversations" activity. Then, they think together about interprofessional resources that could serve students and families during a crisis.

Professional development plan

Stage 1: Engage session

Focus: Collaborate

Step 1: Preparation

Facilitators organize professional learning activity materials. Be sure to supply paper/pencils on tables and a copy of the **Give it a Go Activity: Family Conversations** for each participant.

Step 2: Welcome and community-care warm-up

The facilitator welcomes teachers as they arrive and begins the session by directing a community-care warm-up activity.

Facilitator: *Welcome! It is good to be together this afternoon. I'd like us to begin our session with a "Take Notice" activity. I'd like everyone to take a deep breath or two and relax for a moment. (Pause) Take a moment and think about our team of faculty and staff. Who or what thoughtful act or kindness have you experienced this last week that has gone unnoticed, yet has been a great encouragement to you? It could be something really simple or a very big favor. I'd like to open the floor for us to share or "take notice" of the things adults in our community do that encourage us and support our work.*

*Teachers share * (Allow 4–5 minutes of sharing.)

Facilitator: Thank you for all that you do for our community.

Step 3: Introduction: Relationships

Facilitator: *We begin today by asking you to think for a moment about a really valuable relationship that you have with someone in your life. What are the qualities or characteristics that make that relationship strong? Turn to someone sitting near you and have a brief conversation about those characteristics.*

*Teachers share with a partner *

Facilitator: *I wonder if each of you would simply name, for our whole group, one of the characteristics you and your colleague talked about?*

Teachers share with the whole group

Step 4: Share session goals

The facilitator shares the goals of the session and engages participants in those goals.

Facilitator: *Today we are going to be thinking together about how building collaborative relationships with the families of our learners has the benefit of supporting our students in a time of crisis. Some of the characteristics that you shared a moment ago will likely show* up in our discussions today because our work will focus on three research-informed principles for intentionally building collaborative relationships with families:

1   Parent/caregiver knowledge is needed;
2   Two-way communication is critical; and
3   Teachers take the lead

Facilitator: *To explore the first principle about the need for parent/caregiver knowledge, I'd like to ask you to stand up and create groups of three individuals (wait for the triads to form). Wonderful. Now, I'd like each of you to choose a child in your life that you are going to be describing. This can be your own child, a grandchild, a niece/nephew or the child of a good friend. In your groups, I'd like you to describe some of the unique characteristics of that child and one piece of information that you believe would be important for their teacher to know. (The facilitator circulates among the groups, listening in.)*

 Participant example: *My nephew Paul is extremely creative and shy. I would want his teacher to know that he can engage with other kids when he is encouraged to.*

 Facilitator: *Our first principle for building collaborative relationships honors the role of parents/caregivers and acknowledges that they have important information to share about their child. As teachers, we need their knowledge as we seek to help their child thrive. Families are a child's first, and most important teacher. When families and teachers, both, share the knowledge that they have regarding the child, a mutual respect begins to emerge and that respect paves the way for collaboration.*

Step 5: Two-way communication is critical

Facilitator: *The second principle for building collaborative relationships states that two-way or reciprocal communication is critical. When this type of communication is practiced, it lays the foundation for open communication during a crisis. Families will feel free to share with teachers the needs that are emerging during a challenging time and teachers will have an established line of communication to share critical information and resources.*

 Much of the communication that comes from school is one-way communication, for example, newsletters that are sent to homes. Two-way communication, however, invites those receiving the communication to respond and engage in conversation. I would like each of you to think of at least one example of two-way communication in your teaching practice or in your experiences as a parent with a teacher (pause). Who can share an example?

 Teachers share examples of two-way communication practices

 Often, simply adding an invitation to one of your current communication pieces, inviting a family member to connect, is a starting point for the kind of reciprocal communication that you hope to develop. I encourage you to take one small step to foster more two-way communication with your families/caregivers.

Step 6: Teachers take the lead

Facilitator: *A third principle for us to consider says that "teachers take the lead" in the process of building collaborative relationships. As teachers reach out, they welcome parents into a relationship and affirm that families belong. A teacher's words matter. Words that indicate you believe families have important information to share about the child tells families that you, as teacher, value their perspective. I would like each of you to think about approaching a parent and asking if you might spend a few minutes speaking with them about their child; learning from them about their child and hearing the hopes/dreams they have for their child. What words might you use that would indicate that you value the parent's perspective? There is paper and pencils on your tables. Please write a brief draft of words you might use.*

*Teachers write down words that invite families to a conversation *

Facilitator: *Would two or three of you be willing to share the words you crafted with the group?*

*Allow several teachers to share the words they've written. (E.g. Tony says, "Ms. Jones, I would love the chance to visit with you about John's passion for board games. A conversation with you will give me some ideas for ways to motivate John in our classroom.") *

Facilitator: *These words that you have written will assist you during the next couple of weeks as you have a chance to put into practice the principles that we've talked about today.*

Step 7: Give it a go activity

Facilitator: *During the next couple of weeks, take an opportunity to engage in a brief conversation with three or four of your student's families. These conversations give you the chance to apply what we've talked about in this session. You will "take the lead" by inviting a family member into a conversation. You both will engage in two-way communication, and you will seek to learn from families and affirm that you value them as partners in the education and well-being of their child. These conversations can take place via phone, zoom or in person. Please complete this* **Give it a Go: Family Conversations** *activity prior to our next gathering. At that time, you will debrief your family conversation experiences with colleagues. I'm going to hand each of you the details for the* **Give it a Go Activity** *and I'd like you to read it over.*

Give it a Go Activity: Family Conversations *– Arrange a time for three to four conversations with parents/caregivers of learners in your classroom. Listen to caregivers share about the specific strengths and talents they see in their child. Ask for helpful things they would like to share about working with their child or with their family. Take the opportunity to affirm your desire to work collaboratively with them. You are encouraged to consider visiting with families that represent culturally diverse, minority, special needs, economically challenged, or traditionally underprivileged populations.*

Facilitator: *What questions do you have about this activity you will complete independently?*

Teachers ask questions; clarify their understanding

Step 8: Closure

Facilitator: *Today, we've spent time thinking about the importance of developing collaborative relationships with our families. Hearing the voices of families gives us a deeper window into "who" each student is. These relationships not only enhance our daily work with students, but are vitally important during a crisis. Following a crisis, having established two-way lines of communication will help you to know more about the needs of your students and will enable you to make a difference for children and families.*

Before we leave, I'd like to offer you the opportunity to tell the group something you heard today that is helpful to you or has caused you to think in deeper ways about collaborative relationships with families?

Teachers share with the whole group

Stage 2: Give it a go activity

Step #1: *Facilitators should plan two communication messages to teachers encouraging them to complete their* **Give it a Go Activity**. *The first message should serve as a follow up to Session 1. The second message should be sent a couple of days before* **Reflect: Session 2**. *Messages can be sent via email, text message, or through a short video or voice recording (see the example text that follows).*

Facilitator: Message #1 Example: *Teachers, thank you for your good work in our session focused on enhancing family collaboration. Please make time this week to complete your* **Give it a Go Activity: Family Conversations**. *You will:*

> *Arrange a time for 3–4 conversations with parents/caregivers of learners in your classroom. Listen to caregivers share about the specific strengths and talents they see in their child. Ask for helpful things they would like to share about working with their child or with their family. Take the opportunity to affirm your desire to work collaboratively with them. Consider visiting with families that represent culturally diverse, minority, special needs, economically challenged, or traditionally underprivileged populations.*

Facilitator: Message #2 Example: *Teachers, just a friendly reminder that we will meet together again in a couple of days. You need to be sure to complete your* **Family Conversations: Give it a Go Activity** *prior to our session. I look forward to your reflections on your family conversations.*

Stage 3: Reflect session

FOCUS: Connect

Step 1: Preparation

The facilitator organizes professional learning activity materials. Be sure to have paper/pencils on tables. Additionally, have access to a whiteboard, poster paper or a similar way to record information shared by participants.

Step 2: Share Session Goals

The facilitator shares the goals of the session.

Facilitator: *Our session today is focused on two goals:*

1 *First, we will reflect on your experiences completing the* **Give it a Go: Family Conversations** *activity.*
2 *Then, we will spend a few moments thinking about the opportunity teachers have to serve as connectors to families by exploring resources that could serve students and families during a crisis.*

Step 3: The facilitator begins by asking teachers to form small groups of three to four colleagues. These groups will reflect on their experiences with the **Give it a Go: Family Conversations**. Consider posting the bulleted questions below in the room to give participants a visual to access during their discussion.

Facilitator: *Teachers, while you often are in a position to deliver important information to families; families also have critical information that you need as you serve their child. I hope you enjoyed the chance to be a learner from a handful of the families/caregivers of your students as you completed the* **Give it a Go: Family Conversations**. *Reciprocal communication and relationships with families are foundational to crisis preparedness. I'd like you to have a chance to visit with a small group of colleagues about your experiences with this task. Here are some possible questions to consider as you share: (point to the visual of these questions)*

- *Did you learn anything new about your student?*
- *Did you discover information about the family/caregiver that will impact your work with them?*
- *Did you discover any needs or potential needs the student or family have?*
- *Did you experience any change in attitude or perspective by virtue of this experience? Or did the family member seem to experience an attitudinal change?*

It is important for everyone in your group to get a chance to share. I will let you know when we are halfway through our allotted time so that your group can be sure that all can participate.

*Teachers reflect on their **Give it a Go** *experiences with their small group.**

Step 4: *As facilitator, you will walk around to the small groups listening to their conversations, keeping an eye on the time you have allotted for this activity. When you hit the halfway mark, say the following:*

Facilitator: *Colleagues, we are halfway through our sharing time. Please be sure that everyone in your group has a chance to share their experiences.*

Step 5: *When the sharing time ends, facilitate a whole group sharing.*

Facilitator: *Thanks for sharing with your colleagues. I'd like to invite one person from each small group to share something from their conversation that they believe is important for our whole group to hear or think about.*

One teacher from each group shares. (E.g. Joan said, "I enjoyed a conversation with the mother of my student, Amy. I find it amazing that from a simple conversation, I can feel myself growing in empathy for this family.")

Step 6: The facilitator leads a whole group discussion about family/caregiver needs that the ***Give it a Go: Family Conversations*** *activity revealed. The facilitator records "Needs Shared" on a whiteboard or a computer screen.*

Facilitator: *I'm curious about the student or family/caregiver needs you discovered through your **Give it a Go: Family Conversations**. Let's spend a few minutes, as a whole group, sharing some of these discoveries. I ask that you protect the confidentiality of the family member by not using their name.*

Teachers share needs they discovered with the whole group.

Facilitator: *The research around schools experiencing a crisis or disaster tells us that you, as teachers, are particularly positioned to connect families to resources that are available to support children and families. You have the unique opportunity to be a CONNECTOR. However, to be able to connect folks, you need to be aware of the assets that currently exist in our setting and community. While this might sound like an overwhelming task, I'd like us to put our heads together and see what our team already knows about assets inside our school and local community. We are going to accomplish this by engaging in an activity called "Widening our Circle of Gratitude." Through this activity we are all going to expand our knowledge of the people and services that can make a difference for our children and families.*

Please take a piece of paper and a writing tool from the center of your table. I am going to ask you to think beyond the teaching staff with which you regularly interact. Think broadly about individuals within our school community and our neighborhood community for which you are grateful because of the assets they bring. What contributions do they make that have a positive impact on students and families? I'd like you to write down WHO they are and what ROLE they serve in. Then, write specifically how they contribute to the well-being of children and families (pause and allow time for completing this task). In your table groups, share your lists with one another (facilitator circulates by the groups noting who they have identified).

Teachers share with their groups

I'm going to ask one member of your group to come to our whiteboard and write up the school and community assets your group has identified.

One member of each group writes the groups' contributions on the whiteboard.

Facilitator: *I'd like to invite you to take a look at the assets/resources that have been identified by our group. These resources are available to us to serve students and families.*

Step 5: Closure: The facilitator thanks teachers for their participation. Each school will have access to their own unique assets and/or professionals that can play supportive roles during a crisis. The list that follows is an example of the kinds of individuals that might emerge in the teacher discussion. Note the SBFC professionals that will likely emerge in these discussions. Facilitators can highlight the opportunity for interprofessional work.

- social workers
- counselors

- school psychologists
- school nurses
- special education specialists (occupational therapist, speech therapist, autism specialists)
- student welfare coordinators
- pastors
- youth workers
- athletic coaches
- school administrators

This session is designed to explore, with teachers, the possible assets that already exist in their setting. Teachers can become connectors to these resources. Facilitators may want to extend this work with teachers at a later date, by inviting individuals in to talk, in detail, about what they have to offer in terms of support for children and families.

Facilitator: *Teachers, thank you for your good work as we have enhanced our ability to build collaborative relationships with families and explored how we might be connectors of resources to support the needs of children and families. You play a particularly supportive role during a crisis and preparation prior to such an event provides the foundation that will enable you to make a difference.*

Multicultural considerations

As plans for professional development are drafted, facilitators will want to give attention to how they refer to families, parents, and caregivers. Most of us will tend to look at these constructs through the lens of our own experience. Because we value inclusivity and because we want to support all of our students, we need to keep in mind that there are many different ways to be a family and that those who are parenting children, while having many things in common, are also quite dissimilar. Facilitators should pause from time to time and check the way they reference families and those who parent to be sure their language is inclusive and acknowledges diversity.

In their book, *Equity Partnerships: A Culturally Proficient Guide to Family, School, and Community Engagement* (Clark-Louque et al., 2020), the authors identify a culturally competent school culture as one where "Families and school staff work together to identify and address needs of diverse cultural populations" (p. 17). They further label the "prevention of changes intended to benefit culturally different community and student groups" as an act of "cultural destructiveness" (p. 17). We believe that most teachers want to be culturally competent.

One way to engage teachers in professional development is to appeal to their deeply held values (NAFSCE, 2022). We believe that the opportunity in these sessions to participate in discussions with colleagues regarding ways to move toward more equitable family engagement will be meaningful and motivating to the school community. Making explicit connections between faculty learning, growth, and the healthy development of ALL learners, regardless of background, will foster support and make for a rich professional development experience.

Challenges and solutions

One of the consistent challenges of a one-size-fits-all professional learning session is that not all teachers in attendance have the same teaching situation. At the elementary level, the majority of the teachers in attendance will be teaching in self-contained classrooms with a small number of students served each day. At the secondary level, however, educators often have large student caseloads, teaching many different groups of students each day. Learning specialists serve specialized populations of students across multiple grade levels. Facilitators need to acknowledge these differences during the sessions and encourage participants to apply this work to their particular teaching assignment. Facilitators can choose to differentiate small group work by grouping teachers from similar teaching assignments for discussions. Building collaborative relationships with the families of learners is critically important and applicable for all teachers at all grade levels.

Conclusion

The three-stage professional development plan presented here, **Engage**, **Apply**, and **Reflect**, offers SBFC professionals and school leaders a strong model of professional development. When teachers are provided these opportunities to engage in the "collaborate" and "connect" principles of family engagement, they increase their capacity to successfully facilitate the healthy development and academic achievement of all learners. Growth in teacher-family engagement will lead to schools that, in the event of crisis or disaster, are better prepared to serve students and their families.

Resources

Common Sense Education https://www.commonsense.org/education/top-picks/apps-and-websites-for-improving-parent-teacher-communication
This site is filled with apps and websites for improving parent-teacher communication.
Family Engagement: Resource Roundup https://www.edutopia.org/home-school-connections-resources
This Edutopia website offers tips, strategies and resources to enhance teacher and family engagement.
Greater Good in Education; Science-Based Practices for Kinder, Happier Schools https://ggie.berkeley.edu/
The Greater Good in Education website contains many evidence-based activities designed to enhance teacher and family engagement. Activities incorporated in the ENGAGE and REFLECT sessions were adapted from this resource.

Toolkit of Resources for Engaging Families and the Community as Partners in Education https://ies.ed.gov/ncee/edlabs/regions/pacific/pdf/REL_2016148. pdf

This research-informed resource is filled with ideas that help teachers consider their professional dispositions related to family engagement as well as hands on strategies for collaboration with diverse families.

References

Amatea, E. S. (2009). *Building culturally responsive family-school relationships*. Upper Saddle River, NJ: Pearson.

Buchanan, K. S., & Buchanan, T. D. (2020). Strengthening a collaborative paradigm: Building an Interprofessional skill in emergent teachers. *International Journal for School-based Family Counseling*, 12. Available at: https://www.schoolbasedfamilycounseling.com/articles-by-volume

Clark-Louque, A. R., Lindsey, R. B., Quezada, R. L., & Jew, C. L. (2020). *Equity partnerships: A culturally proficient guide to family, school, and community engagement*. Corwin.

Clark-Louque, A., & Sullivan, T. A. (2020). Black girls and school discipline: Shifting from the narrow zone of zero tolerance to a wide region of restorative practices and culturally proficient partnerships. *Journal of Leadership, Equity, and Research*, 6(2), 1–21. http://journals.sfu.ca/cvj/index.php/cvj/index

Constantino, S. M. (2021). *Engage every family: Five simple principles* (2nd ed.). Corwin.

Darling-Hammond, L., Hyler, M. E., & Gardner, M. (2017). *Effective teacher professional development*. Learning Policy Institute.

Darling-Hammond, L., & Oakes, J. (2019). *Preparing teachers for deeper learning*. Cambridge, Massachusetts: Harvard Education Press.

Epstein, J. L. (2018). School, family, and community partnerships in teachers' professional work. *Journal of Education for Teaching*, 44(3), 397–406.

Gerrard, B., & Soriano, M. (2013). *School-based family counseling: Transforming family-school relationships*. United States: Institute for School-Based Family Counseling.

Le Brocque, R., De Young, A., Montague, G., Pocock, S., March, S., Triggell, N., … & Kenardy, J. (2017). Schools and natural disaster recovery: The unique and vital role that teachers and education professionals play in ensuring the mental health of students following natural disasters. *Journal of Psychologists and Counsellors in Schools*, 27(1), 1–23.

Leibforth, T., & Clark, M. (2009). Getting acquainted with students' families. In E. S. Amatea (Ed.), *Building culturally responsive family-school relationships* (pp. 201–230). Upper Saddle River, NJ: Pearson.

Mutch, C. (2020). How might research on schools' responses to earlier crises help us in the COVID-19 recovery process? Set: Research Information for Teachers. doi:10.18296/set.0169

National Association for Family, School, and Community Engagement (2022). Body of knowledge for family-facing professionals. NAFSCE. https://nafsce.org/page/BoK

22 Strengthening families during a crisis through teacher-parent engagement

Nurit Kaplan Toren and Jaffa Weiss

Overview

This chapter describes how to strengthen parents and families, with the aim of helping them develop skills which will help during crisis. We believe that teachers can initiate such a process, based on parents-teachers trust relationships.

Background

Parents need not possess an academic degree or a license to play their role as caregivers. They practice parenting based on their pre-parental period in life, when they viewed parenthood as children, and read or watched movies about parents-children relationships.

Parents tend to believe that their parenting methods are best suitable for their children and family, and therefore, any criticism, inspection, or even small criticisms or insinuations by others, regarding their parenthood, are seen as putting their competence as parents in doubt. Therefore, teachers should be trained to connect with parents, especially during stressful situations.

However, sometimes the way teachers invite parents to be involved in their child's education and life has a significant effect on both the parents and the child.

Family engagement, which includes parents' involvement in the child's education at home and school, as well as in forming parents-teacher relationships from kindergarten (Ogg et al., 2021) to high school (Kaplan Toren & Seginer, 2015), is essential.

Disasters affect families as well as children. Parents serve as a buffer for the child's stress and have a critical role in disaster response and management (Tambling et al., 2021). Children look up to their parents, searching for cues to act, especially during disasters and stressful situations. How parents function during and after the disaster has a significant influence on how children respond. For example, research has shown an association between parental anxiety and depression and child anxiety and depression (Goodman & Brand, 2011). Moreover, findings reveal a link between parents' internalized symptoms during the COVID-19 pandemic and adolescents' behavioral pattern of

DOI: 10.4324/9781003201977-27

avoidance (Lorenzo et al., 2021). Therefore, healthy family functioning helps children to adopt positive strategies during crisis.

The present chapter focuses on the contributions of teacher-parent positive relationships as a predictor of family engagement and family resilience and suggests methods that teachers can use to support parents before, during, and after a crisis.

Trust between parents and teachers is essential for establishing effective parents' and teachers' partnerships (Adams & Christenson, 1998). Trust has been defined in the context of parent-teacher relationships as "confidence that another person will act in a way to benefit or sustain the relationship" to achieve positive outcomes for students (Adams & Christenson, 1998, p. 6). Parents with higher trust, according to teachers' reports, engage in more parental involvement behaviors than parents reporting low trust (Adams & Christenson, 1998). Additionally, parents' trust in teachers predicts important child outcomes, such as higher credits earned, GPA, and attendance (Adams & Christenson, 2000).

Following the School-Based Family Counseling (SBFC) model (Gerrard & Soriano, 2020), this chapter will focus on both prevention and intervention.

This chapter outlines both prevention and intervention actions. Prevention is any action that helps and strengthens children and adults to cope with life in a positive way and to improve their well-being. Successful prevention activities will be a good basis for an intervention program in times of crisis.

School-Focus			
Prevention Focus	**School-Family Prevention** 1. Getting to know each other - Expectations Management 2. Establishing teacher-parents' partnership - Developing communication channels	**School-Family Intervention** 1. Strengthening parents' self-efficacy 2. Teacher-parents' informal talk	**Intervention Focus**
	Family and Child Prevention 1. Expresing emotions and the awareness of one's strengths	**Family and child intervention** 1. Strengthening parent-child interaction 2. Encouraging a family to function as a unit	
Family-Focus			

Figure 22.1 How to strengthen family competence according to SBFC metamodel

Intervention is taking action to strengthen and protect children and adults, when someone is at risk. Intervention includes a process of identifying that someone is at risk and taking steps to ensure their safety.

Prevention is like preparing for use of your umbrella and coat, whereas intervention is actually using them on rainy days.

In the current chapter, prevention focuses on ways to develop teacher-parent trust relationships and on developing awareness of one's strengths and emotions.

Intervention focuses on ways in which teachers can strengthen parents' self-efficacy, improve parent-child interaction, and encourage a family to function as a unit (Figure 22.1).

Procedure

Part 1: Prevention

A major aspect of strengthening the family is building and promoting trust between parents and teachers. In order to promote that, trust building steps should be taken, starting with the initial meeting between the teachers and the parents and continuing with the period of acquaintance and joint work.

Getting to know each other – expectations management

Aims: To reach an understanding regarding expectations that both parents and teachers have from each other.

To exchange expectations in an accurate and clear manner, which will allow for a follow-up along the way, regarding meeting the expectations.

Target population: parents, homeroom teacher, and teachers

Students' age: from kindergarten to high school

Challenges: The process should take into consideration the age of the students, addressing both the needs of the group as one unit and the needs of each individual in the group.

Activities

In the first teacher-parents meeting, at the beginning of the year (Open House), the teacher will ask each of the parents participating in the meeting, to mention one expectation they have of the teacher in the coming year.

While all the expectations are expressed and noted by all the members of the group, the teacher will write them on the board, for all participants to see. It is recommended that one of the participants takes notes of what was said, for the future use of the teacher. The teacher himself/herself must prepare, in advance, his/her "credo," his/her worldview regarding the interaction between teachers and parents and the importance he/she sees in the rapport between parents and teachers for the well-being of the children.

In the second part of that meeting, parents write down on a sheet of paper their personal expectation from the teacher regarding their own child. Those sheets of papers will be collected by the teachers, to help them create a channel of private dialogue between themselves and the parents and will enable the teachers to treat the children in a way that suits their personal needs.

Establishing a partnership – developing communication channels

END OF THE SEMESTER CONVERSATION BETWEEN TEACHERS AND PARENTS

Aim: To report to the parents about the conduct of their son/daughter during the semester, emphasizing the emotional and social aspects, as well as the successes and difficulties of their child.

Target population: parents and homeroom teacher

We recommend that in upper grades, the students take part in the conversation, or at least a part of it.

Students' age: from kindergarten to high school

Challenges: The level of conversation should be adapted according to the mental maturity of the students.

Based on Barry (2008), here are some tips for teachers to help them communicate with parents:

1　We must remember that parents know their children better than anyone else. Therefore, full attention should be paid to the parents' concerns.
2　In teacher-parents meetings, respect and neutrality are suggested. Use the child's name; refer to him/her as an individual. Address his or her parents by name or by Mr. or Mrs. X. Avoid using words that insinuate blaming the child or his/her parents for the child behavior, which is a result of the child's difficulties and disabilities.
3　Expectations should be clear regarding the goals of the meetings and the role of the experts. When parents are involved in a discussion of the school's program policies, they will have the opportunity to be involved. They will have a level of ownership rather than feeling powerless.
4　Share with parents their child's progress. Don't contact them only when there is a disciplinary problem or decline in achievement.
5　Teachers must admit if they have acted incorrectly. They can say that they are sorry about it and take responsibility.

It is recommended to have a preliminary meeting with the students, asking them to summarize their semester experiences as they write down their answers to a given set of questions (Figure 22.2).

Their answers will be used as a basis for the teacher-parents-student conversation. This should be an opportunity for all participants to get a broad picture of the students' functioning (both academic and emotional) at school.

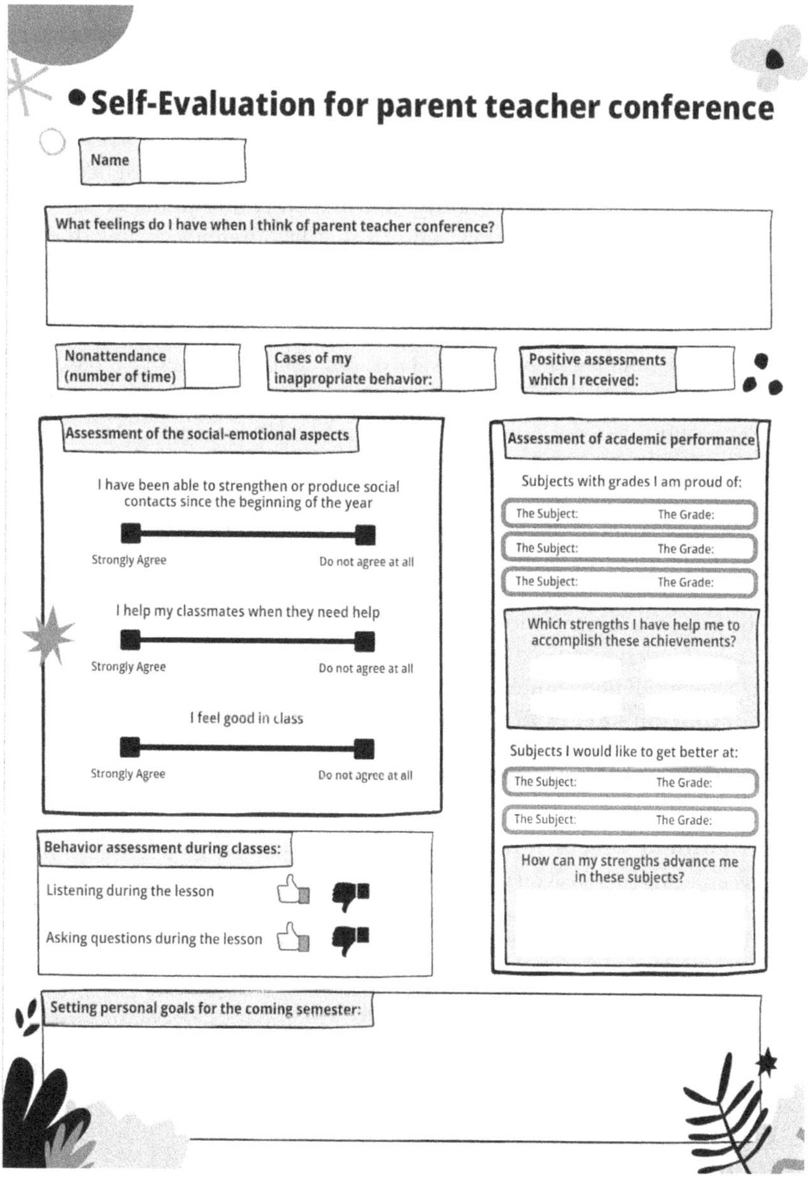

Self-Evaluation for parent teacher conference

Name

What feelings do I have when I think of parent teacher conference?

Nonattendance (number of time):

Cases of my inappropriate behavior:

Positive assessments which I received:

Assessment of the social-emotional aspects

I have been able to strengthen or produce social contacts since the beginning of the year

Strongly Agree   Do not agree at all

I help my classmates when they need help

Strongly Agree   Do not agree at all

I feel good in class

Strongly Agree   Do not agree at all

Behavior assessment during classes:

Listening during the lesson

Asking questions during the lesson

Assessment of academic performance

Subjects with grades I am proud of:

The Subject: The Grade:

The Subject: The Grade:

The Subject: The Grade:

Which strengths I have help me to accomplish these achievements?

Subjects I would like to get better at:

The Subject: The Grade:

The Subject: The Grade:

How can my strengths advance me in these subjects?

Setting personal goals for the coming semester:

Figure 22.2 Self-evaluation for parent teacher conference

A MONTHLY/PERIODIC INFORMATION REPORT SHEET (ON EDUCATIONAL TOPICS AND SOCIAL EVENTS)

Aims: To share information with parents, about curricular and extra-curricular activities, events, and experiences that were part of the educational process in the preceding month/period.

To stimulate the motivation to have a family discussion at home about the learning and educational processes.

Target population: parents

Students' age: from kindergarten to high school

Challenges: to be attentive and hear out the parents' requests and needs.

Activity:

The report sheets will include information about activities which take place in the kindergarten or school, mostly information regarding child developmental psychology and education and tips that help parents cope with daily situations of rearing children. Those sheets can be sent by email, by using cellphone applications, or by sticking them on the wall at a convenient location at the entrance to the kindergarten.

The information sheet should be short and concise and can be based on academic articles or lectures, in order to convey the message, without burdening the parents.

These sheets, which are handed out to parents through the daily routine, can help in the future, if or when required in situations of crisis (as will be discussed later in the chapter on interventions in crisis situations).

Information sheets in kindergarten: A list or a table which conveys information about topics, activities, and events planned for the current week must be placed at a convenient location. While waiting to pick up their children from kindergarten, parents will be able to read and keep themselves updated. The cell phone or email can be used to inform the parents as well.

Information sheets in junior high school and high school: Since we are dealing with more mature students, they may be asked to be involved in the preparation process of the information sheet by adding their photos and sharing their experiences.

Enrichment sheets: It is recommended that teachers prepare a monthly/periodic information sheet on a topic that deals with handling situations concerning students: coping with loss, the importance of sleep at different ages, healthy lifestyle, rules of caution when using mobile and computer applications, etc.

HOME VISITS

Aim: To meet the student, the parents and the whole family in the student's natural environment.

Target population: the whole family

Students' age: kindergarten to high school

Challenges: A home visit has many positive aspects. Most parents and children are excited about the visit and prepare for it with great joy. The problem that accompanies the issue of home visits is that teachers are usually not rewarded for it. Even if there is a benefit for the educational system, it must be taken into account that sometimes, not only the teacher, but also the school mental health professional is required to visit, depending on the socio-economic background of the student. Not every school can afford the expenses.

Moreover, home visits put a strain on the teacher since they take place in the afternoon or the evening, and teachers are not always willing to perform this task.

An alternate option: In light of the difficulty of recruiting teachers for the home visit assignment, and due to the fact that in higher grades, when adolescents do not always feel comfortable to involve their parents in their school life, an alternate method of getting acquainted with the student's home is suggested. Students can be asked to create a short video of their family (Tik-Tok), which introduces the family members and a video or photos of their home. They will later share it with the teacher. At the same time, students can be given the task of photographing places in the school and sharing it with their parents. They can be instructed to take a picture of a place they like at school and a place they do not like and then share it with their parents and maybe, with their teachers and their classmates.

Expressing emotions and awareness of one's strengths

SHARING EMOTIONS

Aim: to develop students' awareness of their emotions and to help them express their feelings, in order to create a basis for dealing with future crisis situations.

Target population: students

Students' age: from kindergarten to high school

Challenges: Not all the students will agree to reveal their feelings in the group. Hence, only those who wish to do so should be required to take an active part in the sessions.

Activities:

Teachers can use various sets of faces/emojis, expressing different emotions, from which the students can choose the one that represents their current feeling. Students, who are willing to share their feelings with the group, will be welcome to do so (Figure 22.3).

FINDING MY STRENGTHS

Aim: To help the student find in their personality, the strengths on which they can rely on in daily life, especially in times of crisis.

Target Population: from kindergarten to high school

Students' age: from kindergarten to high school

Challenges: As children get older, they are less likely to share their personal problems, concerning their lives and personality, with others. Thus, the process should be allowed to take place at an individual level (student with teacher) or in a group, but in writing, allowing only students, who wish to share their thoughts with the group, to do so. The process, even when done only by some students, may be effective for all participants of the group.

Activities:

"Super-me":

Young students will be asked to color on the figure shown in Figure 22.4 parts of their body from which they derive their strength and explain why they chose it and how those parts help them.

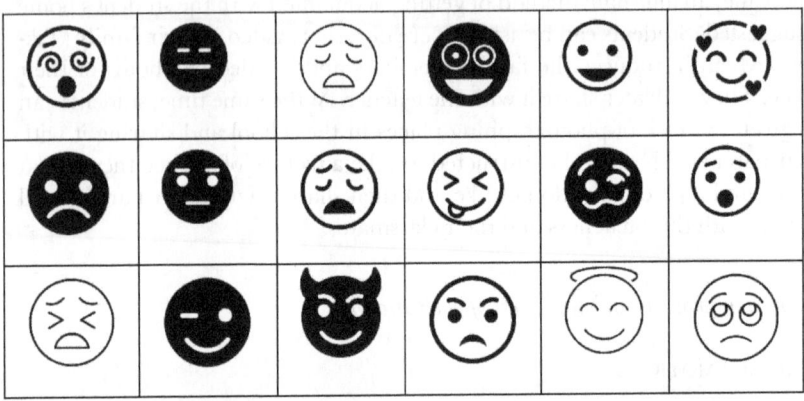

Figure 22.3 Emotions

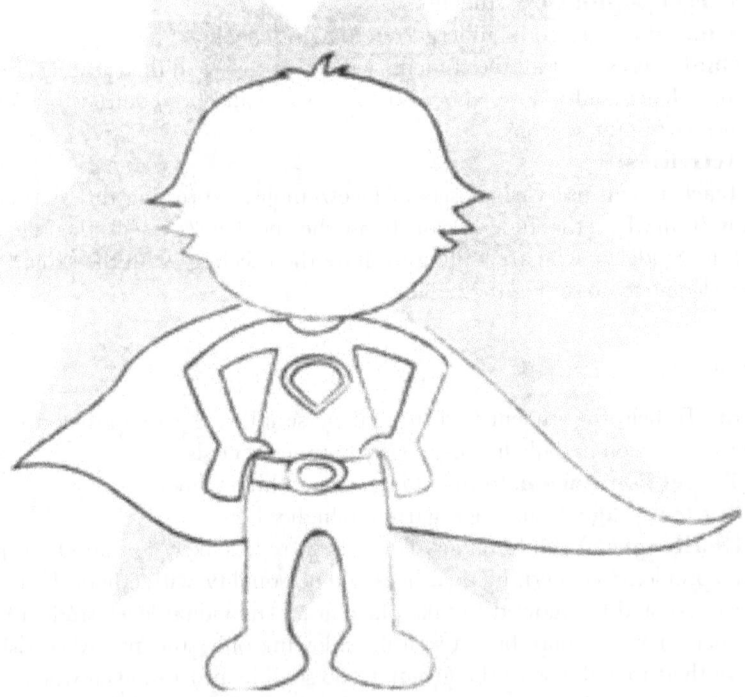

Figure 22.4 "Super-Me"

"Building my Personality":

Each student will answer various questions individually (e.g., traits/abilities in my personality that I am proud of; difficulty I dealt with successfully and how I succeeded) and later in the group, those students who are willing to share their answers will be welcome (Figure 22.5).

It is recommended to inform the parents about those activities (*Sharing emotions* and *Finding my strengths*) and to encourage both students and parents to talk about them.

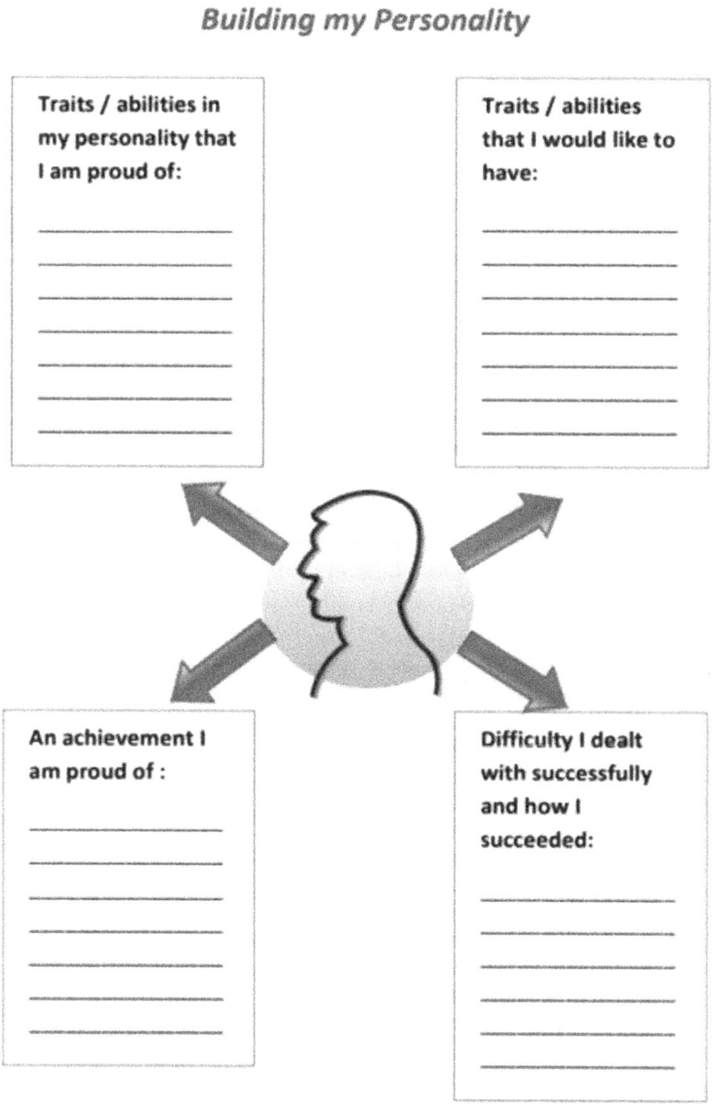

Building my Personality

Traits / abilities in
my personality that
I am proud of:

Traits / abilities
that I would like to
have:

An achievement I
am proud of :

Difficulty I dealt
with successfully
and how I
succeeded:

Figure 22.5 Building my personality

Part 2: Intervention

The intervention takes place in times of crisis. The success of the intervention depends on the effectiveness of the longitudinal prevention process, which provides both students and families with skills and tools to cope with difficulties.

Target population: students and families

Students' age: from kindergarten to high school.

Strengthening parents' self-efficacy

In a stressful situation, such as during a flight, parents should be the first ones to put on the oxygen mask before taking care of their children. In a similar way, in the time of crisis, the teachers' role is to support the parents.

Activities:

(a) Teacher-parents informal talk, initiated on a regular basis, by the teacher, may help the teacher to find out how the parents feel and how family elements in the children's immediate context support or not support effective coping.

Examples of informal teacher-parent conversation questions:

> *Hi Carol* (always contact the parent by his/her first name) *how are you? How are you doing these days? How do you cope with the current challenges? Is anyone helping you? Is there anything you would like to ask or consult with me about? How do you think your child copes with the situation? How do you and your child get along under the circumstances? Was there anything you would have liked to change? Is there anything I can do to help?*

It is not only the contents of the conversation but the teacher's willingness to listen to the parent, which is of great importance.

(b) To empower the parents and to instill a sense of hope and avoid a sense of despair, it is important to help parents to be proactive and not passive.

Teachers can share assignments with parents. For example, if the parents share with the teacher their difficulties with their child (e.g., wetting at night, reluctance to attend an online class, the child's difficulty in getting up in the morning, or the child's anxieties), teacher and parent can think together about possible solutions and set regular meetings for follow-up.

(c) Sharing emotions. The teacher can recommend parents to establish parents' group support on cell phones, or any other social network and application, for correspondence. It can be used for sharing emotions, hopes and reliable information.

Strengthening parent-child interaction

Children might be particularly vulnerable to serious mental health consequences associated with crisis. Parents are the significant figures in the child's immediate environment and they have an important role in supporting their children and being a role model for the child's stress management. Therefore, it is important to help parents to strengthen their rapport with their children.

Contact notebook: Parents and children can keep a notebook in which they exchange messages. For example, each one in his/her turn will write three good things that happened during the day.

Notes with short positive statements: The teacher can recommend to parents to write inspiring and positive notes that will be attached to the refrigerator or put under the pillow or next to the toothpaste (e.g., I love you; Yes, we can!; You look wonderful with the mask (during pandemic); Thank you for helping prepare dinner, etc.). Parents can also write down family jokes or riddles. It should be noted that parents and children should exchange mutual notes.

Encourage a family to function as a unit

Researchers point out four factors in the children's immediate family context of parents, siblings, extended family, and pets, which appear essential to their capacity to cope with a crisis: a sense of protection, reassurance, re-establishment of routines and stability (Mooney, 2017).

Establishment of routines: One of the most popular family routines in Israel is meeting for a family meal at least once a week. The teacher can recommend that parents add a meaning to the family meetings (e.g., each family member will share an amusing incident or a good thing that happened to him/her during the week; each family member will thank someone or something that happened during the passing week; or dedicate an object, real or imaginary to another member in the family).

CHOOSING MY WAY TO COPE WITH CRISIS

"Two roads diverged in a wood, and I took the one less traveled by" (The Road Not Taken, Robert Frost).

Throughout our lives, we take decisions under different circumstances. If we choose one way, obviously, we choose not to use the alternative. The way we choose to deal with crises is also a choice that depends on us. The map called "my way" (Figure 22.6) shows different routes which represent various modes of coping.

This map is given to the students and their families, in order for them to analyze the way each one of them chose to deal with a difficulty/crisis, they had experienced in the past and to hear how others in the family chose to deal with their difficulties/crises.

After the first round, there will be a second round based on the question: If you had encountered the same problem today, would you have dealt with the problem differently? If so, how? And so, it can be seen if the student has changed the way they cope in light of their experience, age and the tools they have acquired over the years.

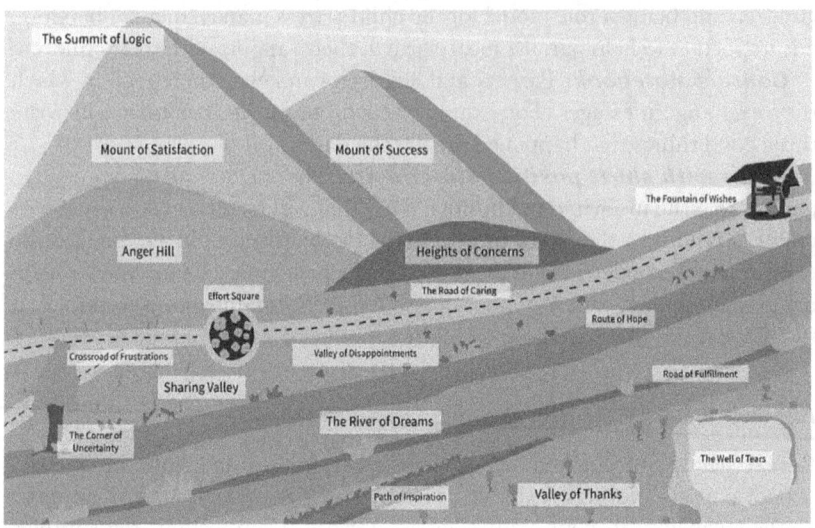

Figure 22.6 My Way

Part 3: Assessment

Evaluation and assessment are an integral part of teaching and learning. They play pivotal roles in determining what is learnt. Evaluation is also known as a powerful means of improving the quality of education. In our case, we recommend assessing the outcomes of both the prevention and intervention programs in creative ways.

The question is how do we know if the prevention or intervention program was successful? Here is a firsthand example for an assessment of teacher-parents-students trust building program.

Along with being a high school principal and as part of my role as a classroom educator, I (JF) hold a concluding meeting of parents and students at the end of each year, where we summarize the year from the perspective of the partnership formed, the collaboration in the educational process, and its contribution to the students' well-being, as well as academic achievements. I remember those meetings as entertaining and creative sessions, which proved to be successful for many years, and I also passed on the idea to other educators at school. I chose the manner of performing the session according to the nature of the parents and students, with the instruction being the same in all cases.

In classrooms, where cooperation with parents was productive, I asked them to bring an object, which in their opinion represented/summarized the parent-student-educator relationship in the past year. In classrooms where the parents cooperated, but were not very active and initiative, I was the one who brought various objects, from which the families chose one. And there are classes, where the teachers themselves were less cooperative, and for them,

I suggested scattering cards on a table in the center of the room with names/ pictures of objects, from which the families could choose the object that described the collaboration in the group over the past year.

I brought simple, small objects which I had found in my house: a stapler, an alarm clock, a calendar, a rolling pin, an eraser, and so on. However, the most exciting moments that I experienced were those in which the objects had been prepared by the parents and children together at home, prior to the meeting. Those, naturally, were parents and children who collaborated remarkably throughout the year.

Examples of items, which were brought by the families to the meeting:

Fruit salad: "You, as an educator, knew how to take various children, with different 'flavors' and different personalities and create from them a delicious and sweet salad."

Cake: "We came to you as a collection of ingredients, different from one another and not united, and you kneaded us like dough, and made a delicious cake whose aroma reaches far." Indeed, this was for a class that received a lot of positive feedback at the school.

Spice basket: A collection of small bags of spices (like tea-bags) in a small basket – "You knew how to unearth various unique features of each student and used them all to create a class of students, who learned and enjoyed their time together side by side in spite of the different flavors."

A small statuette of an owl (symbolizes wisdom and curiosity): "You educated both the children and the parents to be curious, to ask questions, be skeptic when necessary and be interested in different areas of life and not only in the school curriculum." That was a class for which I planned enrichment sessions throughout the year, some of which were attended by parents, who came as lecturers, to share with us their expertise.

As a conclusion, parents' and students' collaboration reflects their good relationships with the teacher, which is the first step in trust building.

Multicultural considerations

Today, in educational systems worldwide, there are students from diverse families that differ in terms of race, language, culture, academic and socio-economic backgrounds, etc. Therefore, teachers who like to engage with families need to be sensitive to differences in culture, values, languages, and various expectations parents may have. Moreover, if teachers and schools wish to respect families and build collaboration with diverse families, they need to use translators for teacher-parents conferences and if needed, to translate materials into different languages (Norheim & Moser, 2020) and invite the families to share their culture with the class.

In addition, the activities that we offer in this chapter should be tailored on the basis of different cultures.

Challenges and solutions

It is well known that some teachers do not think that their role includes working with parents and they do not feel they have the capacity to address the family's needs. This is mainly because they are not trained to work with parents.

In Israel, like in other countries (e.g., Japan), homeroom teachers are responsible for students' emotional and social well-being (Yablon & Itzhaky, 2013), class atmosphere, and academic development. Given that students spend a large amount of time in class, homeroom teachers play a major role in developing students' interpersonal skills (Ito, 2011). We are recommending this program for homeroom teachers. However, we understand that not all countries have homeroom teachers. It is also clear to us that not all teachers and homeroom teachers are trained to work with families. Therefore, we recommend schools to have teacher training related to mental health, behavior management and partnering with parents (Swick, Powers & Doyle, 2020).

Conclusion

There is no official policy regarding teacher-parent communication, and very little has been done in teacher training to raise awareness and foster teachers' motivation toward engaging with parents. However, parental functioning during daily activities and especially in times of crisis, is of great importance for children's well-being and, therefore, it is important that teachers work to strengthen their relationships with the parents and support the parents who are significant figures for the children.

Resources

How to build teacher-parent-child trust see:
Kelly M. S. (2020). How to develop community resources. In B. A. Gerrard, M. J. Carter & D. Ribera (Eds.). *School-Based Family Counseling an Interdisciplinary Practitioner's Guide* (pp. 312–334). New York: Routledge.

References

Adams, K. S., & Christenson, S. L. (1998). Differences in parent and teacher trust levels: Implications for creating collaborative family-school relationships. *Special Services in the Schools*, *14*(1–2), 1–22.

Adams, K. S., & Christenson, S. L. (2000). Trust and the family–school relationship examination of parent–teacher differences in elementary and secondary grades. *Journal of School Psychology*, *38*(5), 477–497.

Barry, M. P. (2008). Parent-professional relationships: It's a matter of trust. *Autism Spectrum Quarterly*, Fall, 36–39.

Gerrard, B. A., & Soriano, M. (2020). School-based family counseling, the revolutionary paradigm. In B. A. Gerrard, M. J. Carter & D. Ribera (Eds.) *School-based family counseling, an interdisciplinary practitioner's guide* (pp. 1–15). New York: Routledge.

Goodman, S. H., & Garber, J. (2017). Evidence-based interventions for depressed mothers and their young children. *Child Development, 88*(2), 368–377.

Ito, A. (2011). Enhancing school connectedness in Japan: The role of homeroom teachers in establishing a positive classroom climate. *Asian Journal of Counselling, 18*(1), 41–62.

Kaplan Toren, N., & Seginer, R. (2015). Classroom climate, parental educational involvement, and student school functioning in early adolescence: A longitudinal study. *Social Psychology of Education, 18*(4), 811–827.

Lorenzo, N. E., Zeytinoglu, S., Morales, S., Listokin, J., Almas, A. N., Degnan, K. A., … & Fox, N. A. (2021). Transactional associations between parent and late adolescent internalizing symptoms during the COVID-19 Pandemic: The moderating role of avoidant coping. *Journal of Youth and Adolescence, 50*(3), 459–469.

Mooney, M. (2019). Children's resilience and mental health in the urban context. In *Handbook of Global Urban Health* (pp. 232–252). Routledge.

Norheim, H., & Moser, T. (2020). Barriers and facilitators for partnerships between parents with immigrant backgrounds and professionals in ECEC: A review based on empirical research. *European Early Childhood Education Research Journal, 28*(6), 789–805.

Ogg, J., Clark, K., Strissel, D., & Rogers, M. (2021). Parents' and teachers' ratings of family engagement: Congruence and prediction of outcomes. *School Psychology, 36*(3), 142.

Swick, D. C., Powers, J. D., & Doyle, C. (2020). How to overcome barriers to SBFC. In B. A. Gerrard, M. J. Carter & D. Ribera (Eds.). *School-based family counseling an interdisciplinary practitioner's guide* (pp. 335–350). New York: Routledge.

Tambling, R. R., Tomkunas, A. J., Russell, B. S., Horton, A. L., & Hutchison, M. (2021). Thematic analysis of parent–child conversations about covid-19: "playing it safe". *Journal of Child and Family Studies, 30*(2), 325–337.

Yablon, Y. B., & Itzhaky, H. (2013). Children's relationships with homeroom teachers as a protective factor in times of terror. *Journal of Social and Personal Relationships, 30*(4), 482–496.

23 Collaborating with immigrant students, school personnel and families in times of disaster

Sudia Paloma McCaleb

Overview

This chapter contains some ideas about how we can begin to build an environment that promotes resiliency and prepare for possible times of disaster by making the school an inclusive welcoming and nurturing environment and also a place where parents are able to share their cultural knowledge with students and teachers. This chapter describes an SBFC School Prevention approach to strengthening school-family relationships.

Background

Immigrant families often live with members of several generations and close together in an apartment with parents working long hours. There may be frequent violence in the neighborhood. A strong sense of trust is developed by families about school and the people who work there and relate to their children. Children are comfortable and their cultures and languages are validated and supported. The parents are also welcomed into the school. When the parents have concerns that they want to discuss with a teacher or SBFC practitioner, the school personnel make themselves available. All school gatherings and potluck dinners happen frequently where parents are encouraged to bring a dish to share from their culture. Group singing is common and an effort is made to sing songs in different languages represented by families at the school. Small parent discussion groups are encouraged and sometimes parents bring an artifact from their culture to share with others and to introduce themselves.

There are many activities that may be implemented to connect the classroom with the family culture and environment. These activities can continue to build parental and cultural understanding at the school. We also need to acknowledge that this nurturing environment does not exist everywhere and it takes commitment to make this happen.

Immigrants have come to this country for many different reasons such as because of environmental, economic and political disasters in their own countries. Sometimes, they are welcomed here and in other times they are not. Sometimes, they are stopped at the border and other times they are held in

DOI: 10.4324/9781003201977-28

prison-like conditions. Sometimes, their children are taken away from them and other times they have sponsors who take care of them once they arrive. Some immigrants arrive as students with student visas and are registered at universities. Many immigrants are here without proper paperwork and live with the constant fear that they will be picked up and deported. Many leave their children behind, while others have citizenship papers or TPS (Temporary Protected Status) or have married an American (sometimes for love and others for a financial relationship to help then to stay in the country).

In any case, all have some strong attachment or love for their country of origin. I remember the first song I learned when I was learning Spanish at the age of 12 and it has always stayed in my mind and I continue to sing it. It is also a song that is sung in bars and other gathering places by lonely male immigrants...La Cancion Mixteca

> *"Que lejos estoy del suelo donde nacido..imensa nostalgia invade mi pensamiento...y al verme tan solo y triste cual hoja al viento..Quiero llorar, quiero morir de sentimiento." (How far I am from the land where I was born...an enormous nostalgia invades my thoughts...and when you see me so lonely and sad like a leaf floating in the wind...I want to cry, I want to die from those sentimental thoughts).*

Another one is Linda Oaxaca that has the lines

> *Oaxaca vives en mi y yo por ti doy la vida...oye la voz de mi angustia, que llora y que canta queriendo volver..Linda Oaxaca de mi alma no quiero morirme sin volverte a ver. (Oaxaca you live in me and I give my life to you...Listen to my voice of anguish that cries and sings of wishing to return..Beautiful Oaxaca of my soul I do not want to die without returning to see you.*

Many of these expressed feelings can be contagious to the children. The children can feel the pain of their parent's longing and may not even know the home country, if they were born in the USA.

Some adults have left their country because of droughts and are no longer able to farm. Some have left because of flooding and have lost their homes and livelihoods. Some have experienced tsunamis, rising sea levels and others severe temperature changes or melting glaciers all making it difficult to continue farming. These cause economic hardships. In some countries like El Salvador, Mexico and Honduras, the USA has "dumped" a lot of their industrially and genetically grown food which is supported by the US government subsidies. These foods sell for cheaper in those countries making it difficult for traditional farmers to continue to support themselves through farming. So, it becomes an economic migration. They can no longer support their families. Haiti has experienced floods, earthquakes and political turmoil (the latter unfortunately supported by the USA). El Salvador had many years of civil war (unfortunately also supported by the USA) when people arrived in the USA from fear of death at home.

There are many reasons why immigrants have arrived in our communities. Most have been uprooted by some kind of disaster, so how can schools, teachers and SBFC professionals support families when everyone is experiencing disasters? In California, wild fires have become common and the threat of earthquake is often present. There is always a prediction that the "big one" will be here soon. Students are best served in times of disaster if they have a resilient foundation and there is a strong connection between home and school and when teachers and SBFC practitioners are working together with the children and their families.

Procedure

This section describes ten activities that a teacher or SBFC practitioner can use to strengthen school-family relationships. In these school-family activities, classroom teachers and SBFC practitioners engage in early sit down (tea or coffee) dialogues with immigrant parents. The teachers and SBFC practitioners express a desire to know and understand the parent's culture and home country experiences. Some sample starters that can be used to engage parents:

What kinds of learning have you experienced?

1   What do you remember learning in your home or community that was of great value?
2   Do you remember people in the family or community that were considered wise? What kind of wisdom did they possess and how did they share it?
3   Do you remember your earliest memories of learning how to read?
4   What kinds of involvement did the adults (maybe your parents) have with the schools?
5   In what ways does your child's school experience enter into your home now?
6   What differences do you see between home and school learning and in what ways do you see the two merging?
7   How do you believe there could be more cooperation between the home and the school? What are you, or maybe other parents, willing to do to help this to happen?
8   What does your family enjoy doing together here?
9   What do you miss most from your country or home community?

Families building together

Parents often express the desire to do "fun" things together. This often becomes watching TV together or playing Nintendo games. I wanted to create an activity to do together that could include dialogue, creativity and literacy development. This activity engages the senses and builds family solidarity and accomplishments.

1 Put together a box/small suitcase of objects: little trains, railroad tracks, cars, wooden buildings, animals, people and trees.
2 Add to the box a large format blank page journal or writing book and a camera that takes pictures. The picture can also be taken by a parent's cell phone and forwarded to the teacher who can eventually have the photos printed.
3 Children take turns bringing home the box. They are asked to build a scene together with other family members, create a story (imaginary or real), write the story in the journal, and take a photo of all the people who helped build the scene.
4 The photo is eventually printed and pasted on the blank page in the box.
5 It becomes a class book of family stories which gets read frequently by the students and taken home for parents to see what others have done.
6 There may even by a family night where families come to the classroom and share the stories with each other, reading them out loud.

A book for peace

The goal for creating this book is to find words or short phrases that concretize the feelings and ideas of peace for the students and their family members.

1 Have students take the opportunity to visualize what peace means for them. Many of the ideas will easily lend themselves to illustration. Students will come to understand that peace is something we can all feel or create in our own lives.
2 Encourage students to express their own relationship to the concept of peace as this will allow them to carry these concepts into a broader framework – hopefully into global peace dimensions.
3 This book may be divided into two sections. The first part is written by the students and the second part by the parents.
4 Begin by leading a group discussion about what peace means to each of us personally (peace in your home, peace among nations, a world at peace or peaceful co-existence).
5 Ask students to choose one word that represents peace for them and to illustrate it for their own book about peace.
6 Ask parents to send in their word or phrase and ask them to illustrate it themselves or have their own child illustrate it for them.
7 Put together a group book about peace for the classroom library.

This book may be extremely appropriate during the winter holiday season when the words, "Peace on Earth and Good Will Towards All," are commonly heard. These words may have no meaning unless there is time to talk about the concepts. One time when the parent's words came back they included words like "reconciliation" and "communication." With older students, you may want to learn about the areas of the world that are not at peace and try to explore and understand what the existing problems are. The concept of restorative justice can be introduced to involve students in related class-room activities and in solving problems with their peers. Teachers or SBFC can facilitate problem solving circles with students involved in a conflict and solve it together and an apology can be given to those who have been hurt or offended. Students can also learn about organizations, like the United Nations and World Without War that are working for world peace and community groups that are working for local peace.

The most frightening time in my life

Fear is a common feeling in most children and young people's lives. Adults may consider a child's fear unimportant or irrational, but for the child it seems very real and may cause great anxiety. This can take the form of fear of strangers, the unknown, new situations or bad dreams. Some children's fears prevent them from learning.

During the month of October, around Halloween and Dia de los Muertos (the "Day of the Dead," a Latin American holiday where families welcome back the souls of the deceased for a brief celebratory reunion), young children tend to cling to their parents for safety and for reassurance that what is happening is just pretend. Activities associated with these holidays can help students face fears while being guided by a skilled teacher or SBFC practitioner.

When parents take the time to share recollections of some of the frightening times they have experienced in their own lives, children become more aware of fear as an acceptable human emotion.

Classroom steps:

1 Begin a discussion with the children about what images they see, especially in October, that are scary to them on the streets, in stores, on television or even at school.
2 Make a list of fears on the board and see which ones are common or more repetitive.
3 Have a discussion about ways children have dealt with their fears. Do they believe their fears are real and justified or with some new knowledge these fears could go away?
4 What do the children believe are fears that their parents have?
5 Send a note or letter home to parents and explain that you have been speaking about fears in the classroom (especially during this Halloween season) and would like parents to share some fear that they have had in their lives, or a scary moment and maybe how they overcame their fear.

6 Parents also can show their children that with time they will outgrow their fear too.

7 Also, on the paper that accompanies the letter, parents are asked to draw a picture of their fear for the children to return to school and become part of a book, "When We Were Young We Were Scared Too."

8 The book goes into the classroom library and will be looked at and read by the students. To be continually reminded that "our parents used to be afraid too" validates the student's own fears and reassures them that they too will outgrow their fears.

Words of advice from our parents

The transmission of values has been at the core of every civilization. Students need to know what their elders consider important and what expectations their elders have for them. What words of wisdom do parents feel obligated to pass on? Sometimes, we ask parents to share and illustrate proverbs that they grew up with and that they share with their children. Some examples that have come back are:

What you may not like in others may be in your own house.
If lemons fall from a tree on your head learn to make lemonaide.
Everyone reaps what they sow.
The devil knows more because he is old and not because he is the devil.
If you keep your mouth closed then the flies won't come in.

The shrimp that sleeps gets carried by the current

1 One idea is to send a letter home to parents and ask them to pretend they must go on a journey in which they are not sure when they will be returning (maybe visiting a sick relative in their home country). Ask them what advice they would give to their children before departing?

2 As the students bring back the responses (written or orally shared) have a group discussion about their parent's words. Were they surprised? Were they aware of their parent's values before and how they expected their children to behave?

3 Let students talk about the similarities and differences about parental expectations and if they feel they can meet those expectations.

Some parents have become very emotional about this question. Some confided that they started to cry but, in the end, felt it was important to think about and share with the children. The creation of this book made parents feel that how they felt was important to the teacher and it also gave the students the opportunity to read the parent's words again and again and to continue to see how loved they are and to know that their teachers also care about what their parents feel.

Singing with children

Songs can have a calming effect on children and adults. It is possible to open the day with some songs when the parents are dropping off their children and invite them to join in morning songs. One that is quite popular is "May There Always Be Sunshine."

> *May there always be sunshine, may there always be blue skies, may there always be mama (papa, grandma, sister, auntie, teacher) may there always be us.*

You can also sing this song in Spanish. Another popular one is the "Rainbow Song."

> *Just like a beautiful rainbow, smiling at skies that are grey. Come our girls and our boys bearing food sharing joys with the children in lands far away. I see in that beautiful rainbow, the flags of all nations unfurled. I hear song and mirth I see peace on Earth in that wonderful, beautiful, marvelous, glorious rainbow around the world.*

We have a bag of colored scarves and at the end the children toss their scarves up in the air to show the colors of the rainbow or dance with them. You can also use pieces of colored paper. "You are the One Your Mommy Loves" (or Daddy, Papa, abuela, auntie)

> *You are the one Your Mommy Loves, you are the one your daddy loves, you are the one we all do love the sweetest one in town. Up in the morning, break of day, into your clothes and out to play, breakfast somewhere along the way, bouncing up and down.*

Of course this song can include many movements. "We Are a Family Under One Sky"

> *We're all a family under one sky, we're a family under one sky..we're people, people.. we're animals, animals, we're flowers and birds in flight.*

Children and parents like singing together and it is a cheerful and also calming way to start a new day.

Childhood friendships

Parents usually have very fond memories of their childhood friendships. Maybe they were friends they walked with down the country road to school each day. Sometimes, they were strong friendships with their own siblings. Sometimes, parents express fears that their children will form friendships that will lead them down the wrong path. When parents share childhood memories with their own children, they are creating the possibility for increased closeness in the relationship. This is also true when teachers and SBFC practitioners learn about the friendships parents had as children. It allows them to be more empathetic and to understand some of the parent's histories and even anxieties.

1 Ask children to help make a list, as a group, as you write on the board, what qualities would they like or are important to them in a friend.
2 Have them draw a picture of a good friend and write something about them. Why are they a special friend and what do they like doing together?
3 Send a note home to parents asking them to talk to their child about a good childhood friend. What was special about the friend. What did they like to do together? They can also draw a picture and write something about the friend on the page.
4 Create a book that combines the children's pictures and the parent's pictures.
5 Have discussion with the class about what they see in the book. In what ways are the parent's friendships similar or different than their children's friendships?
6 Let the children take turns bringing home the book and sharing it with their parents.
7 Ask parents to share their reactions/observations with their children and then the children can share in class their parent's reflections based on the book.
8 Were they surprised at the generational differences or similarities about friendships?
   Once again, teachers and SBFC practitioners taking time to discuss friendship, reach out to parents and show interest and caring about friendship, is an important aspect for building trust.

School gardens

Growing food at a school can be exciting and also help to share healthy eating and cooking with students and their families. We live in a culture that offers so many unhealthy eating options and lots of junk food varieties for children. I have also experimented with in-class gardens with a drip system hooked up. We had a weekly salad eating day and we added grated carrots and cheese. Some parents asked me, "My child loves the salads he is eating in the classroom. Can you teach me how to make a salad?"

1 Parents, students and teachers can work together to build a simple outdoor planter box.
2 Seeds or small seedlings can be purchased at a local nursery and planted in the box. Easy-to-grow examples are lettuce, tomatoes, chard, zucchini, string beans, peas and artichokes.
3 Students can have a watering schedule to keep plants moist.
4 Crops are harvested at different times and recipes can be created for eating each new crop.

5   Students can take home some of the vegetables to share with family.
6   A harvest meal can be planned in the classroom and parents invited and even requested to bring a dish to share.
7   Photographs can be taken of each stage of the project: from building the box, to planting the seeds, to watering, to harvesting, to eating. The photographs can be organized and a text written to tell the story. The story can be placed on the hall wall outside the classroom for others to see and get new ideas.

Tile mural project

A tile mural can be amazing, but also a bit complicated. Each child can contribute a painted tile to the project.

1   Decide on a theme for the tile mural. We have used the theme of "I have a dream" from Martin /Luther King's speech. We have also worked with an ocean theme, where each classroom does a different area: the sandy beach, the underwater crustaceans, the big swimming fish, etc. Students may also paint something that represents a part of their culture or home country that they wish to show.
2   Purchase enough unfinished tiles for each child in the project and some tile paints.
3   Have a discussion of the theme of the mural and generate ideas with students.

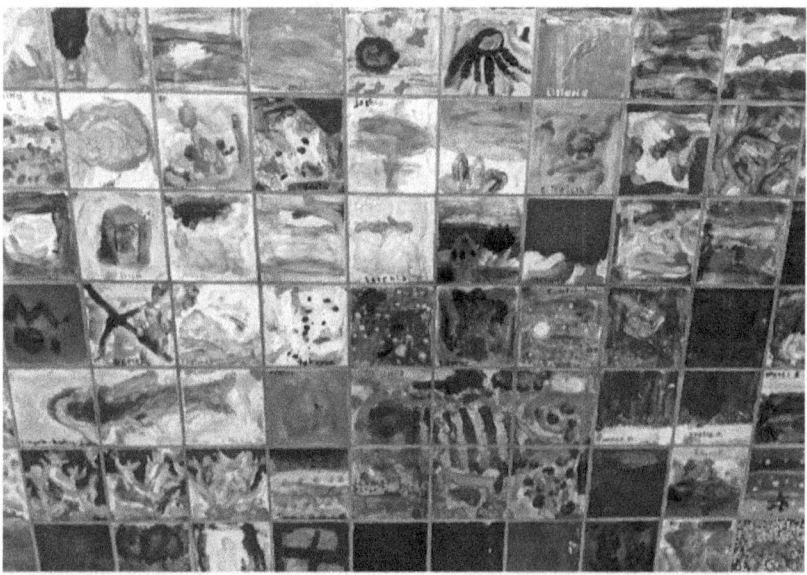

Figure 23.1 Example of a tile mural project

4 Decide on a painting day.
5 Bring tiles to a place that does the firing of student tiles.
6 When tiles are fired, invite parents to help with a day for affixing the tiles to the wall and another day for grouting.
7 When the mural is complete, celebrate as a community event with songs and even a cake with candles. A sample mural is shown as Figure 23.1.

A mural like this can help families to feel a further sense of belonging with the school.

Multicultural considerations

Often the immigrant experience has been one of a singular culture or language: their own. They are unaccustomed to being with, working with or living in the same community with other cultures and languages. A natural response can be shyness, avoidance or fear. The teachers and the SBFC professionals in a school can work together to help families to get to know each other, and learn about and appreciate each other's cultures. Within classrooms, students develop friendships across cultures and teachers can use books/stories that depict the lives of people in different cultures. Some schools host multicultural pot luck dinners so families can enjoy the experience of sharing food from their culture and tasting the food from others. It is also possible to learn some words and greetings from a variety of languages present in the school. The more that schools stress and work on inclusion, the better prepared everyone will be to live in a multicultural society.

Challenges and solutions

Not all schools are culturally and linguistically welcoming environments. Sometimes school administrators are unaware of what they need to do to make this happen. They may not have skills in a second or third language and may have a difficult time relating to parents from another culture. Workshops and discussions can be facilitated by teachers and SBFC professionals who are committed to making schools inclusive and know the benefits to learning and to mental health.

Conclusion

When immigrant families feel that the school and the people who work there, including teachers, SBFC practitioners and administrators really care about them, culturally, linguistically, and experientially, it creates more trust between the family and the school. During times of disaster, this is extremely important for keeping everyone safe. Administrators and staff should expect that the school will become a hub for services such as food distribution, temporary shelter, and information about coping with stress, and information about important events. For the school community it can become a center of messaging and coordination of volunteer activities. These activities can occur spontaneously during a disaster, but if plans are made in advance, they will provide a deeper level of emotional and physical support. Parents are seen and not invisible. A joint staff and parent and student disaster planning committee will demonstrate to all involved that the school is a place that the community can look to during a real disaster. Such a committee will provide another opportunity for bonding between the school community and another aspect of resiliency. Integrating experiential activities between the school and the classroom not only can build literacy and critical thinking skills, but a widespread feeling of general security and being part of the multicultural multilingual school community.

Resources

Delpit, L. D. (2006). *Other people's children: Cultural conflict in the classroom.* The New Press.
Lisa Delpit poses an urgent question: Why do we have such a hard time making school a happy place for poor children and children of color?
Giroux, H. A. (2007). *Border crossings: Cultural workers and the politics of education.* Routledge.
Henry Giroux has expanded his field of vision, demonstrating that a critical pedagogy has implications for all of cultural and social differences.
Horton, M., & Freire, P. (1990). *We make the road by walking: Conversations on education and social change.* Temple University Press.
Miles Horton and Paolo Freire help us to see that ordinary men and women can be helped to learn to take control over their own destinies and to create a humane, democratic and just society.
Igoa, C. (2013). *The inner world of the immigrant child.* Routledge.
Cristina Igoa presents the immigrant children's stories in an easily and readable and understandable fashion and is clearly inspired by her pupils at the same time she is an inspiration to them. The book offers a lot to teachers and SBFC who are faced with increasing diversity in schools.
McCaleb, S. P. (2013). *Building communities of learners: A collaboration among teachers, students, families, and community.* Routledge.
Sudia Paloma McCaleb present of the dangers inherent to traditional schooling processes and examines some compelling alternative possibilities. It serves an important function of bringing the abstract rhetoric of critical pedagogy alive in real classrooms.
Nieto, S. (2015). *The light in their eyes: Creating multicultural learning communities,* tenth anniversary edition. Teachers College Press.
Sonia Nieto In lucid and engaging prose, communicates how educators, SBFC and policy makers can ensure how all children can experience personal affirmation and powerful learning at school.
Nieto, S., & Bode, P. (2017). *Affirming diversity: The Sociopolitical context of multicultural education.* Pearson.
Sonia Nieto's book provides a comprehensive framework for analyzing the multiple causes of school failure among subordinated groups of students, and on the basis of this analysis, suggests creative intervention strategies that are supported by research and theory.

Skutnabb-Kangas, T. (1981). *Bilingualism or not: The education of minorities.* Multilingual Matters.

The book deals with bilingualism, particularly as it relates to migrants and indigenous communities. It also analyses controversies about the education of migrants and minorities and places them in the wider political context.

24 Intimate parenting to build family resilience

Zipora Shechtman

Overview

School personnel provide a variety of services to teachers and students, but parents are often left out. This is surprising considering the important role that parents hold in their child's growth and well-being. Parents' role becomes more complicated at times of crisis, such as war or COVID pandemic. Parents are often challenged by their children because of personal difficulties, and even more so at time of crisis. The level of loneliness, anxiety and depression increase for both children and parents; parents are confused, angry and helpless, reacting in rejection, criticism, anger, and disappointment, while the children need the opposite reaction – warmth, love, empathy, appreciation, and trust. Children depend on their parents' emotional support, particularly at difficult times. Both parents and children need a feeling of emotional closeness and a sense of intimacy in their relationship, however, this is not the case for many of them, as many parents find it difficult to handle themselves intimately. As the parent-child relationship is key to the child's emotional, social, behavioral, and academic success, parents must be assisted, and school is an ideal place to do so. The School-based family counseling (SBFC) model suggests a comprehensive view of services that should be provided by school professionals, including parent education, support group, consultation, and counseling groups, which are still quite rare. Among those services counseling groups to develop parent-child intimate relationship, will be the focus of this chapter. At times of crisis Intimate relationship in the family is a must.

Background

All parents face challenges with their children, some occasionally; yet, many others struggle constantly. At times of crisis, those challenges become overwhelming leaving the parents frustrated and helpless. Here are some voices expressed by parents:

> *"It kills me to see him struggling with distant learning. He is a poor student in normal times, and now is a complete failure. I really worry about his future"* (a mother of a boy with learning disabilities).

DOI: 10.4324/9781003201977-29

I am so embarrassed with his behavior; it seems that he has no control of himself. He lost the only friend he had, and I am stuck with him 24-hours a day. I avoid contact with people, even family, and end up in total isolation

(A mother of a child with ADHD)

"He is so restless, angry and aggressive. I know he needs to feel secure but I cannot give him the warmth he needs. He makes me so mad, which brings out the worst of me. I often lose it and react violently to him, but then I feel stupid and frustrated (a Father of a child with a behavior disorder).

It appears that children present a wealth of problems, leading parents to feel stressed, worried, anxious, ashamed, helpless, and dissatisfied with their own dysfunction. These emotions lead to negative reactions to the child. Parents react with anger, rejection, and punishment (Weiner et al., 2016), while these children particularly need attention, warmth, and love.

Effective parents develop a strong sense of attachment with their child from a very early stage of child development. A secure type of attachment helps children to develop trust in self and others, sensitivity and empathy, and pro-social behavior. Some parents are not consistent in their attachment to their child, which leads to an anxious attachment style, resulting in self-doubts and social anxiety. In the worst case, when parents are not able to develop a sense of trust in the child, he or she develops an avoidant attachment style, resulting in the child's lack of self-trust and trust of others, and a tendency to avoid people, be lonely, highly withdrawn or aggressive and violent (Cassidy & Shaver, 2018).

In later stages of the child's development, parents' reaction to their children's emotional state become important, affecting their social and emotional functioning. Parents, who are attuned to the child's emotions, listen to the child with interest and empathy, show love and respect, help the child to develop self-confidence, pro-social behavior, a sense of well-being, and personal growth. However, parents, who are impatient, disrespectful, harsh, and aggressive, lead children to develop a sense of mistrust, suspicion, and defensive behavior (Eizenberg et al., 1996; Gershoff et al., 2018).

Some parents simply lack an understanding of the children's need and many others lack the skills to react properly. Here is a simple scenario.

A mother and her 3-year old daughter are back from a long walk. At a certain point the child sits down on the street announcing that she is not going to continue walking. The mother, who is a few steps ahead, asks her several times to get up and on her constant refusing continues walking. The child bursts into crying, but remains sitting.

I am confident that no physical harm would be done to the child; however, the scenario could have developed very differently if the mother would stop and talk about the child's feelings. Is she tired, angry, frustrated? This was a wonderful, but missed, opportunity to express understanding, become emotionally close, and develop a language of feelings. The way the scenario ended for the little girl left her sad, frustrated, and anxious.

It seems obvious that parents can learn to be more effective; however, the question is: Who should provide the parenting services and what should be the goal for intervention? I suggest that schools should take the lead, with the goal of developing intimate parenting.

School as the provider of service to parents

School-based family counseling (SBFC) is a comprehensive model to improve services in school and includes parent education. However, in most cases, the school system refrains from including services for parents, either because they are too busy with services for teachers and students, or because they don't perceive parent education as part of their tasks. Yet, as we know that parent functioning is directly related to the child's behavior, emotional state, social behavior, and learning (Patterson, 2002), ignoring parent involvement in school is wrong and must be changed. The SBFC model includes a double focus: school and family, and a double level of intervention in each: prevention and intervention (Gerrard et al., 2019). The model suggests psychoeducation and guidance groups for students and teachers on the prevention level, and counseling/psychotherapy and crisis intervention on the intervention level, services that are provided in most schools. The family focus includes parent education and support groups on the prevention level, and family counseling, parent consultation, and group counseling at the intervention level, most of which are not performed in the school system.

Unfortunately, parents are left alone to meet their challenges with their children. Children suffer from isolation, rejection, shaming, and violence in school. Many show anxiety and depression symptoms, all increased during the last two years during the COVID pandemic. Parents are helpless, preoccupied with their own struggle, and many cannot effort private help. School is the most convenience place to reach out to parents and should include all the services suggested in the SBFC model. In this chapter, I focus on group counseling, with the goal of increasing parent-child intimate relationships.

The goal for intervention: intimate parenting

Intimate parenting seems to be the answer to many parents because it focuses on relationships. Positive relationships have the power to prevent conflicts, minimize difficulties, and empower people, because they are built on love, trust, loyalty, and honesty, all blocks to build an emotionally close relationship. We are familiar with the term intimacy related to opposite-sex relationship but intimacy does not necessarily have to involve sex. It does exist also in other relationships, for example, in close friendships. Sharabany (1994), in her research on intimate friendship, identified eight major components:

emotional closeness, sense of confidence, uniqueness and privacy, trust and loyalty, sensitivity and spontaneity, empathy and understanding, giving and accepting, and mutual interest. In an intimate relationship, one feels comfortable to be authentic, show his/her negative parts such as fear, shame, and guilt, and still be loved. Such relationships build self-trust, and trust in the world, and are the best buffer to a sense of loneliness. Why not think about child-parent relationships in the same way? Parents should be the persons with which children can share emotions, thoughts, experiences, and secrets. Parents need to be the first that children can consult with when pleasant and unpleasant situations come up. Here are two opposite scenarios:

> *Gale was 15-years old when she became pregnant. She was an excellent student in high school and a very thoughtful person when she met her criminal boyfriend and believed she could save him. She shared with her parents the news and they totally accepted her. They made a plan to get rid of the boyfriend and helped her go through the childbirth. No blame or threat was expressed to her. They ended up raising the newborn and Gale went back to school, became a lawyer, and remained close to her parents.*
>
> *Dinna started dating boys at the age of 15 and returning home very late. A psychologist suggested letting her stay out the next time she is late. The next time was a cold and rainy night and the parents indeed didn't open the door. She begged for a while, they heard her saying-"what kind of parents do not let their daughter in during such cold", then disappeared. Five years later, they reported that they did not see her since that night and have no idea where she is.*

These are two extreme examples of educated parents who established very different ties with their teenage daughters. However, most close relationships are expressed in many simple ways: sharing a dream, a disappointment, a fear, or a failure, without being interpreted or criticized, or asking for something or expressing a happy moment. Intimacy is expected from both parties. Parents need to set conditions for the child to feel safe but also to model intimacy by sharing their experiences, frustrations, and failures. Ann Griffin in her book *When all is said* (2019) tells about an old successful man who writes a goodbye letter to his son, telling him for the first time that he was dyslexic and could not read. Throughout his life, he rejected his son, never enjoyed his son's visits, and never read the articles his son wrote. Their relationship could have been so much different if only he could admit to his learning disorder earlier.

To be an intimate parent one needs to be connected to his/her inner emotions and own the language necessary to express emotions. Therefore, in the approach used here, the focus of treatment is on emotions, using the Emotion-Focused Therapy (EFT) developed by Less Greenberg (2002). The EFT process of treatment includes exploration of emotions and cognition, and developing insight, which may lead to change in behavior. Such processes can best be learned in a group format, as the group process requests intimacy and effectively develops intimate skills.

Evidence base of EFT groups with parents

Four large-scale studies investigated the impact of the suggested treatment on parents. We investigated the suggested group counseling treatment compared with psychoeducational groups, which are more commonly used (Shechtman & Gilat, 2005). Results indicated the reduction of parental stress and improved child perception only in the group counseling. In the psychoeducational groups, mothers' stress actually increased. Moreover, outcomes were also gathered for fathers who were not involved in treatment. These showed that only fathers related to the group counseling shown improvement on both measures. Finally, to understand the process, we asked parents about the therapeutic factors that were helpful to them. The most frequently mentioned factors were group support and interpersonal learning. Taking all these outcomes together suggests that emotion-focused groups for parents are effective.

Another study compared group intervention with individual intervention using the same EFT treatment (Danino & Shechtman, 2012). We found improvement in both interventions compared to control no-treatment. However, group treatment showed a stronger impact on reducing parental stress, while individual treatment showed better outcomes on parent responses to children's experiences.

A third study investigated a comprehensive set of outcomes on children of parents involved in group counseling (Ziperfal & Shechtman, 2017). Based on self, teacher, and parent reports, outcomes indicated improvement on children's emotional states and behaviors, with a lasting effect of close to one year. In this particular study, we also investigated processes that lead to change. The three most frequent processes that parents mentioned included: change in perception, development of self-awareness, and improved parent self-esteem (in this order). Examples of parent statements illustrating this are shown below.

> *The meetings helped me see the positive side of my child. I am now less stressed and anxious.*
>
> (perception change)

> *I know that I have to be more patient with him, so now when I want him to do something I go up to him, touch him, and softly ask him to do it.*
>
> (change in self-awareness)

> *Before the group I felt that I am the worst mother on earth. Now I am more confident. I think that my daughter is lucky to have me as her mother.*
>
> (change in self-esteem

Procedure

Group interventions vary from educational groups, through counseling groups to therapy groups. Psychoeducational groups basically involve teaching and guidance. These are helpful with providing knowledge and information to improve parent functioning. They are less effective with parents who face heavy challenges, which require self-understanding and motivation to make change in their own behavior. Counseling groups aim to promote self-development and psychotherapy groups aim to promote personality change. Counseling and psychotherapy groups are frequently psychodynamic-oriented; they are provided in small groups in which the unique therapeutic factors (e.g. cohesion and interpersonal learning; Yalom & Leszcz, 2016) are used frequently. Group members develop close contacts with each other and provide high quality support and feedback. Members share personal information and feelings which intensify intimacy. Members assist each other and learn from others. All these factors help people grow emotionally and change. In our past research, we found that intimacy skills developed in group can be transferred to people outside the group.

Psychotherapy groups are process-oriented, typically non-structured, yet comprising some major themes, and develop in three stages: the beginning, working, and final stages.

The beginning stage

At the beginning stage we establish a sense of trust and create a therapeutic relationship between group members and with the counselor. We use activities for "breaking the ice," getting acquainted, agreeing on the goals of the group, and establishing norms of emotional expressiveness and mutual support. For example: a father is describing himself as the center of any group, taking the role of the happy "clown." He is talking on a very superficial level without realizing that he is taking up the time of the group. A question from a group member: "*But how did you feel as a clown?*" leads him to focus on emotions. First he said: "*I need to think about it*" and later "*I was quite sad. I guess I did it to gain attention.*" In this case, the group helped him to comply with the group norm to speak on an emotional level.

The working stage

The working stage is geared to help parents become more intimate with their children.

The themes involve:

- empowering the parent
- the parent as a child
- the current relationship with the child
- empathy in the relationship
- getting closer to the child
- realistic expectations
- issues to be fixed in the relationships

The first session of this stage focuses on parents' strengths. Parents come to the group with a strong sense of failure. Starting with a positive approach empowers parents, increases self-efficacy and self-esteem. For example, group members are asked to give themselves an award for parenting. One mother says that she cannot find anything positive in her parenting; she is angry, restless, stressed, and impatient. She leaves the group quite unhappy. A day later, she posts her award on the group WhatsApp:

> *When I was thinking about myself in privacy I realized that I could identify many positive aspects of my parenting: I care about my children, I gave up part of my career to be with them, I manage to help them with their homework, I devote time to play with them, and I express my respect to them, most of the time.*

This is a good start to think about necessary changes.

From positive self-perception, we move to parent self-understanding, including parents' past influences. Usually, we are acting spontaneously on messages from past generations without realizing their strong impact. Sometimes, they are quite harmful. A mother confesses to the group that she hits her five-year-old daughter, explaining that it is an automatic response: "this is how I grew up" she explains. This requires change, which was later achieved.

After concepts and feelings about self are explored we move to understand the child, and his/her difficulties. The goal at this point is to develop empathic skills of listening and understanding.

One mother puts out a long list of complaints about her 12-year-old daughter. "She doesn't like my food, my style of dress, my questions. I feel rejected by her, which makes me angry and leads to frequent fights." Exploration of the situation reveals that the mother is over-controlling and highly critical. A deeper level of emotional exploration suggests that the mother envies her daughter for the way she looks as a teen: well dressed and young. This self-understanding changed the way the mother perceived the situation. She decided to let go of her super control, and was able to see her daughter as a growing woman and be proud of her. Self-understanding in its deepest level enables parents to become closer to their child and make a change in their own behavior.

To help parents engage in the therapeutic process we use therapeutic devises from the arts in psychotherapy: art therapy, bibliotherapy, phototherapy, therapeutic cards, and therapeutic games. For example, we showed a picture of a tree broken by the wind, a mother said "this is how I feel at the end of the day," which led to a process of self-expression, exploration of the emotions involved, and alternative possible behavior. In another session, we read a poem about social support. One mother confessed that she has a hard time getting support, which led to discussing trust and how to facilitate it. In another case, we shared family photos. One mother shared a photo in which her challenging child was absent. She explained that the child was restless and therefore was asked to leave the picture. She looked at the picture sadly then said: "I am so sorry we gave up on him so easily, he must be very hurt." The next session we wrote letters to the children. This mother used the opportunity to express her sadness and ask for his forgiveness.

The final stage

The final stage of the group process is short, but very important, as it accumulates all the learning achieved to be practiced in future difficult moments. First, we summarize individual achievements (what we have learned and how we have changed), then we identify personal goals for the future (what we still need to work on), and finally we say good bye to the group. This last step is very important because it is an opportunity to accumulate a lot of emotional support that will stay with group members long after the group terminated.

The process lasts about 15 weekly sessions, of one and one-half hour each, led by one or two trained therapists.

Multicultural considerations

Israel is a pluralistic society, with the majority holding an individualistic cultural orientation. However, we also have groups of orthodox populations, Arab and Druze, who hold more traditional and collectivistic perceptions, who may be less open to emotional therapy. One of our studies was carried out with Druze mothers. The study investigated the impact of emotion-focused treatment on 50 Druze mothers of children with ADHD, in a single village (Shechtman & Birani-Nasaraladin, 2006). Twenty-five mothers were involved in treatment compared to 25 no-treatment mothers. Results indicated very positive outcomes for treatment mothers. The parents improved in their reaction to children and children showed a decrease in anti-social behaviors.

Based on these results, we concluded that this treatment is effective with parents.

Challenges and solutions

Parents are unique participants in the EFT group. They do not perceive themselves as clients; thus, they often don't understand why and how they have become the focus of treatment. They came to the group as naïve parents, egger to receive help in coping with their children. They expect group therapy to "fix" their child, without understanding that they themselves are the solution to the problem. This discrepancy between their expectation and the reality of the group process is difficult for many parents, leading to a high level of resistance. Group therapists must be attuned to such difficulties, explain the type of intervention offered, reduce the level of anxiety, establish a contract based on trust and understanding, and throughout the group process keep a balance between counseling and guidance.

Another challenge is conducting such groups in the school, where parents may know each other. EFT requires relatively higher levels of self-disclosure, which may be more demanding when people are familiar with one another. Yet, school is the most convenient place to bring parents to therapy, as they may never reach out to therapy in another place. There are several ways to overcome such difficulties. First, it is preferred to compose the group by parents from different classrooms, which will reduce the chances that people know each other. Second, therapists need to discuss with parents the fear of sharing personal information vs. the emotional burden of keeping secrets. Finally, therapists must focus on a positive and supportive climate, which may eventually reduce the level of fear and shame.

Conclusion

In most counseling interactions with parents, the goal is to educate and guide parents to cope more effectively with their children. In contrast, the current group counseling intervention is aimed to develop a style of life based on parent-child intimate relationships. Intimate relationships are built on love, empathy, and support – the most important blocks for children at time of crisis and disaster. When stability and security are gone, parents' emotional closeness becomes the major source of confidence for the child. To achieve this goal the target of treatment is the **parent not the child**. We do not intend to fix the child but rather change the parents, as this would lead to change in parent-child relationships, and eventually lead to change of the child. Once parents are freed from anger, frustration, and guilt, they may let go of self-criticism and find a more empathic path to communicate with their children. Therefore, the beginning of treatment is aimed to develop parents' positive self-perceptions, then to self-explore overt and covert emotions which block the path to constructive communication. Understanding one's feelings will lead to insight, and eventually to change.

Group counseling is the most effective mode of intervention as it is based on processes of intimate relationship. Involvement in the group process requires a sense of trust, self-disclosure, empathic listening, understanding others, and helping others. Group members feel that they are "in the same boat." They identify with the experiences of other parents, develop an altruistic need to help others, and are supported by others. All these processes contribute to an improved self-concept and better understanding of others. The parents also develop improved skills of listening and providing feedback. These are processes that empower people, improve their emotional state, and also teach interpersonal skills. Such skills gained through experiential learning become part of a person's behavior and can be transferred to their relationships with their children.

Parent EFT group counseling is cost effective and is congruent with the SBFC approach. Emotion-focused groups are psychologically positive-oriented; thus, they lead to parental self-growth and cannot be harmful. Based on our clinical experience and research, we can suggest that these groups are safe and helpful. Considering the central role parents play in children's functioning and the limited services parents can receive, such groups should be part of school services in all schools.

Resources

Greenberg, L. S. (2002). *Emotion-focused therapy: Coaching clients to work through their feelings.* Washington, DC: American Psychological Association.
This book is the basis for Emotion Focused therapy. It includes the theory and clinical application.
Shechtman, Z. (2020). Intimate parenting: Empowering parents in counseling groups (in Hebrew). Israel, Tzameret.
This book outlines the rationale of EFT and how to apply it to group counseling. It includes descriptions of clinical processes, illustrations of interventions, and research results.
Yalom, I. D., & Leszcz, M. (2020). *The theory and practice of group psychotherapy* (6th Ed.). New York: Basic Books.
This book is the "bible" of any group work. It provides the important curative factors which lead to group success. It includes the theory of group work and a wealth of research.

References

Cassidy, J., & Shaver, O. R. (2018; 3rd ed.) (Eds.), *Handbook of attachment: Theory, research, and clinical* applications. New York: Guilford.
Danino, M., & Shechtman, Z. (2012). Superiority of group counseling to individual coaching of parents of children with learning disability. *Psychotherapy Research, 22,* 592–603.
Eizenberg, N., Fabes, R. A., & Murphy, B. C. (1996). Parents' reactions to children's negative emotions: Relations to children's social competence and conforming behavior. *Child Development, 67,* 2227–2247.
Gershoff, E. T., Good, G. S., Miller-Perrim, C. L., Holden, G. W., Jackson, Y, & Kazdin, A. E. (2018). Strength of the causal evidence against physical punishment of children and its implications for parents, psychologists, and policymakers. *American Psychology, 73,* 626–638.
Gerrard, B., Carter, M., & Ribera, D, (Eds.) (2019). *School-based family counseling: An interdisciplinary practitioner's guide.* Routledge.
Greenberg, L. S. (2002). *Emotion-focused therapy: Coaching clients to work through their feelings.* Washington, DC: American Psychological Association.
Patterson, J. M. (2002). Understanding family resilience. *Journal of Clinical Psychology, 58,* 233–248.
Sharabany, R. (1994). Intimate friendship scale: Conceptual understanding, psychometric properties, and construct validity. *Journal of Social and Personal Relationship, 15,* 449–470.
Shechtman, Z., & Birani-Nasaraladin, D. (2005). Treatment of aggression; the contribution of parent involvement. *International Journal of Group Psychotherapy, 6,* 93–112

Shechtman, Z., & Birani-Nasaraladin, D. (2005). Treating mothers of aggressive children: A research study. *International Journal of Group Psychotherapy*, 56, 93–112. doi: 10.1521/ijgp.2006.56.1.93

Shechtman, Z., & Gilat, I. (2005). The effect of group counseling on parents of a child with learning disabilities (LD) as compared with an NLD sibling. *Group Dynamics: Theory, Research and Practice*, 9, 275–286.

Weiner, J., Biodic, D., Grimbos, T., & Herbert, D. (2016). Parenting stress of parents of adolescents with attention-deficit disorder. *Journal of Abnormal Child Psychology*, 44, 561–574.

Yalom, I. D., & Leszcz, M. (2020). *The theory and practice of group psychotherapy* (6th ed.). New York: Basic Books.

Ziperfal, M., & Shechtman, Z. (2017). Psychodynamic group intervention with parents of children with ADHD: Outcomes for parents and their children. *Group Dynamics: Theory, Research, and Practice*, 21, 135–147.

Part VI

Community intervention

25 Addressing the aftermath of violence in a school context

An SBFC approach

Maria C. Marchetti-Mercer

Overview

This chapter will describe a series of therapeutic interventions that can be applied when working with a school where an incident of violence has taken place. It will focus on the fact that a school must be viewed as a multi-layered and complex system and different levels and forms of therapeutic interventions will therefore be necessary to address the potential trauma experienced by all those involved. This fits in with the principles of School-Based Family Counseling (SBFC) which integrates school and family counseling using a systemic approach. The intervention model which is proposed is based on work done in South Africa but can easily be applied to other cultural contexts. It is hoped that the proposed approach will be useful not only to SBFC practitioners but also other mental health professionals who in the sphere of their work may be called upon to provide trauma counseling in an inherently complex environment, such as a school, in the aftermath of violence. It is of paramount importance that an attitude of respect for the knowledge and resilience of the school and all its different members be fostered during the entire process.

Background

The therapeutic intervention described in this chapter is based on work done in South Africa. While South Africa has not generally experienced the kind of school shootings that seem to take place frequently in countries such as the United States, it does regularly witness high levels of violence in the context of schools. These include armed robberies, kidnappings and other forms of violence perpetrated by teachers on pupils and vice versa. However, addressing all the types of violence that can take place within a school system is outside the scope of this chapter which will rather focus on an example of a time-limited intervention following a specific incident of violence. From a therapeutic perspective, the focus will not be so much on the nature of the incident per se, but rather how it impacts the different subsystems and role players that make up a school system. A different type of intervention may be required depending on whether the School-Based Family Counseling (SBFC) practitioner is already employed by the school or is invited from the outside

DOI: 10.4324/9781003201977-31

following a specific incident of violence. Given the complexity and size of a school system, the approach that is described would be better implemented if a team of professionals is deployed.

The following important principles have to be considered as part of this intervention:

1 The role of the SBFC practitioner
2 The different levels of intervention required
3 The relationship with the different role players

The role of the SBFC practitioner

In the instance where the SBFC professional enters the school system as an outsider, certain factors must be considered. First, the SBFC practitioner's own perceptions about what the client (the school system) may need which may in fact differ from the client's needs. Second, the SBFC practitioner's own views on how people react to trauma are largely informed by their own training and prevailing theories on trauma (Marchetti-Mercer, 2013).

It is therefore recommended that when devising and planning an intervention for a complex community such as a school, SBFC practitioners enter from a position of "not-knowing" as advocated by post-modern writers such as Anderson and Goolishian (1992). From this perspective, the client system must rather be seen as a collaborator in the process of healing rather than a passive recipient of help. Failure to consider this may potentially lead to more trauma (Marchetti-Mercer, 2013).

The different levels of intervention required

The SBFC approach emphasizes working with children in the context of family, school, peer and community systems using a family systems theoretical orientation (Gerrard, Carter & Ribera, 2019). The intervention discussed in this chapter uses this theoretical lens emphasizing the fact that any incident of violence in a school system has ramifications for the whole school system, as well as outside people such as parents and the larger community.

The relationship with the different role players

The SBFC professional will have to interact with all the different role players all with diverse experiences and needs. These may include school administrators, teachers, students, janitors, parents and other members of the community. Different types of relationships will have to be fostered and developed. An attitude of respect for the different types of knowledge that each groups can contribute must be maintained.

Procedure

The procedure described below is an example of a short-term crisis intervention where the SBFC practitioner is required to be very active providing both information and emotional support (Carson, Butcher & Mineka, 1996). Consequently, there is also a time limit to the intervention which must be communicated to the school from the beginning.

This procedure is based on work done by a team of South African therapists comprising two senior psychologists and 12 graduate psychology students. See information in Box 25.1 for more details on the specific case study. While a specific procedure is being described, the intervention may have to be tailored according to the needs of the client system.

Box 25.1 Case study involving school violence

On a Monday morning, an elementary school in a rural area outside Tshwane (South Africa) was the target of an attempted robbery when a number of armed men tried to rob a cash-in-transit van that was being used to courier money from the school premises. In South Africa, money is often transported in such security vehicles. More than ten armed men appeared at the school entrance in five cars and threatened the security guards who had come to collect monies from the school financial department. A small war, as described by onlookers, ensued and more than 60 shots were fired between the security guards and the robbers who were carrying AK 47 and R 5 rifles as well as pistols. The robbers managed to take 30 money trunks from the van, which were fortunately later recovered by the police. One of the robbers was shot at the scene of the crime, while his accomplices, although managing to flee at the time, were later apprehended by the police. In the meantime, the school principal, learning of the commotion, grabbed a pistol from his office and also came running to the scene. The school secretary immediately phoned the police who reacted promptly, resulting in the subsequent swift apprehension of the robbers. This was not the first example of attempted robbery at this particular school but other incidents had taken place without violence. A large number of the children directly witnessed the shooting as the grade one and two classes (six- to seven-year-olds) faced the grounds where the shooting took place. Initially, many of the youngsters said that they thought the noise came from fireworks but they later realized that it was a serious shooting.

Fortunately, the teachers reacted quickly and got the children to lie down on the floor, thus preventing injury. The shooting was also heard by the children in the other classes but they did not register what was happening and were merely overwhelmed by the noise. Parents were immediately informed of the incident and many of them rushed to the school to take stock of what had happened and to take their children home. The incident made headline news in most local newspapers.

In the aftermath of the shooting, the school became the focus of a lot of media attention as well as falling under the eye of community leaders and politicians. This event seemed to highlight the vulnerability of rural schools, many of which are fairly isolated and lack proper security (Marchetti-Mercer, 2013).

Step 1: Initial contact with the school client

The first point of entry into the school is usually through the school administrators. Identifying the contact/referring person/ body is important as well as determining their expectations of the therapeutic process. Whoever seeks out psychological assistance will have already made a certain assessment of the situation, as well as have certain expectations of the SBFC professional. It is essential to engage respectfully and listen carefully. It is also important to remember that school administrators may also have been significantly impacted by the trauma which will need to be addressed therapeutically.

Important therapeutic considerations

There is a real danger that when "experts" move in after members of a particular system have suffered a traumatic experience they may create additional trauma by emphasizing the helplessness and the neediness of the clients. This may inadvertently communicate that there is something wrong with the client and that the therapist is the only one who can "fix" it, taking away their sense of empowerment and ignoring their inherent resilience.

It is important to maintain by a strong element of "therapeutic flexibility" when entering a complex system such as a school in order to address the needs of the clients as those which may emerge during the therapeutic interventions. If one's initial therapeutic plan is too rigid and too prescriptive they may eventually be rejected (Marchetti-Mercer, 2013)

Step 2: Identifying different levels of intervention

During this phase, it is important to identify the different groups that need psychological assistance. This may involve the individual(s) directly impacted by the violence as well as other groups in the school system (this may involve other students, teachers, administrative staff, janitors and parents). Again, the SBFC professional will have to adapt their therapeutic plan depending on the situation.

The different phases described below are based on the needs of the participants of the case study described in Box 26.1.

Step 3: Group debriefing with children

In our case, the first level of intervention was with the children who had directly witnessed the shooting incident. We decided to use a group debriefing intervention, given the limited resources and time limitation. Group interventions may be useful in these kinds of situation where a large number of people need to be assisted within a limited time frame.

The aim of our intervention was as follows:

a   Allow the children to express their feelings regarding the shooting incident in a non-threatening context.
b   Allow them to regain some sense of control over their environment.
c   Normalize the experience as a group by allowing them to see that their classmates had experienced similar feelings of fear and anxiety.

Pynoos and Eth (1986) argue that allowing the child to develop an increased sense of security, competence and mastery following a traumatic event is regarded as a desirable goal of trauma work with children. It was decided to use a developmentally appropriate therapeutic technique such as art (in this case drawings) which would allow the children to express their feelings around the shooting in a non-threatening manner. The SBFC professional may choose other techniques as long as it is developmentally appropriate.

Each child was given the opportunity to draw a picture of what had happened and given a chance to talk about his/her picture to the rest of the class. Team members provided each child with a lot of positive reinforcement throughout the process. In the second part of the intervention, each child was asked to draw a picture describing what they would do if they were the chief of the police to make the school safer for the children. The aim of this exercise was to give the children a sense of empowerment making them feel involved in the decision-making about safety in schools. Significantly, the drawings revealed similar recurring trends such as big policemen with large guns, fierce police dogs, high fences around the school building and so forth.

The teachers also assisted during this process and the team gave them a lot of positive reinforcement for the very quick way in which they had reacted in order to protect the children. The teachers were in fact very distressed after the incident as they had feared for their own as well as the children's safety. However, they had responded quite effectively and managed to keep a reasonably calm atmosphere.

Important therapeutic considerations

In a context where both children and teachers have been impacted by violence, the emotional needs of the teachers may be underestimated. The teachers tried to protect the children and took a lot of initiative trying to appear strong for the sake of the children. We noticed that the teachers had been deeply affected by the incident as it had impinged on their sense of safety at their place of work. They seemed to be experiencing a wide range of feelings such as fear/anxiety as well as anger at having been a target of violence. In situations like this, it may be appropriate to offer teachers individual psychological follow-up.

Step 4 Individual assessment of children not directly involved

While not everyone may be directly involved, a violent act in a school system may also impact other students (for example, students who did not witness the violence). It is important to identify these and teachers may be a useful referral source. In our case, the therapeutic team offered psychological assistance to other children in the school based on recommendations from the teachers.

There are different ways in which this can be done and it will be up to the SBFC practitioner to decide on a suitable type of assessment. In our case, the student members of the team evaluated a number of children through diagnostic interviews and projective techniques such as the Draw-a-Person test or the Kinetic Family Test and then made recommendations for further counseling if deemed necessary. This process took place for an entire week. Following the incident, a number of children also refused to come to school and parents contacted members of the team for advice as to how address the problem.

Important therapeutic considerations

In our case, we soon realized that many children were being referred for assessment whose difficulties were in no way related to the shooting. It became evident that the school and parents had decided to make use of the psychological services which were being made available to them as there was no permanent counseling support available at the school. Given the time limit of the team's presence in the school, we eventually had to refer the children to an outside counseling center. Again what is highlighted here is the fact that the needs of a community may be different than what envisaged by the SBFC practitioner and that during the therapeutic process they must be able to adapt the therapeutic plan to the clients' needs.

Step 5 Group Intervention with teachers and other school workers

The next part of the intervention should be aimed at addressing the needs of the teachers. As mentioned earlier, in our case, the teachers seemed to have experienced a serious crisis related to their role as caregivers. Moreover, they no longer experienced their place of work as safe. In our case, it was useful to hold group sessions with teachers led by two co-therapists. The value of group therapy is widely recorded in the literature, for example, Yalom (1995) and may be an important way for teachers to share their own feelings with one another and ultimately normalize their own experiences of the event.

We also ran a group for the different workers in the school, comprising janitors and cleaning staff as we feared that these groups of people may often be overlooked. In our case, these workers were mainly African who were not very fluent in English. Consequently, the group was led by a therapist fluent in an African language, thus allowing participants to speak in their mother tongue.

Important therapeutic considerations

It is important to create a context where teachers also have the chance to express their feelings surrounding the incident. In our case, the groups were open and discussions around their feelings regarding the shooting took place. The level of emotional intensity seemed to differ from group to group and we observed interesting gender difference where male teachers tended to underplay the emotional impact of the incident. It was also essential to provide a space for other workers in the school where their experiences could be acknowledged and respected. Gender and power differences prevalent in a school system must be considered in the course of the therapeutic intervention.

Step 6: Involving the parents

In line with the underlying philosophy of the SBFC model, which aims to engage parents and families as partners with the SBFC professional (Gerrard, Carter & Ribera, 2019), it is essential to involve parents as part of any therapeutic intervention. Furthermore, specifically involving parents in the therapeutic process following trauma experienced by their children is of paramount importance (Leibowitz, Mendelsohn & Michelson, 1999; Udwin, 1993).

In order to engage with the parents as a group, a parents' evening or session can be organized in order for parents to share their concerns and pose any questions to the SBFC professional(s). Thereafter, individual time can be allocated if parents want to have a more in-depth consultation.

The focus of such an intervention should be mostly psycho-educational providing as much information and tools to parents to assist and support their children. Drawing up an information sheet listing the different symptoms of Post-traumatic Stress Disorder (PTSD) may be useful as it will make parents aware of the possible symptoms of PTSD that their children may experience later on. In our case, we also provided them some guidelines on how to deal with their children in a psychologically supportive manner with children.

Important therapeutic considerations

We experienced a poor turnout at the parents' evening which was a source of disappointment for the team which had put in a lot of preparation for the event. One of the reasons for this was possibly the fact that the event had been organized for the evening and given issues of security and the geographical position of the school, it was difficult for parents to attend. This is once highlighted the fact that in the course of such a complex intervention, the therapist(s) may have devised a certain therapeutic plan without considering the needs and challenges of the clients. Furthermore, in the case of the parents who did attend, many of the queries were not directly related to the shooting incident. Again, this highlighted the fact that this was a school community which needed psychological services well beyond those dealing with the aftermath of the shooting incident.

Step 7: Exiting the school system

Any therapeutic intervention will require a proper termination strategy. This intervention will require reflection on one's own role as a therapist especially following such an emotionally and time-intensive intervention. This may be inherently challenging for the SBFC professional who may feel that they have not done "enough" for their clients. This may be exacerbated by factors such as the nature of the initial trauma or perceived resources available to the school.

Important therapeutic considerations

As part of the termination strategy, it is important to emphasize the inherent resilience of the school system and how different groups can provide support to each other going forward.

Multicultural considerations

This intervention was developed within the South African context which differs greatly from other parts of the world. It is however a context which by definition is highly multicultural not only because of different ethnic and racial representation but also because of its linguistic diversity.

Schools across the world may differ in terms of their heterogeneity but we can assume that any SBFC professional would expect to work with a reasonably diverse population when entering a school system. A therapeutic stance of respect and listening to the needs of the various client populations, which have been highlighted in the procedure section, are indispensable in this therapeutic experience. Developing a "not-knowing" and respectful attitude may be the most important tool available to the SBFC practitioner as they engage with diverse client systems.

Challenges and solutions

Entering a school system following an episode of violence may be challenging for the SBFC practitioner depending on the nature of the event. In our case, fortunately no one was seriously injured nor killed, but should this be the case, the trauma that the SBFC professional(s) may have to address will be significant and may require adaptations to this procedure.

A number of specific challenges should be considered:

1　The relationship with the school
　　SBFC practitioners must be cautious not to enter the school system as "experts" as this may communicate to the members of the school that they are helpless and unable to deal with the aftermath of the experience. Often,

theories of trauma debriefing are prescriptive and encourage therapists to follow specific guidelines when dealing with clients. However, when using such interventions, the therapist must be careful not to exacerbate feelings of powerlessness and rather emphasize a process of co-operation and co-creation between therapists and the school system.

2   The relationship with the family and community

Violent school events often cause great shock to communities as schools are traditionally perceived by parents and society as secure nurturing environments. When these safe havens are violated, this impacts not only the school system but also the larger communities within which schools operate.

The therapeutic plan should therefore be guided by the school community which consists of staff and students as well as parents. A high priority should be the involvement of the families as this is the context into which children have to return, and this can certainly aid the therapeutic process. The family remains the primary context within which the child functions: traditional views of family therapy have always emphasized that any therapy aimed at a child must always take place in the context of the family or at least be mindful of the family system (Minuchin, 1974).

When working with a school exposed to trauma, it is therefore essential to work with children in the context of their family as befitting an SBFC perspective. It can be argued that an important mediating factor in children's responses to trauma is the family context of the child and especially the parent's reaction to the traumatic event (Stallard & Law, 1994).

3   The relationship between the school and the families

Exposure of a school system to a traumatic event may deeply influence the relationship between the school and the families of the children. In the specific case discussed here, many parents directly or indirectly blamed the school for poor security measures which may have placed their children at risk. Although these accusations proved to be unfounded, they may rather have been a reflection of the deep emotional distress experienced by parents following their children's traumatic event.

These feelings may however hinder the healing process as children may find themselves in the middle of conflict, given they are dual members of both the school and family systems. Feeling torn between these two may place additional emotional demands upon the children.

In the aftermath of school violence, much emphasis may be placed on the children's experiences while disregarding the feelings and experiences of the teachers and other staff members. This may lead to teachers resenting the families' negative feelings even more. Teachers' perceptions and role definitions as caregivers are also deeply affected by the trauma and must be addressed. They may question themselves as to whether or not they had acted responsibly or if they could have done more to protect the children from possible harm. In a situation where children have been hurt or died, teachers may even experience a strong sense of survivors' guilt in addition to feeling that they had not done enough to protect the children.

Conclusion

Entering a school system following an incident of violence poses many opportunities but also challenges to the SBFC professional. A school is a complex system comprising a number of different subsystems. An SBFC theoretical lens lends itself well to the kind of multi-layered intervention which is described in this chapter as it emphasizes the relationship between school, children and parents. It also highlights how psychological healing can take place at the interface of these relationships.

Resources

Raubeson, Merryl E. (2013). Learning from art therapists: Strategies for treating children with PTSD. Masters Thesis, Smith College, Northampton, MA. https://scholarworks.smith.edu/theses/607
This is a thesis that looks at the work of practicing art therapists providing interesting examples for SBFC working with traumatised-youth
St. Thomas, B., & Johnson, P. (2002). In their own voices: Play activities and art with traumatised children. *Groupwork: An Interdisciplinary Journal for Working with Groups, 13*(2), 34–48.
This is a very useful article highlighting some useful therapeutic techniques that can be used with children who have been exposed to trauma.
van Westrhenen, N., Fritz, E., Vermeer, A., Boelen, P., & Kleber, R. (2019). Creative arts in psychotherapy for traumatized children in South Africa: An evaluation study. *PloS one, 14*(2), e0210857. https://doi.org/10.1371/journal.pone.0210857-
This article describes therapeutic work done with traumatised children and evaluates this manner of intervention.
World Health Organization. (2019). School-based violence prevention: A practical handbook. World Health Organization. https://apps.who.int/iris/handle/10665/324930.
This is a very comprehensive and practical guide to both prevention and intervention when it comes to school-based violence.

References

Anderson, H., & Goolishian H.A. (1992). The client is the expert: A not-knowing approach to therapy. In S. Mc Namee & K. Gergen (Eds.). *Social construction and the therapeutic process* (pp. 25–39). Sage.
Carson, R.C., Butcher, J.N., & Mineka, S. (1996). *Abnormal psychology and modern life.* (10th ed). Harper Collins College Publishers.
Gerrard, B., Carter, M. & Ribera, D. (Eds.) (2019). *School-based family counseling: An interdisciplinary practitioner's guide.* Routledge.
Leibowitz, S., Mendelsohn, M., & Michelson, C. (1999). Child rape: extending the therapeutic intervention to include the mother-child dyad. *South African Journal of Psychology, 29*(3), 103–108.

Marchetti-Mercer M.C. (2013). Therapeutic interventions following an incident of violence in a school: a South African case study. Chapter 46. In B. Gerrard & M. Soriano (Eds.), *School-based family counseling: Transforming family-school relationships* (pp. 518–528).Createspace. 978–1490934822

Minuchin, S. (1974). *Families and family therapy*. Harvard University Press.

Pynoos, R.S., & Eth, S. (1986). Witness to violence: the child interview. *Journal of the American Academy of Child Psychiatry, 25*, 306–319.

Stallard, P., & Law, F. (1994). The psychological effects of trauma on children. *Children in Society, 8*, 89–97.

Udwin, O. (1993). Annotation: Children's reactions to traumatic events. *Child Psychology & Psychiatry & Allied Disciplines, 34*(2), 115–127. https://doi.org/10.1111/j.1469-7610.1993.tb00974.x

Yalom, I.D. (1995). *The theory and practice of group psychotherapy* (4th ed.). Basic Books.

26 Community-based psychosocial intervention for child protection in disaster

Shayana Deb, Sibnath Deb, and Anjali Gireesan

Overview

Children are precious resources for any society and quality care and support facilities are prerequisite during early childhood. During any crisis or disaster, a large number of children experience various forms of challenges and become vulnerable to neglect, physical abuse, sexual abuse, poverty, psychological trauma and family violence. A good number of children also become orphans at the time of crisis. Community-based psychosocial intervention is found to be very beneficial for the protection of the rights of the children and ensuring their safety, in addition to providing support to their families. This chapter discusses community preparedness for responding at times of crisis and the role of the SBFC practitioner as a facilitator is very crucial under such situations.

Background

Disasters and/or crises in life are normal phenomena for various reasons. It can happen in any society and at any point of time. It does not affect the ordinary chores of perennial survival but influences every individual psychologically, physically, socially and economically. The response of every individual during a crisis situation is different. Some people cope well with stressful situations, while some feel extremely helpless and look for support.

Like most countries, India has encountered several natural disasters in the past. These include the Super Cyclone in Orissa (1999), the Earthquake in Gujarat (2001), the Tsunami in the Indian Ocean (2004), the Kashmir Earthquake (2005), severe floods in north and north-east India and the recent disaster, christened Himalayan Tsunami (2013) in Uttarakhand, Floods in Chennai (2015) and Floods in Kerala (2018), to name a few. All these natural disasters adversely affected normal life and caused the death of many people. At the same time, India also witnessed several man-made disasters like the Gujarat riots (2002), bombings in Mumbai (2006) which killed several people and damaged a number of buildings in different locations, Mumbai terrorist attack (2008), continuous armed conflict in Kashmir, riots in Orissa (2008), incidents of riots and ethnic violence in Assam and the Delhi riots

DOI: 10.4324/9781003201977-32

(2020), which disrupted daily activities. Of late, the COVID-19 pandemic, a biological disaster, affected the entire world and for the last 19 months all educational institutions are closed for the safety of all stakeholders.

People belonging to the lower social strata experience maximum hardship during any crisis due to lack of resources, poverty and poor social network (Hallegatte et al., 2020). Children become the worst victims of any crisis and/ or disaster and become vulnerable to various risks, as they depend upon others and are not matured enough to cope with the situation (Bhadra, 2016; Muzenda-Mudavanhu, 2016).

Disaster has high association with child protection in any society. It poses security threats, disrupts normal life and isolates people from their near and dear ones and the community. Children experience violence both within and outside the family. The closure of educational facilities and the loss of family members ultimately disconnect the children from their school and peer group members. Protection of children after the disaster is a challenging issue and it requires partnership with allied agencies for providing holistic services to the children and their families. At times of crisis, the SBFC practitioner should join hands with the community-based organizations for addressing the issues and challenges faced by the children at the community level.

The immediate crisis which arises after the disaster includes lack of safe shelter, lack of safe drinking water, food crisis and medical challenges, disruption of educational and social life and post-traumatic stress which needs immediate attention of community-based organizations.

Community-based psychosocial support facilities for child safety: evidence-based experiences

Lindqvist et al. (2002) examined the outcome of the World Health Organization's (WHO) Safe Community model, with respect to child injuries and observed that introduction of an injury prevention program based on WHO's Safe Community model worked well in reducing the risk of child injury. In another community-based intervention program, an effort was made to examine the effectiveness of the step-by-step program, in which mentors worked with parents affected by Fetal Alcohol Spectrum Disorder (FASD) on a one-to-one basis and found it to be beneficial (Denys et al., 2011).

In an intervention in Kanyakumari, India immediately after the Tsunami, people were rescued and put in a safe shelter. In the relief camp, the volunteers started working with the children to facilitate care and support. Within a few days, the local non-government organizations (NGOs) of the area were contacted by the volunteers. They also contacted the respective government officials, authorities of local schools and child care providers of the Integrated Child Development Scheme Centres, namely Anganwadi Workers, and many health workers were also identified. Subsequently, psychosocial support services were arranged by the local NGOs and the government staff, who were directly working with the survivors in the relief camps and temporary shelters. The psychosocial support services helped the children to deal with their traumatic experiences and regain self-confidence to start a new life. These activities also protected the affected children from any further psychological harm and abuse at a time when the nurturing and protective environment was completely destroyed by the Tsunami (NIMHANS & WHO, 2006; WHO, 2006; NIMHANS, 2007).

The school recovery program in the Tsunami-affected areas of Kanyakumari District in India, developed by the American Red Cross-India Delegation team, in association with the Indian Red Cross local (IFRC, 2008; Bhadra & Pratheepa, 2009), was found to be very beneficial to bring the school back to the normal functioning stage with the help of teachers, parents and students representatives. The broad objective of the school recovery program was to create a child-friendly space, developing a sense of place in the schools and safe school protocol, in addition to helping school children to gain resiliency to deal with future challenges.

Children living along the borders of India suffer from anxiety and fear because of cross-firing between two countries. It is very challenging to address the issue of security threat, which is common to people as well as children. Often, schools are taken by the armed forces which affect the education of the children (Kousar & Bhadra, 2021). However, a time bound intervention conducted with a few children in five schools in Kashmir, with an objective to provide psychosocial support, enhance resilience and take safety measures, was found to be beneficial in relieving their stress, as they were allowed to express their feelings through storytelling, drawing and role-play. At the end of the intervention, most of the children were found to be relaxed, which was evident from their countenance and overall body language (Bhadra & Dyer, 2022).

In order to deal with the emotions of students going to school, college and university, online mode of lecture on issues like "COVID-19: A Time to be Resilient" by experienced mental health professionals was found to be beneficial, in order to guide students to follow all safety measures, be resilient in a crisis situation, focus on online education and not to view news related to COVID-19.

Evidence clearly demonstrates the benefits of community-based intervention programs to support children and their families in crisis, through participatory community engagement approach, thus prioritizing their needs and providing need-based services.

Procedure

Identifying community leaders like public representatives, at the local and state levels, spiritual leaders, juvenile justice welfare committee members, medical officers, child protection officers, mental health professionals, personnel working in different residential institutes for children, NGO personnel working with children at the grassroots levels, school teachers, school counselors and relevant government officials is the first step for planning and designing community-based intervention services for child safety, at times of crisis. It can be done with a particular group of community members like child protection officers or medical officers alone, but organizing a multidisciplinary community-based training program, by inviting professionals from various sectors, would help to better understand the issue and the role of each category of professionals and the necessity for coordination and partnership, in order to adopt a holistic approach and deliver better services to children. The steps which are involved in this process include secondary research, recruitment, need assessment, designing a multidisciplinary training program and planning, implementing as well as evaluating the training program (Figure 26.1).

Step I: Secondary research

The objective of secondary research is to gather information about strategies adopted for community-based intervention programs, organized in the past for addressing emerging issues at the community level, in particular, about various child protection schemes in different locations and their effectiveness. Review of secondary information will be useful for the SBFC practitioner in developing the outline of the community-based multidisciplinary training program, which will protect children at times of crisis.

Step II: Recruitment

Selection of community leaders for community-based multidisciplinary orientation programs on child protection at times of crisis is an important step to identify the community leaders who are child-friendly, sensitive to children's issues and concerns, passionate about working with children in difficult circumstances and possess past field experience. Considering the above criteria, community leaders from different categories should be identified by the SBFC practitioner through a snowball technique and their written informed consent needs to be obtained for participation in the training/orientation program.

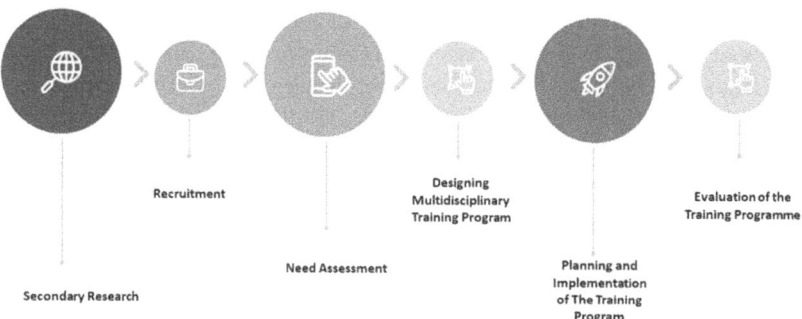

Figure 26.1 Steps involved in planning/designing a community-based intervention program

Informed consent forms should also have the provision to take their consent for their participation and availability in ensuring child safety at times of any crisis in the community. This approach will help the SBFC practitioner to remain prepared with community volunteers for any challenge, for the greater interest of the children.

Step III: Need assessment

Understanding the knowledge, attitude and perception of community leaders about child rights, child safety, present status of children in the local community, their vulnerability toward risk, legislative measures for child protection, government policies and programs for healthy child development and welfare of children, as well as role of different stakeholders at times of disaster and crisis are essential in designing multidisciplinary orientation programs by the SBFC practitioner, for child protection. This exercise will also help the SBFC practitioners to understand the needs of the community leaders, in terms of information about child protection in crisis, design need-based training programs, and come out with a road map for different stakeholders regarding working together to help disaster victim children and their families, through proper linkages and coordination.

Step IV: Designing a multidisciplinary orientation/ Training program

Analyzing the data of need assessment as an effective orientation/training program should be designed for disaster preparedness. Disaster preparedness is very important for prompt response at times of crisis. Specific orientation/ training programs include having a multidisciplinary orientation/training program, for community leaders, on child protection in crisis and children's vulnerability to neglect, abuse and maltreatment.

Step V: Planning, implementation and evaluation of the training/orientation programs

The SBFC practitioner should develop a brief leaflet with detailed information about the need to organize such a training program, its objective, the methodology to be followed and the target group of the training program, the date and time of the program and it should also be circulated among a selective group of community leaders, for their inputs and be finalized, based on their inputs. It is important to decide the duration of the training program based on the needs. Ideally, such types of training programs should be organized in a convenient location with proper sitting arrangements and audio-visual facilities, either on holidays or during the evening, as every potential community leader will have their own schedule of daily activities. Organizing training programs as per the convenience of the target groups will ensure more and effective participation in the training programs. Nevertheless, an effort should be made to organize a full day training program, continuously for two or three days, with the consent of the participants and a follow-up or refresher training, after a month or two months, if possible. Mixed-method and participatory approaches should be followed in organizing the training program. For example, a few lectures should be arranged by the experts on basic concepts and for sharing of available evidence, followed by questions and answers and group activities on various themes. However, the SBFC practitioner should design the training program based on the needs of the target group and the facilities available in the local community.

Any intervention or training program should be subjected to evaluation, for examining its effectiveness. It could be done by following qualitative or quantitative data collection methods, before and after the training program. The SBFC practitioner may develop simple questionnaires with both closed and open-ended questions to capture the views and opinions of the participants. Analysis of pre- and post-training data will be an eye opener for the SBFC to understand the effectiveness of the training and in designing future intervention training programs based on the valuable inputs.

An example of a three-day multidisciplinary training on child protection in crisis and disaster

Objectives of the training

- Discussing the safety of the children in crisis situations, the specific role of different stakeholders and interconnection among the stakeholders.
- Assessing the basic needs of the children and their families at times of crisis.
- Developing a program for psychological and medical support, safe shelter and other basic needs.
- Coordination and monitoring of the progress of various intervention activities.

An Example of a program schedule

The tentative program schedule is subject to modification, based on the needs and the local situation. There are seven steps involved in organizing the training program (see Table 26.1). These include warm-up sessions, discussing the rules for the training, sharing basic information about child safety in crisis and evidence related to successful case studies, group activities, sharing the outcome of group exercises, developing a road map for the multidisciplinary team for their role in crisis, summarizing the learning experience and evaluating the training by the participants.

Step I: Warm-up: The first day of the training program should start with a warm-up session, immediately after the brief inaugural function, and explaining the objectives of the multidisciplinary training program meant for

Table 26.1 Examples of training topics and methods

	Tentative topics to be covered	Methods to be followed
Day 1:	Child vulnerability in crisis	Lecture by an expert, followed by an interaction
	Basic information on need for child protection	Lecture by an expert, followed by an interaction
	Role of agencies and caregivers at times of crisis	Group Exercise and Sharing of the Outcome of Group Exercise
	Coordination among different agencies	Group Exercise and Sharing of the Outcome of Group Exercise
Day 2:	Nature of basic services to be provided: safe shelter, safe drinking water, sanitation facilities, food, clothes, medical care, safety, organizing social and cultural programs, games, sports and group activities	Group Exercise and Sharing of the Outcome of Group Exercise
Day 3:	Need for Monitoring of services	Lecture by an expert
	Follow-up and/or after care services	Lecture by an expert

the community leaders, for ensuring psychosocial and general support facilities. To begin with, self-introduction can be the starting point, which will familiarize the participants with each other. Thereafter, the facilitator of the training program, i.e. the SBFC practitioner, can ask four to five participants from different categories to share their personal and professional experiences regarding case studies, with regard to child safety or child vulnerability, and writing few safety measures for children, which will, in turn, set the tone of the training program.

Facilitator: *Welcome, esteemed participants of the three-day multidisciplinary training program. The broad objective of this training program is to exchange our views about child protection in crisis situations and develop a road map by defining clearly the role of each one of us as a professional to address their issues holistically. We are going to start todays' training with a warm-up session with a self-introduction, followed by sharing some of our experiences about child vulnerability in crisis. Thereafter, participants may be asked to write what they think could be the best five safety measures for children during any crisis, based on personal experience. Five minutes time should be given for the same.*

Community leaders complete the activity

Facilitator: *Thank you participants for sharing your experience and thoughts on issues which are highly interesting and are eye openers for us. Thereafter, participants may be asked to share any specific issue and/or concern about issues related to the training, so that during the training, the same can be addressed.*

Step II: Discussing the Rules of the Training: It is very important to share the rules of the training program with the participants to ensure smooth implementation of the training program as per the program schedule.

Facilitator: *Now I am going to share certain rules of the training program with all of you. They include (i) asking questions or clarification of any issue during the training program, one by one, (ii) respecting the views of others, while responding to any issue, (iii) no cross talk during the lecture session of training, (iv) not referring to any discussion or point raised by anybody outside the training program and (v) attending all the sessions of the training. I hope it is clear to everyone. However, feel free to ask any questions related to the rules of the training program.*

Step III: Sharing the Basic Information about Child Safety in Crisis and Related Evidence: The resource persons will deliver lectures using a PowerPoint presentation, to appraise the participants about child safety issues in crisis and the risk factors related to neglect, abuse and maltreatment, based on latest available evidence and positive case studies pertaining to the effectiveness of training programs.

Facilitator: *I think it was a very enlightening session for all of us and we have developed a better understanding of the issue. I am sure all of you will agree with me. I would urge some of you to share your views about the sessions.*

Participant 1: *It was a very informative session.*

Participant 2: *Latest evidence shared by the resource person was enlightening for us.*

Participant 3: *Now we have a clear picture about the present status of the children and their vulnerability in crisis.*

after lunch

Step IV: Group Exercise: Now we are going to have four group exercises by dividing the participants equally in four groups. The objective of the group exercise and the brainstorming sessions is to discuss certain pertinent issues related to child safety at times of crisis, i.e. (i) examining the situation and deciding upon the immediate care and support services, in terms of general and psychosocial support facilities, for the children and their families, (ii) role of different categories of community leaders for service delivery, (iii) method of coordination among different categories of community leaders and (iv) close monitoring of service delivery and safety of the children. For group exercises, one hour of time should be given. One person will be the team leader, which will be decided by the group members and finally at the end of the group exercise, they will write the outcome of the exercise in a chart paper for presentation.

Facilitator: *How was the exercise? How do you feel now after having a brainstorming session? I saw that all of you were actively engaged in the discussion and exchange of views and ideas.*

Step V: Sharing Outcome of Group Exercise and Developing a Road Map for the Multidisciplinary Team: The next session is about sharing the outcome of group exercises with other team members. After the presentation of each group, there will be discussions, inviting any question and/or queries for clarity of the issues and then coming to a unanimous understanding. All the chart papers will be preserved for summing up the information of all the groups.

Facilitator: *It was a wonderful session where we could see the innovative ideas and suggestions of each group, related to each topic. Now, I thank all for providing a better understanding about our role in child safety, during any crisis.*

Step VI: Summarize the Learning Experience: In this session, the participants will be asked to reflect upon following questions one by one:

> *What did he/she learn or relearn?*
>> *How can a community leader use what he/she learned in the field?*
>> *How active was the participant during the training?*
>> *What is the feeling now after attending the training?*

Facilitator: *I would urge one or two from each group to share your experience of the group exercise.*

Participant I: We could learn from each other during the group exercise.

Participant II: The group exercise helped me to possess better clarity about our role in the crisis, to ensure safety for every child.

Participant III: Now the method of coordination during any crisis is very clear to me.

Participant IV: The need for monitoring the progress of intervention programs at the community level, during the crisis, and its importance, has been realized by all of us.

Step VII: After Care Support Facilities: Once the crisis is over, there is a need to follow up with the families to understand their issues and concerns, if any, and provide them support, in terms of referral, so that their issues are addressed. After care is very essential in helping families to settle down and take care of their children's welfare.

Facilitator: *I think all of you are clear about the need for after care facilities. If any of you have any queries, feel free to ask or if there exists any incident that you would like to share from your experience, you are welcome.*

Participant I: I was involved in after care services for flood victim families and could see the helpless conditions for some families, after the immediate rescue operation. There were arrangements of safe drinking water, medicine and even food.

Step VIII: Evaluate the Training by the Participants: Any training program should be subjected to evaluation by the participants at the end, using different methods. It might be a pre- and post-method or a post-only assessment following the training. For example, using a semi-structured questionnaire, the organizer can ask each participant to share their views about the training. Some of the questions could be (i) How did you find the overall training? (ii) How were the resource persons? (iii) Which part of the training did you find interesting and beneficial? (iv) Which part of the training was not effective? (v) Any suggestions for improvement of future training programs? (vi) Did the organizer contact you well in advance and make necessary arrangements? (vii) How was the venue and food? (viii) Do you think the duration of the training should be for more days?

Facilitator: *Thanks for giving your frank views about the training. It would help us to understand the effectiveness of the training and to design future training programs effectively.*

Multicultural considerations

Any disaster management program should be developed after keeping cultural diversity in mind. Normally, people of different religious, cultural and social backgrounds live in the same community and their knowledge, cultural beliefs and practices about child rearing are different and even, it might be totally different from the SBFC professionals. In India, most of the schools do not have SBFC services. In some private schools, one or two mental health professionals are appointed and in most cases they are untrained. The objective of appointing mental health professionals in private schools is to attract more students and in reality, most of them are engaged in other official work. SBFC is new in India and it requires attention of the policymakers, so that there is a circular from the respective government authority to appoint SBFC practitioners for every school.

Nevertheless, multicultural considerations demand attention in designing community-based intervention programs and are also important at the time of the implementation. Prior to designing any intervention program, an effort should be made to understand the cultural beliefs and practices about child welfare in the community and accordingly, an intervention program must be designed for the community. Training programs should be organized in the local language, so that community members understand the issue better and also, they can express their opinion while undergoing the training or orientation program. Efforts should be taken to engage concerned government officials in the training program, as they are the key persons for the implementation of various child welfare schemes in the community. In general, after the sanction of any project, very few government officials, who are closely associated with the program, monitor the implementation process. Therefore, this issue requires attention in the training program. Myths about gender role need to be emphasized in the training programs for parents, i.e. both the parents should play equal roles in quality upbringing of the children and ensuring child safety.

Challenges and solutions

Any disaster causes several challenges for the common people. People from marginalized communities, especially women and children, become the worst victims of disaster. However, in Table 26.2, a number of steps are suggested for addressing various challenges.

Table 26.2 Challenges and solutions

	Possible challenges	Solutions
1	Shortage of trained manpower at the community level	Organizing multidisciplinary training programs and creating trained manpower
2	Assessing the magnitude of the damage caused by the disaster	Rapid assessment of any disaster by a group of experts is essential to understand the nature and extent of damage for planning and designing appropriate intervention programs.
3	Reaching out to disaster affected families and children in remote areas.	Efforts should be taken to divide the responsibility among various voluntary organizations to reach out to the unreached, for delivering need-based support services.
4	Providing immediate relief.	Disaster preparedness would help to render immediate rescue operation services.
5	Coordinating with various agencies interested in providing relief aids, to ensure smooth relief services to disaster victims.	At times of crisis, various national and international organizations are willing to deliver support services to victims, in terms of providing resources like medical care, food and medicines. Local government and/or administration should take the lead role in coordinating and receiving the resources and utilizing them for the services of humanity, through proper monitoring mechanisms.
6	Ensuring safety for all disaster affected children	Close monitoring of rescue and rehabilitation programs are essential by the training community leaders, who might engage the elderly people of the local community and non-government organizations working with children and youth volunteers.
7	Addressing mental health needs of the disaster affected families and their children because of shortage of trained manpower.	This is a common challenge for resource constrained countries. However, psycho-educational approaches can be created, i.e. giving basic training on group counseling to youth possessing graduation level education.
8	Organizing cultural, sports and culture-specific group activities for the children	In some locations, it might be difficult to organize social and cultural programs. Considering the local facilities, some social and cultural programs may be organized, which will be stress relieving and will help children and their families to develop a sense of belongingness.
9	Fund constraints for the overall welfare of children	Through the internet, one should look for philanthropic organizations who fund during crisis situations, in addition to contacting the Disaster Management Organization of the local government.

10	Monitoring of the regular progress of community intervention	Monitoring and follow-up is overlooked on most occasions. This issue needs attention in any community-based training program, to ensure smooth progress of intervention programs or rescue and rehabilitation programs.
11	Follow-up and connecting children who lost their parents or their close ones	Along with close follow-up of after care services, an effort should be taken to locate the parents and connect the children with parents, with the help of local Police.
12	Providing on-going psychosocial support to children, who are highly traumatized and lost their parents.	A separate trained team should work for on-going mental support services to help traumatized children or these children should be referred to trained professionals.

Conclusion

Community preparedness for community-based psychosocial intervention, in addition to addressing general needs of the disaster victim families and children, should be given special emphasis in every society by the local administration to address the emerging challenges at the time of crisis or disaster. A participation approach, involving all key leaders of the community, including respective government officials, local public representatives, parents and school teachers, in addition to others, as cited before, would help to face the challenges, to ensure protection of children from adversities and also to support their family members. However, there are various challenges in addressing child safety and their familial issues. One of the major challenges is coordination between the rehabilitation and the resettlement process. This can be handled by inviting participation of all the community leaders to address the issues affecting welfare of children until the community resumes normal life.

Resources

Alisic, E. (2012). Teachers' perspectives on providing support to children after trauma: A qualitative study. *School Psychology Quarterly, 27*(1), 51–59. https://doi.org/10.1037/a0028590
This article based on qualitative study gives a better understanding to adopt a tailored made approach for providing training to the school teachers for providing support to children with trauma.
Protection of Children during the Coronavirus Pandemic (v.1)1 https://www.unicef.org › media › file › Technical…
This document highlights the issues to be taken care of for protection of children during any pandemic.

Toros, K. (2013). School-based intervention in the context of armed conflict: Strengthening teacher capacity to facilitate psychosocial support and well-being of children. *International Journal of Humanities and Social Science, 3*(7), 228–237.
This article provides evidence regarding the positive outcome of strengthening teacher capacity through school-based intervention programs to extend psychosocial support to the children in armed conflict situations.

UNHCR. (1994). *Refugee children: guidelines on protection and care.* Geneva: UNHCR.
This document provides broad guidelines for protection of rights of refugee children.

Ventevogel, P., Ommeren, M. v., Schilperoord, M., & Saxena, S. (2015). *Improving mental health care in humanitarian emergencies.* Bulletin of the World Health Organization, 666-666A.
This document talks about improving mental care support services at times of crisis and/or emergencies.

Winthrop, R., & Kirk, J. (2008). Learning for a bright future: schooling, armed conflict, and children's well-being. *Comparative Education Review, 52*(4), 639–661. https://doi.org/10.1086/591301
Although school is regarded as a platform for addressing children's well-being, there is also evidence indicating schooling can jeopardize children's well-being as highlighted by this article.

Yahav, R. (2011). Exposure of children to war and terrorism: A review. *Journal of Child & Adolescent Trauma, 4,* 90–108. DOI:10.1080/19361521.2011.577395
This review-based article provides evidence of children's remarkable resilience in the face of life-threatening events.

Yasan, A., Saka, G., Ertem, M., Ozkan, M., & Ataman, M. (2008). Prevalence of PTSD and related factors in communities living in a conflictual area: Diyarbakir case. *Torture, 18,* 29–37.
This article demonstrates the prevalence of traumatic life experience of children living in a conflictual area which will be eye opener for the community leaders to design appropriate mental health intervention programs.

Additional Resources

WHO. (2003). *Information series on school health document: The physical school environment: An essential component of a health-promoting school.* Geneva: World Health Organization.

WHO. (2005). *The physical school environment, as an essential component of health-promoting school.* Geneva: World Health Organization.

WHO. (2006). *Psychosocial support for tsunami affected populations in India.* New Delhi: Non-Communicable Diseases and Mental Health Cluster, WHO Country Office, India.

References

Bhadra, S. & Dyer, A. R. (2022). Resilience and well-being among the survivors of natural disasters and conflicts. In S. Deb & B.A. Gerrard (Eds.). *Handbook of health and well-being: challenges, strategies and future trends* (pp. 637–668), Singapore: Springer Nature.

Bhadra, S., & Pratheepa, C. M. (2009, November 8, 9). *Strengthening communities and recovery through psychosocial support.* Retrieved June 26, 2013, from National

Institute of Disaster Management: 2nd India Disaster Management Congress: http://nidm.gov.in/idmc2/PDF/Presentations/Psycho_Social/Pres3.pdf.

Bhadra, S. (2016). Psycho-social support for protection of children in disasters. In Deb (Ed.). *Child safety, welfare and well-being* (pp. 259–278). New Delhi: Springer.

Denys, K., Rasmussen, C., & Henneveld, D. (2011). The effectiveness of a community-based intervention for parents with FASD. *Community Mental Health Journal, 47*(2), 209–219.

Hallegatte, S., Vogt-Schilb, A., Rozenberg, J., Bangalore, M., & Beaudet, C. (2020). From poverty to disaster and back: A review of the literature. *Economics of Disasters and Climate Change, 4*(1), 223–247. DOI: 10.1007/s41885-020-00060-5

IFRC. (2008, July 21). *Federation-wide tsunami semi-annual report 2004–2008: India appeal No. 28/2004.* http://reliefweb.int/report/india/federation-wide-tsunami-semi-annual-report-2004-2008-india-appeal-no-282004.

Kousar, R., & Bhadra, S. (2021). Border conflict: understanding the impact on the education of the children in Jammu region. *Journal of Peace Education, 18*, 48–71.

Lindqvist, K., Timpka, T., Schelp, L., & Risto, O. (2002). Evaluation of a child safety program based on the WHO safe community model. *Injury Prevention, 8*(1), 23–26. DOI: 10.1136/ip.8.1.23

Muzenda-Mudavanhu, C. (2016). A review of children's participation in disaster risk reduction: opinion paper. *Jàmbá: Journal of Disaster Risk Studies, 8*(1), 1–6. DOI:10.4102/jamba.v8i1.218

NIMHANS. (2007). Conference on psychosocial care and mental health services in disasters. *Summary report and recommendations of the national conference on psychosocial care and mental health services in disasters* (pp. 1–46). Bangalore: NIMHANS.

NIMHANS and WHO. (2006). Psycho-social support in disaster: Proceedings and recommendations of NIMHANS-WHO India workshop. *Psycho social support in disaster* (pp. 1–12). Bangalore: NIMHANS and WHO India Country Office.

27 How to develop a volunteer global psychological first aid organization

The Disastershock Global Response Team

The DGRT Team: Olufunke Olufunsho Adegoke, Nyna Amin, Priti Bhattacharya, Sagar Bhattacharya, Karen Buchanan, Tom Buchanan, Lina Cuartas, Sibnath Deb, Samantha Gaiera, Damian Gallegos-Lemos, Karin Dremel, Brian A. Gerrard*, Peter Geiger, Judith Giampaoli, Suzanne Giraudo, Garry Hung, Masamine Jimba, Lenka Josifkova, Eileen Klima, Celina Korzeniowski, Linden Koshland, Robyne Le Brocque, Zarielle Lis, Reji Mathew, Aimee McConneloug, Avery Meadows, Amirhossein Montazeri, Julie Moravcová, Toni Nemia, Molouwa Olapegba, Ilene Naomi Rusk, Sue Linville Shaffer*, Jacqueline Shinefield, Marissa Sogliuzzo, Bridget Steed, Emilia Suviala, Harmony Tryon, Nurit Toren, Talia Vivrett, Tara Vivrett, Ava White

*Principal authors of this chapter.

Overview

This chapter describes the eight principles used to develop the Disastershock Global Response Team (DGRT) during the period 2020–2022. The principles are illustrated with examples from the DGRT during two important disasters: the COVID-19 pandemic and the War on Ukraine.

Background

The Disastershock Global Response Team (DGRT) is a volunteer humanitarian relief organization that provides psychological first aid in the form of resources for coping with disaster-related stress. These are available free

DOI: 10.4324/9781003201977-33

on the website disastershock.com. The DGRT is a Special Interest Group of the Oxford Symposium in School-Based Family Counseling. The Oxford Symposium in School-Based Family Counseling is an international association of scholars and practitioners from 20 countries who are committed to the promotion of School-Based Family Counseling (SBFC). SBFC is an integrated systems approach to helping children succeed academically and personally by the combination of mental health approaches that link family and school. The Symposium members meet yearly at Brasenose College, Oxford and other international locations to present research on SBFC. This research may be found in the *International Journal for School-Based Family Counseling*, the Proceedings of the Oxford Symposium in School-Based Family Counseling, and in several books written mainly by Symposium members.

The DGRT emerged out of a Symposium Special Interest Group called the Disaster Coping Resources Team (DCRT). The DCRT was a ten-member team which met monthly from 2016 to 2019 and developed a website with resources to help families, schools, and children cope with disaster-related stress. One of these resources was a manual titled *Disastershock: How to Cope with the Emotional Stress of a Major Disaster* (hereafter referred to as Disastershock).

Disastershock is a brief (54-page) manual containing 20 practical strategies for parents and caregivers to help lower their stress, as well as the stress of their children, following a major disaster (see Figure 27.1).

Disastershock was written in 1989 following the Loma Prieta earthquake in San Francisco. It has been distributed free worldwide for over 30 years to support communities dealing with a wide range of disasters, including the 1989 Loma Prieta earthquake in San Francisco, terrorist attacks (New York, Brussels, Paris, Lahore, San Bernardino, Egypt: Al-Rawda), Parkland school shooting, Manchester bombing, flooding (Houston), hurricane (Puerto Rico, Florida Panhandle), fire (California and Australia), tsunami (Sumatra, Indonesia; Tonga), and volcanic eruption (Guatemala). Recently, it was updated to include the COVID-19 pandemic. Disastershock has been endorsed by mental health experts around the world.

In March, 2020, when it became evident that a dangerous pandemic was underway, two co-authors of Disastershock – Brian Gerrard and Sue Linville Shaffer – reconnected with each other after 35 years and decided to form a team that would translate *Disastershock* into as many different languages as possible and then distribute e-copies free. During the next three months, a global team of 101 persons from 26 countries was formed and given the name Disastershock Global Volunteer Team (DGVT). By September, there were 26 translations of Disastershock available free for download at the team's website disastershock.com. In September, 2020, a smaller team (of about 30 persons) called the DGRT was formed to carry on additional projects: refinement of the website, development of a Disastershock manual for school personnel, a Tip Sheet project for developing single sheet handouts containing useful tips for coping with disaster-related stress, videos for dealing with disaster stress, a Disastershock Facebook page, and a research project called the Ways of

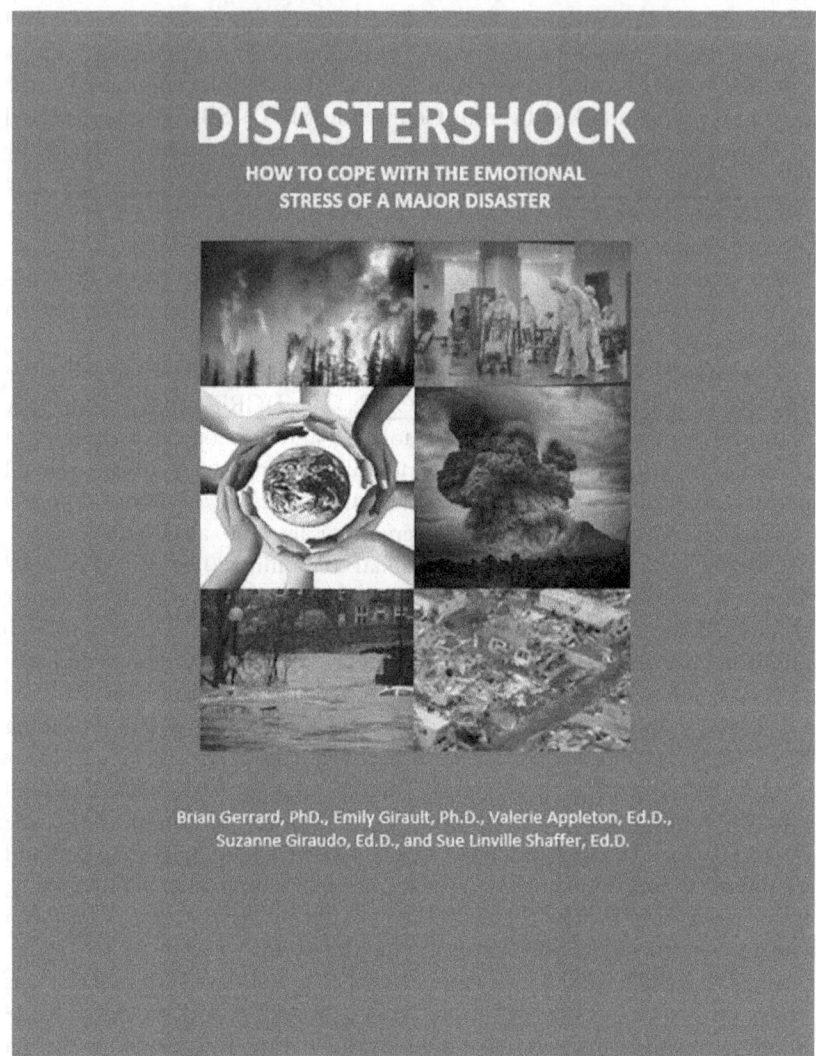

Figure 27.1 Disastershock: how to cope with the emotional stress of a major disaster

Coping with the COVID-19 pandemic which involved interviews with persons in 12 different countries. Figure 27.2 shows the timeline during which these projects were carried out.

In March, 2022, we sent an email to James Elder, the UNICEF Representative to Ukraine, describing our program and seeking advice on how we could best share our coping materials with Ukrainian refugees. In his response, he said: "Kudos…to the Disastershock Global Response Team" and offered a helpful suggestion. Because we are an organization that is particularly focused on helping children, we particularly valued Mr. Elder's comment coming from a UNICEF representative. In an anonymous survey we conducted in July, 2021, DGRT members evaluated the extent to which they felt we were achieving our mission by answering this question: "To what extent do you think the Disastershock Team fulfilled its mission of developing coping resources for persons affected by disaster?" Figure 27.3 shows that 80% of respondents assigned a rating of 8 or higher on a 1–10 scale with 1 = Low, 10 = High.

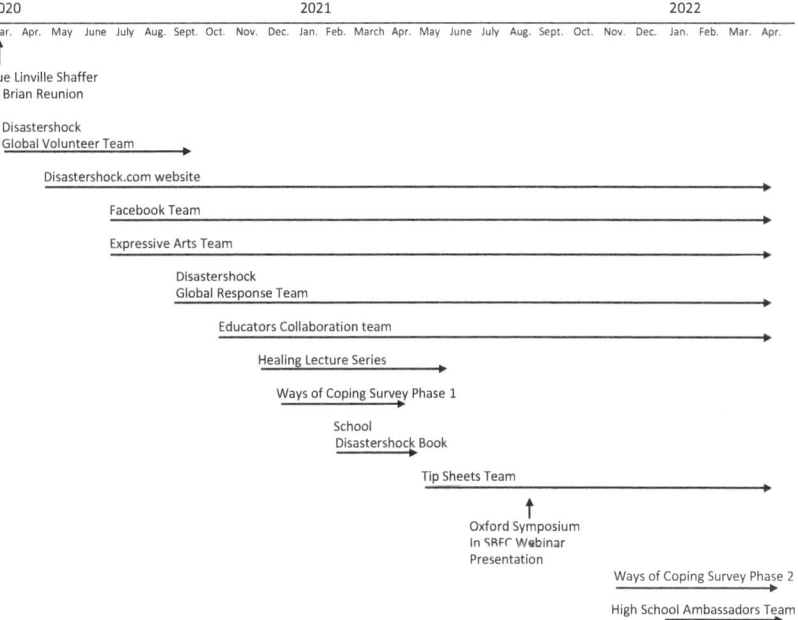

Figure 27.2 Timeline for the Disastershock team

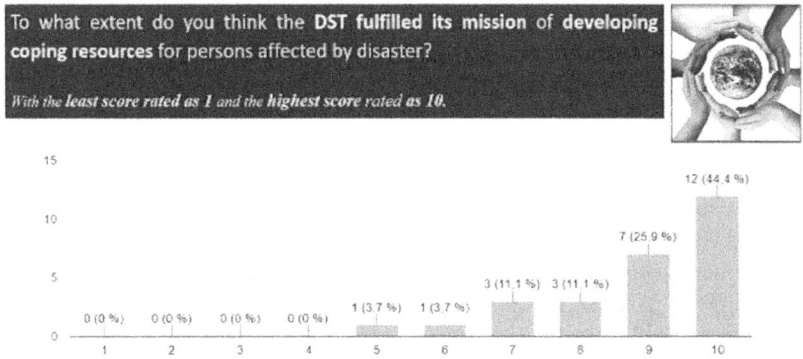

Figure 27.3 Bar graph showing extent to which members believed the DGRT was fulfilling its mission

As of this writing, the DGRT members are actively involved in developing and sharing coping resources with the millions of Ukrainian refugees displaced by the Russian invasion of Ukraine. Both Disastershock manuals have been translated into Ukrainian and the languages of other countries to which the refugees are fleeing.

In the Procedure section that follows, we will describe the eight principles that we used in developing the DGRT and to which we credit our success as a volunteer humanitarian relief organization.

Procedure

The principles are as follows:

Principle 1: Develop a Helpful Psychological First Aid Product
Principle 2: Have an Effective Leadership Team
    Principle 2A: Maintain Team Cohesion
    Principle 2B: Maintain Task Focus
Principle 3: Build a Diverse Team
Principle 4: Meet on a Regular Basis
Principle 5: Develop Sub-Teams Based on Interest and Ability
Principle 6: Be Flexible
Principle 7: Be Open to Feedback
Principle 8: Highlight Successes and Express Gratitude for Contributions

Principle 1: Develop a helpful psychological first aid product

The team initially focused on the *Disastershock* manual. The *Disastershock* manual has a number of unique characteristics. First, it contains numerous best practices approaches, such as cognitive-behavior therapy evidence-based strategies, for helping adults and children to lower stress (see Box 27.1 for a description of the table of contents).

Second, the strategies are described in simple concrete language that are easy for a parent to use with a child or themselves. Instead of offering general advice like "Practice deep breathing to lower your stress," there is a step-by-step description of how to do deep breathing (see Box 27.2).

You should now be breathing slowly and deeply. If you wish, you may extend your breathing intervals to 6, 7, 8, 9, or 10 seconds. Remember to stop if you feel uncomfortable at any time. Practice this deep breathing for at least five minutes. You can use this method whenever you feel tense – when you are alone or in public.

Mental health experts from around the world have endorsed *Disastershock* as a valuable resource for coping with disaster-related stress (see Box 27.3). Everyone who was invited to join the Disastershock team was able to view Disastershock online at disastercopingresources.com (the website for the DCRT) and later online at disastershock.com. We frequently received compliments on

Box 27.1 *Disastershock* **Table of Contents**

TABLE OF CONTENTS

Box 27.2 Method 1: Deep breathing

Method 1: Deep breathing

This is the procedure of reducing tension in your body through practicing slow, deep breathing. This is a method you can use any time you feel tense or anxious. It is best practiced sitting or lying where you will not be disturbed. If you feel uncomfortable at any time, stop the exercise.

Let's try it.

Take a slow, deep breath through your nose for two seconds: 1–2.

Now hold your breath for two seconds: 1-2 and let it out slowly through your nose for two seconds: 1–2.

Now repeat, breathe in for two seconds: 1 -2, hold for two seconds: 1 -2, breathe out for two seconds: 1 -2.

Now go to three seconds: Breathe in: 1 -2–3. Hold: 1 -2–3. Breathe out: 1 -2–3. Now repeat: breathe in: 1–2-3. Hold: 1 -2-3. Breathe out 1–2-3. Now continue deep breathing with a 3 second interval until it feels comfortable.

When you feel ready go to 4 seconds. Breathe in 1–2–3–4. Hold 1–2–3–4. Breathe out 1–2–3–4. Now repeat: Breathe in: 1 2–3–4. Hold 1–2–3–4. Breathe out: 1–2–3–4. That's excellent.

When you feel ready, try 5 seconds

Box 27.3 What mental health experts say about Disastershock: How to cope with the emotional stress of a major disaster

The value of this relatively brief book lies in its comprehensive and down to earth nature. Comprehensive in its coverage of a wide range of strategies to manage emotional stress, as well as its focus on helping children of different ages relax and cope with emotional stress. It is down to earth in that all activities suggested are practical and easy to put into action – especially when you are right there, shocked and tense. A book to have on your shelf for when the unforeseen strikes.

—Hans Everts, PhD, Emeritus Professor Counsellor
Education, Faculty of Education, University of Auckland,
Auckland, New Zealand

This is one of the most useful books that I have used in my 28 years as a professor of family therapy and 34 years as a licensed psychotherapist. It is highly informative about the conditions of trauma and its effect on a wide

variety of clients. **More importantly, it has many useful and effective techniques for minimizing the development of Post-Traumatic Stress Disorder (PTSD) in children and adults. It has stood the test of time because of its utility, and it is an important foundation for training practitioners in the treatment of diverse trauma.**

—Michael J. Carter, LMFT, PhD, Associate Professor, Department of Special Education & Counseling, Charter College of Education, California State University, Los Angeles, Los Angeles, California

A must-have resource for disaster management agencies, workers and victims of natural and human catastrophes. A compact manual, it provides practical information for mental and emotional recuperation to cope with the aftermath of life-threatening events and situations.

—Nyna Amin, PhD, Associate Professor: Curriculum Studies, University Distinguished Teacher, School of Education, University of KwaZulu-Natal, Durban, South Africa

This is an excellent book and a much needed one as it provides a simple and practical guide to handling emotional shock from disaster. Children are voiceless in time of disaster and the impact can be lifelong. I congratulate the authors for making a difference by sharing their skills and techniques in empowering children and youth.

—Professor Cecilia L.W. Chan, Ph.D., R.S.W., J.P., Si Yuan Chair Professor in Health and Social Work, Chair and Professor: Department of Social Work and Social Administration, The University of Hong Kong, Hong Kong (SAR)

Disastershock draws on informed practical interventions for both adults, children and therapists to better navigate the minefield of emotional stress. The book provides many effective tools that can be interwoven into any therapist's existing conceptual framework.

—Huda Ayyash-Abdo, PhD, Associate Professor of Psychology, Department of Social Sciences, Lebanese American University, Beirut Campus, Lebanon

This book (manual) is brilliant in its clarity and simplicity, with easy to follow evidence-based procedures on how parents can immediately help their child/children facing a major disaster. Although addressed specifically to parents, this comprehensive resource is also enormously helpful to professionals involved in providing compassionate care and healing to children experiencing emotional stress especially following a disaster. I will certainly continue to talk about, and recommend, this invaluable resource rich book to my mental health colleagues, friends and family.

—Teresita A. Jose, Ph.D., R. Psych.,
Psychologist, Calgary, Alberta

In a simple and sensitive way, the authors of this book supply the readers with tools to help them cope with difficult moments. They give the readers a feeling that they are not alone in this world. Their message is very clear: the authors believe in you! They trust your power to overcome any disaster whether you are an adult, a parent or a child. Therefore, they help the readers to identify responses to disaster shock and encourage the individual to act in order to reduce stress. The authors expose us to variety of stress reduction methods and give us a sense of mastery and control of our life especially in time of crisis. This book conveys a message of optimism: the majority of adults and children can cope with fears and anxieties which follow a disaster. The solution is in our hands! I highly recommend this book as part of our disaster preparatory kit.

—Nurit Kaplan Toren, PhD, Associate Professor,
Department of Learning, Instruction,
and Teacher Education, Faculty of Education,
University of Haifa, Haifa, Israel

This handbook is an excellent resource for any counsellor or therapist who works with clients who have experienced a major disaster. Although the authors focus on disasters such as terrorist incidents, earthquakes, train or car accidents, I believe this manual can be utilized with lesser fearful or frightening exposure to trauma. Recently in the United Kingdom we have had the Grenfell fire disaster, 'scary clown' social media anxieties, in addition to terrorism in the UK and Europe where children and young people have been exposed to shocking and graphic news reports. This has been difficult for many children and parents. This is a superb and practical guide with advice and strategies drawn from evidence based theory and practice. I believe this book will help parents, teachers, and counsellors to support children's emotional and psychological resilience. There are clear pragmatic strategies to address the shock to adult witnesses or survivors of a wide range of challenging shocks or disasters. I will be circulating this excellent and informative guide to 300 school based counsellors and 1200 volunteer counsellors all over the United Kingdom and I believe it will be useful to schools parents and counsellors who are confronted by clients who have experienced the trauma of shock or disasters.

—Stephen Adams Langley, PhD, Senior Clinical Consultant, Place2Be, London, United Kingdom

Disastershock from the persons who did the initial 26 language translations. We felt that having a valuable psychological first aid product to distribute was a significant factor in attracting volunteers.

Principle 2: Have an effective leadership team

The DGRT is led by Sue Linville Shaffer, EdD, LMFT and Brian Gerrard, PhD. Both Shaffer and Gerrard have extensive successful leadership experience in administering mental health organizations. Shaffer taught for 25 years in the Counseling Psychology Department at the University of San Francisco and was the Director of Clinical Services for Kara, a nonprofit grief counseling agency providing grief and trauma support to individuals, families, and children in Palo Alto, California. She was an active member of the Advanced Critical Incident Stress Management Team Bay Area (CISM), facilitating debriefings and crisis interventions in varied settings, including schools, agencies, and workplaces Bay Area wide. She is a 2021 graduate of the Applied Compassion Academy at Stanford University. Shaffer has maintained a private practice in marital and family therapy for 30 years and specializes in working with families who have suffered grief and traumatic loss. Gerrard is the Chief Academic Officer for the Western Institute for Social Research, Berkeley, California and was formerly the Chair of the Counseling Psychology Department and the Executive Director of the Center for Child and Family Development at the University of San Francisco. He is also the Chair of the Board of Directors for the Institute for School-Based Family Counseling and the Director of the Oxford Symposium in School-Based Family Counseling. Both Shaffer and Gerrard have extensive experience teaching in the field of marital and family therapy at the University of San Francisco.

Having developed these combined leadership skills over many years made it easy for us to provide leadership to the Disastershock team. Although we reconnected after no contact for 35 years, we quickly formed a strong and supportive friendship which was evident to all team members.

During the DGVT phase (March–July, 2020), we had leadership support from six persons:

> David Shoup, PhD, who played a critical role in setting up a Google Drive location to monitor the development of translations, helped format most of the translations, and acted as our computer tech adviser.
>
> Seth Hamlin, who helped set up our original disastershock.com website, so important in sharing our disaster coping resources.
>
> Rebecca Li, who helped us think about organizational structure and facilitated Gerrard to give a coping seminar to the staff of a California state branch.
>
> Julie Norton, LMFT and Bridget Steed, LMFT who helped develop an Expressive Arts and Recovery page on the website.
>
> Lina Cuartas, who developed our Facebook page and made daily uploads to it.

Their willingness to play an active leadership role inspired us and helped us to quickly develop our translations and the website. During this period, we were meeting on zoom weekly and exchanging emails daily.

During the DGRT phase, our leadership support team consisted of:

Lina Cuartas: Coordinator Facebook

Bridget Steed: Coordinator Arts & Recovery

Jackie Shinefield: Coordinator Tip Sheets

Bridget Steed and Reji Mathew: Coordinators Website Development

Brian Gerrard: Coordinator Educators Collaborative Team

Coordinator Ways of Coping Research Team

Eileen Klima: Coordinator Ambassadors Team

Shaffer and Gerrard actively encouraged members to take on leadership roles. We gave equal emphasis to maintaining group cohesion and focusing on tasks. The 9-9 Managerial Grid leadership model (Blake & McCanse, 1991) which emphasizes a high concern for people and a high concern for production is consistent with our leadership philosophy (see Figure 27.4).

Principle 2A: Maintain team cohesion

We maintained team cohesion in several ways. First, we would spend at least 20 minutes at the beginning of each zoom meeting doing a "Brief Member

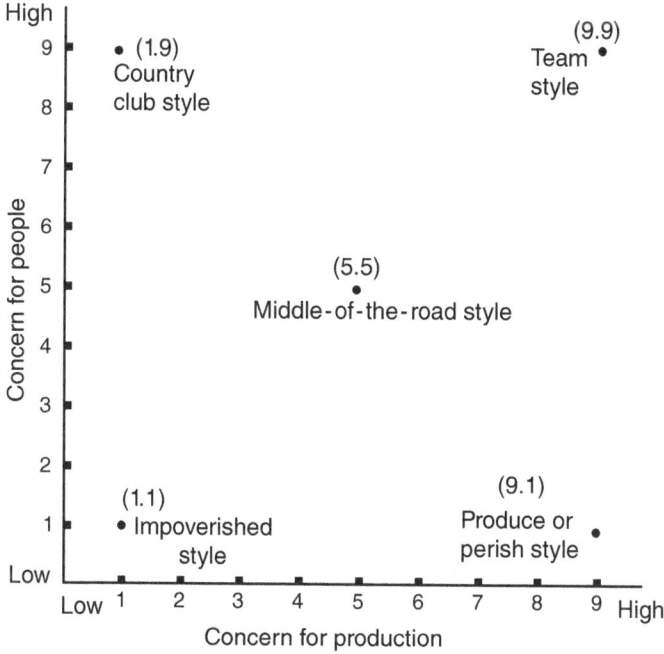

Figure 27.4 The managerial grid

Check-in." During the check-in, we would ask members to briefly introduce themselves and then report on how they were coping with the pandemic (or more recently the War on Ukraine). These personal check-ins were led by Shaffer who has a very warm engaging style that makes members feel valued. She would occasionally vary how she did the check-in. For example, on one occasion, she asked everyone to share what was going on in their lives by describing what was a "Rose, a Thorn, and a Bud" (i.e. a Positive, a Challenge, and an emerging Positive) in their week. On another occasion, she asked everyone to share something really enjoyable they had done during the week. These regular personal sharings built strong group cohesion over time and provided group support that was important because of the stress everyone was feeling due to the growing number of cases and deaths caused by the COVID-19 pandemic.

Group cohesion was also facilitated by the decision to limit zoom meetings to 1 hour. This was our acknowledgment that most of our members were involved in frequent zoom meetings during the week and that lengthy zoom meetings ran the risk of facilitating member "burn-out." When a member reported some achievement, such as completion of a Disastershock language translation, we would congratulate them at a zoom meeting and also in an email.

Principle 2B: Maintain task focus

A strong task focus was maintained by devoting 40 minutes of our 1-hour zoom meetings to forming smaller teams with specific tasks. At each general DGRT meeting, each team would report on task accomplishments. An effort was made to encourage all team members to participate on a team or a specific task. Some examples are described below.

The Educators Collaboration Team consisted of ten persons from the USA, Argentina, Japan, Israel, Australia, and Canada. This team developed the Educators Resource pages and wrote a second Disastershock book: *Disastershock: How Schools Can Cope with the Emotional Stress of a Major Disaster. A Manual for Principals and Teachers* (see Figure 27.5 for a description of the Table of Contents). The book describes how teachers can develop a trauma-sensitive classroom for students affected by a disaster. Each team member contributed a section to this 75-page book which has been translated into Ukrainian, Polish, and Hungarian and is being sent to Departments of Education in Poland, Hungary, and other countries where Ukrainian refugee students are entering local schools. This team is also designing a teacher survey assessing how teachers coped with the pandemic.

Another example is the Tip Sheet Team which has developed single-page Tip Sheets that are decorated with art while containing practical tips for lowering disaster-related stress (see Figure 27.6).

The Ways of Coping Research Team conducted interviews with persons in 12 different countries and investigated best practices for coping with the pandemic. This study was written up in the 2021 Proceedings of the Oxford Symposium in School-Based Family Counseling. This team is also doing a follow-up large-scale survey to investigate hypotheses developed in the earlier study.

At this writing, all team members are involved in sharing Disastershock resources over the internet with Ukrainian refugees displaced by the War on Ukraine.

An important factor with the all-volunteer DGRT members is that their tasks are all related to helping children and families cope with disaster-related stress. Since all the DGRT members are themselves exposed to stress during the pandemic and the War on Ukraine, they all have a deeper empathy for the suffering of those who experienced job loss, death of a family member, or separation of family members. Two of our members each had three family members die of COVID. During our zoom meetings, we heard frequent reports from members in other countries report on the devastating effects of the pandemic when few masks or vaccines were available. We were all deeply moved by a member who tearfully reported on seeing Ukrainian refugees in desperate condition entering her country. Because of the international nature of our membership, we frequently felt like we were taking the pulse of the planet during our meetings. These were important factors in motivating DGRT members to work at challenging tasks.

TABLE OF CONTENTS

Figure 27.5 Table of contents for Disastershock: how schools can cope with the
emotional stress of a major disaster

Principle 3: Build a diverse team

The original DGVT consisted of 101 persons from 26 countries (see Box 27.4).
This team developed 26 translations of the main Disastershock book within
four months. This success was due to the cultural diversity of the team. Half

the members (51) were from different countries than the USA. Twenty-one of the members living in the USA were from other countries or had dual citizenship. The DGVT was so highly diverse that we frequently felt like a mini-United Nations when we would meet. The majority of our members were female (73) which is a reflection of the tendency for females to be more prevalent in the helping professions (the most frequent profession of members was mental health). We were able to assemble this diverse team rapidly through Shaffer's involvement with the Applied Compassion Academy at Stanford University whose membership consisted of students from around the globe, and through Gerrard's international contacts with members of the Oxford Symposium in School-Based Family Counseling.

Box 27.4 Disastershock Global Volunteer Team

As of this writing July 25, 2020 this 101-person team representing 27 different countries volunteered their time to translate Disastershock into 20+ different languages and to help distribute Disastershock around the world during the 2020 Covid-19 pandemic. Our team is still growing, and other people are joining the team to expand the reach of this effort. Please continue our work by sharing Disastershock with others and check our website to see how you can help: www.disastershock.com

Olufunke Olufunsho Adegoke –
  Nigeria
Bhavna Agarwal – USA/India
Nyna Amin – South Africa
Parto Aram – USA
Vince Nyabunga Arasa – Kenya
Huda Ayyash-Abdo – Lebanon/
  USA
C. Jaya Sankar Babu – India
Liat Ben-Uzi – Israel
Helena Berger – Czech Republic
Priti Bhattacharya – India
Sagar Bhattacharya – India
Sandra Sanabria Bohórquez –
  Colombia/USA
Nagaraj Boobalan – India
Antoine P. Broustra – USA
Wei-Yi Chin – Taiwan

Julia Lam Iok Chu – China
Andrea Circella – Italy
Alexandre Coimbra – USA/
  Brazil
Lina Cuartas – Columbia/USA
Carmen E. Dawson – USA/
  Philippines
Sibnath Deb – India
Shuyu Deng – China
Karin Dremel – USA
T.R.A.Devakumar – India
Elena Dvortsova – Russia
Susanne Ebert-Khosla – USA/
  Germany
Xinyue Fan – China
Yohko Fick – Japan
Damian Gallegos-Lemos –
  Ecuador/Spain

Brian Gerrard – Canada
Suzanne Giraudo – USA
Elaine Gouvêa – USA/Brazil
Seth Hamlin – USA
Aan Hermawan – Indonesia
Van Van Hoang– Vietnam
Ming-Kuo Hung – Taiwan
Lenka Josifkova – Czech
   Republic
Motoko Katayama – Japan
Tatiana Khalaf – Lebanon
Sheena Kim – USA
Celma Kirkwood – USA/Brazil
Joanna Wong Pui Kei – China
Sheena Kim – USA
Valerie Leong Pou Kio – China
Celina Korzeniowski – Argentina
Geliya Kudryavtseva – USA
Olga Kuznetsova – USA/Russia
Amy Lang – USA
Jia Rebecca Li – USA
Chung-Jung Lin – Taiwan
Akiko Lipton – Japan
Lucía Lemos – Ecuador
Marizela Maciel – USA
Elizabeth Moon – USA
Susie Montermoso – USA/
   Philippines
Christine Nazareth – USA/
   Brazil
Julie Norton – USA
Sawyer Norton – USA
Yasemin Özkan   Turkey
Francesca Pagano – USA/
   Brazil
Kiran Pala – USA
Marie-Claude Parpaglione –
   Italy/France
Amy Paul – India
David Paul – India
Joseph Puthussery – USA

Barbara Piper-Roelofs –
   Netherlands
Eliana Ponce de Leon Reeves –
   USA
Célia Queiroz – USA/Brazil
Jen Raynes – USA
Andrea Riedmayer – Germany
Karin Rohlfs – Germany/USA
Ilene Naomi Rusk – Canada
Nihal Sahan – USA
Marie-claude Sannazzari –
   France
Rama Saripalle – USA/India
Erwin Schmitt – Germany
Heike Schmitz – Germany/USA
Meryem Danışmaz Sevin –
   Turkey
Sue Linville Shaffer – USA
Ratnesh Sharma – USA
Jacqueline Shinefield – USA
David Shoup – USA
Alena Skrbkova – Czech
   Republic/Belgium
Bridget Steed – USA
Zhenrong Su   China
Leena Sujan – USA/India
Emilia Suviala – USA/Finland
Ning Tang – China
Shruti Tewari – USA/India
Svetlana Tikhonova – USA/
   Russia
Lucia Pavia Ticzon – Philippines
Armin Touserkanian – Iran
Ludmila Vasilyeva – Russia
Raymond Vercruysse – USA
Justin Wilson – Canada
Yuen Wu – China
Pınar Kütük Yılmaz – Turkey
Philip C. H. Yuen – China
Jiayuan Zhang – China
Ruoyun Zhu – China

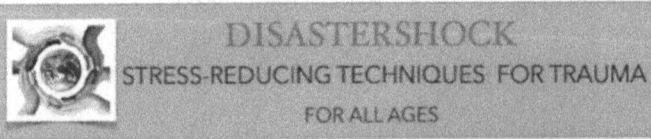

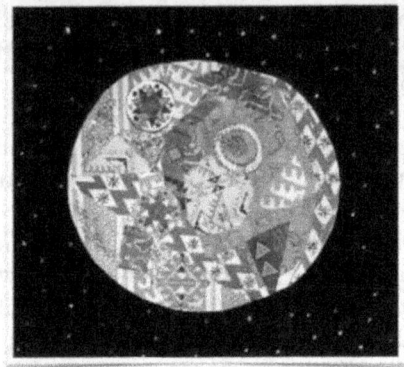

DEEP BREATHING

For Adults:

Take a slow, deep breath through your nose for two seconds: 1 - 2.

Now hold your breath for two seconds: 1 - 2 and let it out slowly through your nose for two seconds: 1 - 2.

Now repeat, breathe in for two seconds:

1 - 2, hold for two seconds: 1 - 2, breathe out for two seconds: 1 - 2.

Now go to three seconds:

Breathe in: 1 - 2 - 3. Hold: 1 - 2 - 3. Breathe out: 1 - 2 - 3. Repeat.

Now continue deep breathing with a 3 second interval until it feels comfortable.

Over 5 minutes, extend your breathing intervals to 4, 5 or 6 seconds. Remember to stop if you feel uncomfortable at any time. You can use this method whenever you feel tense.

For Young Children:

Imagine you have a bubble bottle and a wand.

Take the wand and blow the biggest bubble by taking a deep breath in and blowing slowly with the bubble to create your big bubble.

Ask the child to do this for 3 minutes.

EXPRESSIVE ARTS

1) Draw a picture that represents how you feel. What does your anxiety look like?

2) Dance or move your body in a way that expresses your emotions. What does your anxiety feel like?

3) Write a story or poem about your worries and fears. What does your anxiety sound like?

4) Act out your anxiety using costumes and props. How does your anxiety present itself?

Visit www.disastershock.com for more free resources!

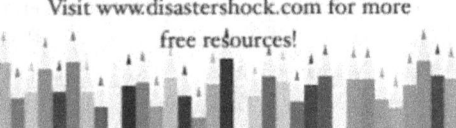

Figure 27.6 Example of a Tip Sheet

Principle 4: Meet on a regular basis

Meeting on a regular basis was very important because few of the team members knew each other. During the DGRT's first year (2020), we met weekly for one hour on Saturday mornings. Beginning in 2021, we switched to having a General meeting once a month but having smaller team meetings weekly or bi-weekly. Having these regularly scheduled meetings helped us to get to know each other and form friendships.

Principle 5: Develop sub-teams based on interest and ability

As we entered our second year of the pandemic (2021) and had achieved our goal of developing 26 Disastershock translations, Shaffer and I encouraged the formation of seven smaller teams where members could develop their specialized interests. These teams consisted of:

1 *Facebook Team*: This team made weekly postings on our Disastershock Facebook page (see Figure 27.7).
2 *Arts & Recovery Team*: This team developed extensive pages demonstrating expressive arts approaches for reducing trauma (see Figure 27.8).
3 *Tip Sheets Team*: This team developed single sheets that could be used as handouts. On each sheet are practical strategies for parents and children to lower stress (see Figure 27.6). Recently, we added QR codes that when scanned link to a Disastershock book (see Figure 27.9 for a Ukrainian Tip Sheet).
4 *Educators Collaborative Team*: This team developed the manual: *Disastershock: How Schools Can Cope with the Emotional Stress of a Major Disaster* (see Figure 27.5). They meet every two weeks at different times to accommodate members living in different parts of the world.
5 *Ways of Coping Research Team*: This team interviewed persons in 12 different countries during December, 2021–March, 2020 in a pilot study to develop hypotheses about best practices in dealing with the pandemic (see Figure 27.10). In a follow-up to their pilot study, the team is conducting a large-scale survey using refined questions developed from the pilot study.
6 *Disastershock Ambassadors Team*: The Ambassador team, formed in 2022, consists of ten high school students from Nigeria, Czech Republic, and the USA. The Ambassadors meet weekly and during March–April, 2022 were actively involved in distributing Disastershock psychological first aid materials to Ukrainian refugees. Students at Cal Poly Humboldt University made a short, very moving video in which four of the Ambassadors explained why the Disastershock program is important. This may be viewed on our Disastershock website (https://www.disastershock.com/general-5).
7 *Website Development Team*: This team played a critical role in professionalizing the appearance of our website disastershock.com. The coordinators for this team are accomplished artists and used their artwork to beautify the website.

The value of forming these smaller teams is that they enabled members to specialize in particular areas of interest and work independently.

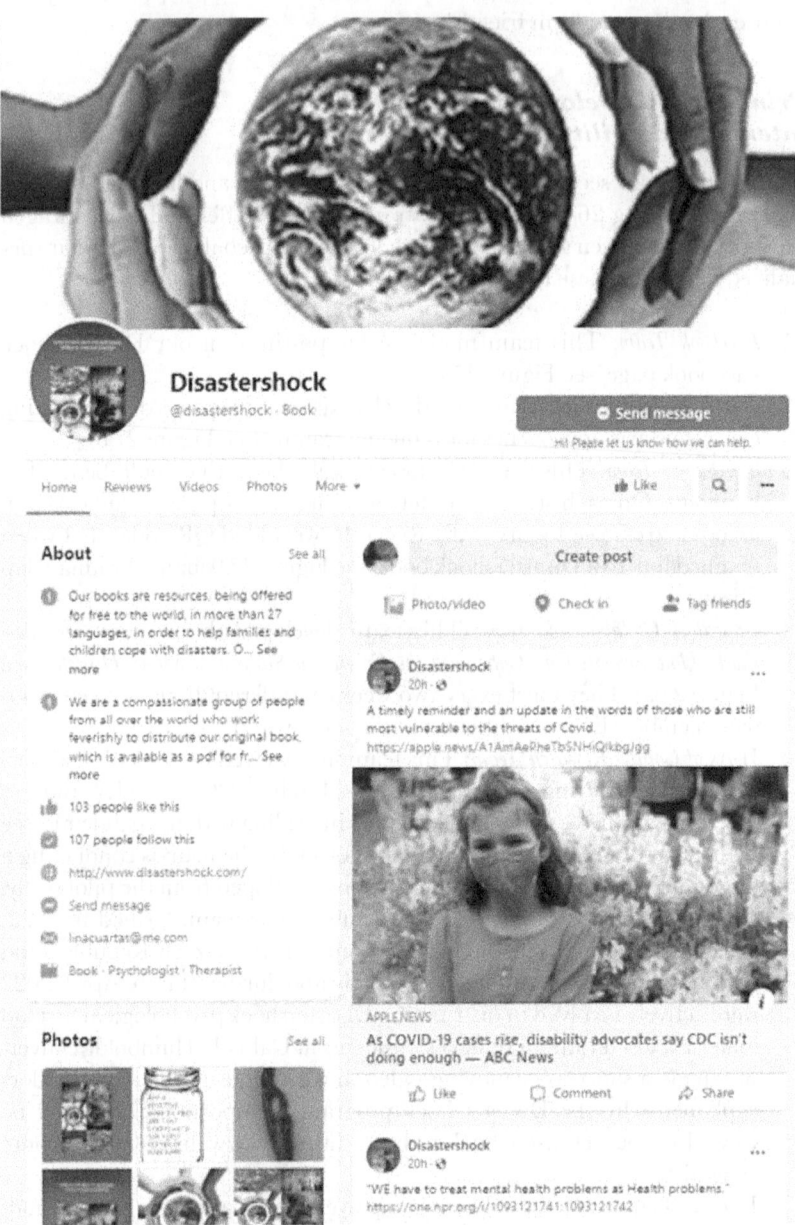

Figure 27.7 Disastershock Facebook page

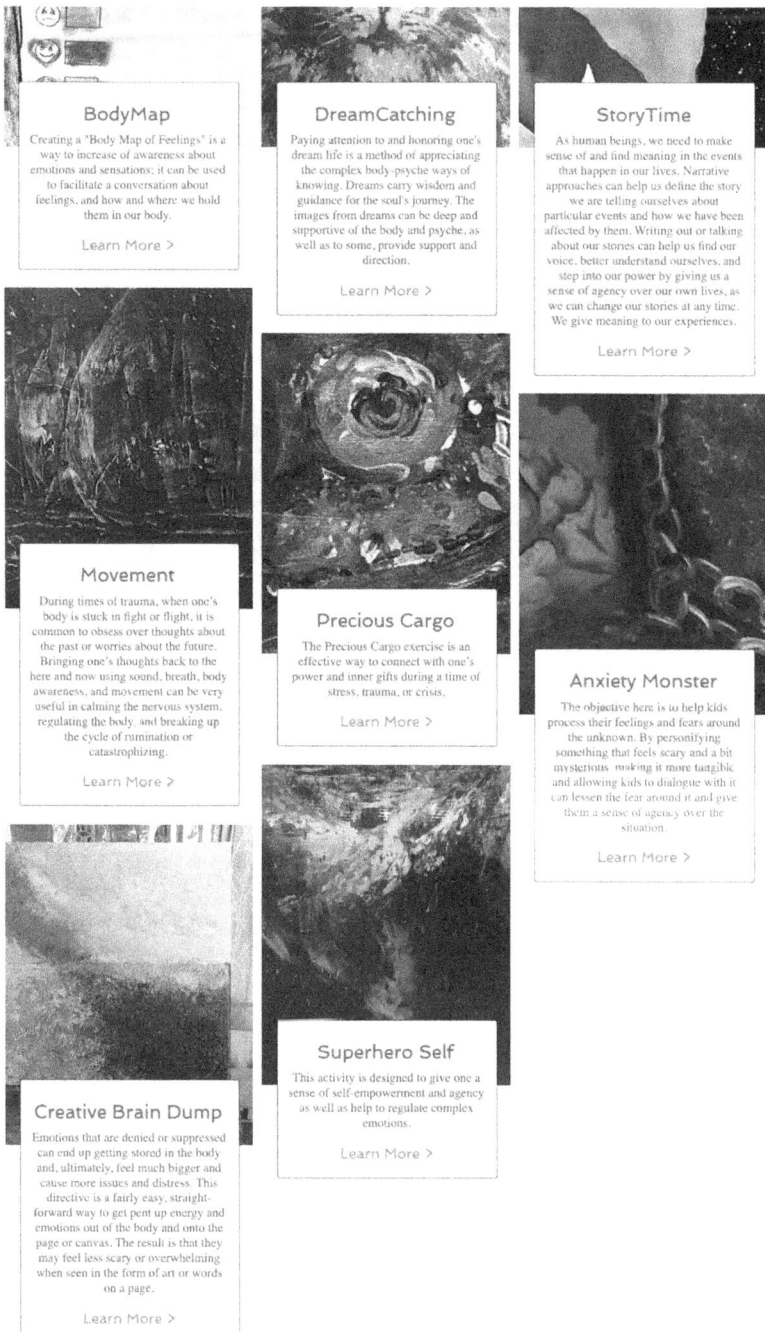

BodyMap

Creating a "Body Map of Feelings" is a way to increase of awareness about emotions and sensations; it can be used to facilitate a conversation about feelings, and how and where we hold them in our body.

Learn More >

DreamCatching

Paying attention to and honoring one's dream life is a method of appreciating the complex body-psyche ways of knowing. Dreams carry wisdom and guidance for the soul's journey. The images from dreams can be deep and supportive of the body and psyche, as well as to some, provide support and direction.

Learn More >

StoryTime

As human beings, we need to make sense of and find meaning in the events that happen in our lives. Narrative approaches can help us define the story we are telling ourselves about particular events and how we have been affected by them. Writing out or talking about our stories can help us find our voice, better understand ourselves, and step into our power by giving us a sense of agency over our own lives, as we can change our stories at any time. We give meaning to our experiences.

Learn More >

Movement

During times of trauma, when one's body is stuck in fight or flight, it is common to obsess over thoughts about the past or worries about the future. Bringing one's thoughts back to the here and now using sound, breath, body awareness, and movement can be very useful in calming the nervous system, regulating the body, and breaking up the cycle of rumination or catastrophizing.

Learn More >

Precious Cargo

The Precious Cargo exercise is an effective way to connect with one's power and inner gifts during a time of stress, trauma, or crisis.

Learn More >

Anxiety Monster

The objective here is to help kids process their feelings and fears around the unknown. By personifying something that feels scary and a bit mysterious, making it more tangible and allowing kids to dialogue with it can lessen the fear around it and give them a sense of agency over the situation.

Learn More >

Superhero Self

This activity is designed to give one a sense of self-empowerment and agency as well as help to regulate complex emotions.

Learn More >

Creative Brain Dump

Emotions that are denied or suppressed can end up getting stored in the body and, ultimately, feel much bigger and cause more issues and distress. This directive is a fairly easy, straight-forward way to get pent up energy and emotions out of the body and onto the page or canvas. The result is that they may feel less scary or overwhelming when seen in the form of art or words on a page.

Learn More >

Figure 27.8 Examples of expressive arts activities

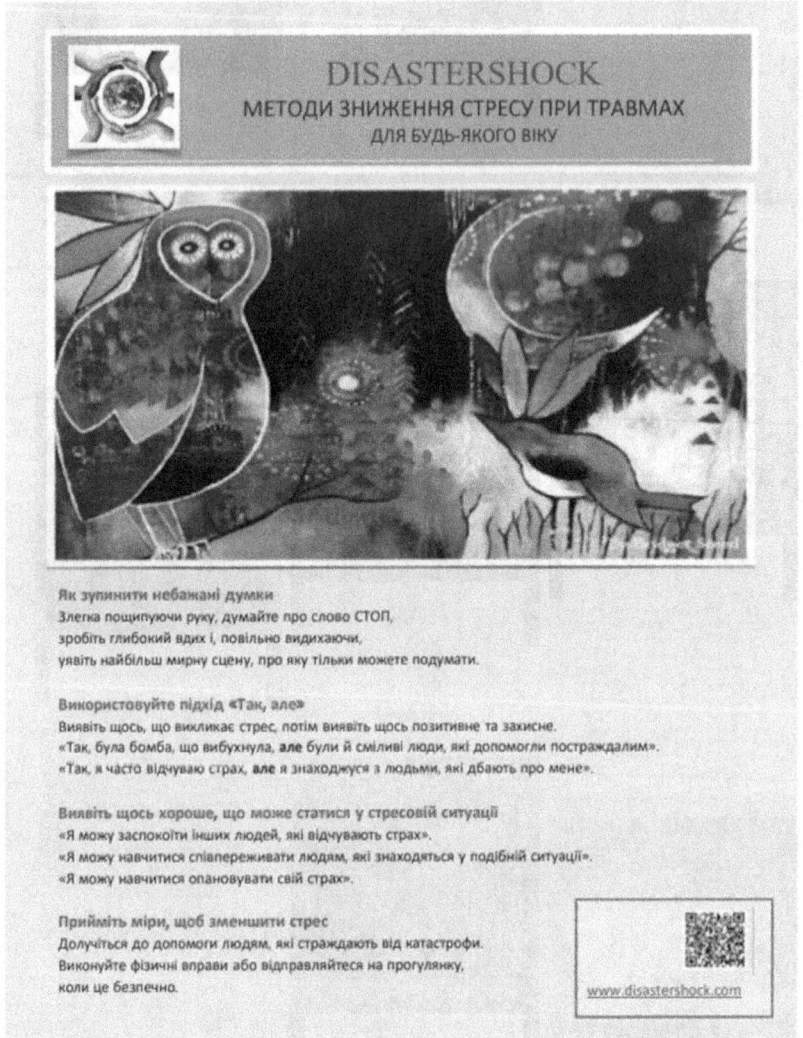

Figure 27.9 Ukrainian Tip Sheet with QR code

Principle 6: Be flexible

This is a very important principle when working with volunteers, especially volunteers who are working professionals. With an employee, one can more easily ensure compliance with an assigned task. This is not the case with volunteers who for various reasons may not be able to follow through with an assignment. Therefore, Shaffer and I, and the other team leaders, would use a "light paintbrush" approach when requesting assignments. We were always

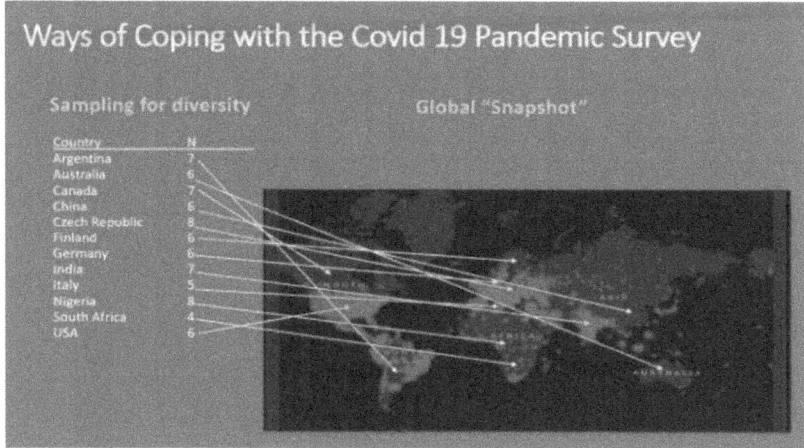

Figure 27.10 Countries sampled in the ways of coping study

willing to modify our approach if someone was unable or unwilling to take on a task. Because all of us were subject to the stress of the COVID-19 pandemic and the horrific images of desperate refugees in Ukraine, we were aware that burn-out from pandemic fatigue was common and could affect anyone. If, for example, a translator was unable to complete a Disastershock translation, we would quickly find someone to help complete the translation rather than pressure the original translator. Additionally, we frequently expressed our appreciation for what each person was able to accomplish, honoring the effort that they put in.

Early on, we decided that we would not try to "capture" volunteers and we communicated to everyone – especially the translators – that they could decide whether they wished to continue with the DGVT after they completed their translation. As early as April, 2020 we began describing the DGVT as having time-limited assignments and that volunteers were free to depart at any time. We formalized this by announcing in July, 2020 that beginning in September, 2020, the DGVT would change its name to the DGRT for members who wanted to continue with distributing the Disastershock translations and helping develop new programs. This acknowledged that not everyone desired a permanent, or long-term, commitment and yet were very interested in a short-term involvement helping others.

Principle 7: Be open to feedback

This principle involves openness to constructive criticism. It is a more difficult principle to implement especially if you believe that you are doing a great job and someone says: "Wait a minute." In our roles as directors for the DGRT,

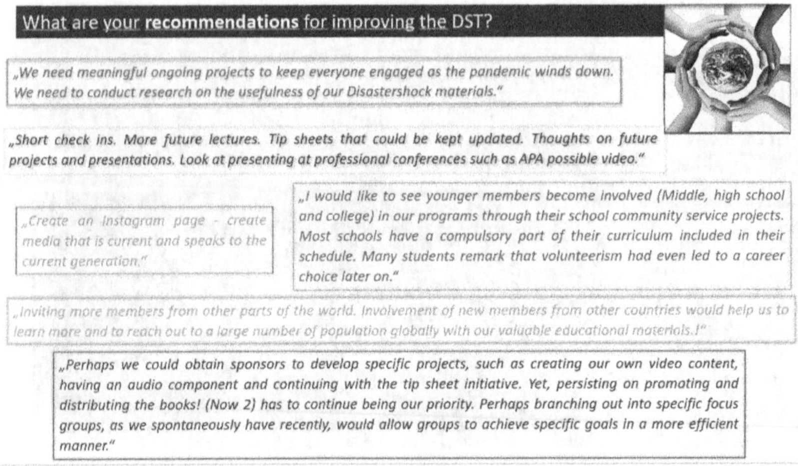

What are your recommendations for improving the DST?

„*We need meaningful ongoing projects to keep everyone engaged as the pandemic winds down. We need to conduct research on the usefulness of our Disastershock materials."*

„*Short check ins. More future lectures. Tip sheets that could be kept updated. Thoughts on future projects and presentations. Look at presenting at professional conferences such as APA possible video."*

„*Create an Instagram page - create media that is current and speaks to the current generation."*

„*I would like to see younger members become involved (Middle, high school and college) in our programs through their school community service projects. Most schools have a compulsory part of their curriculum included in their schedule. Many students remark that volunteerism had even led to a career choice later on."*

„*Inviting more members from other parts of the world. Involvement of new members from other countries would help us to learn more and to reach out to a large number of population globally with our valuable educational materials.!"*

„*Perhaps we could obtain sponsors to develop specific projects, such as creating our own video content, having an audio component and continuing with the tip sheet initiative. Yet, persisting on promoting and distributing the books! (Now 2) has to continue being our priority. Perhaps branching out into specific focus groups, as we spontaneously have recently, would allow groups to achieve specific goals in a more efficient manner."*

Figure 27.11 DGRT member recommendations for improving programs

Shaffer and I strived to be constantly open to inviting feedback from each other and the team leaders on how to best accomplish tasks. In one instance, we developed a Tip Sheet with a QR code that when scanned was supposed to access a Disastershock manual. However, the QR code instead accessed an advertisement. Feedback about this was critical to correcting the QR code so that it only accessed the Disastershock manual. One of our colleagues pointed out that we were spending so much time on personal check-in that there was little time left for discussing tasks. Consequently, we limited personal check-ins to one minute for each person.

In July, 2021, we conducted an anonymous survey of members and received valuable feedback that members felt we were achieving our mission (see Figure 27.3) as well as valuable suggestions for improving our programs (see Figure 27.11). Seven of the eleven recommendations have already been implemented (see Table 27.1) and we have plans to implement the remaining suggestions once our "all hands on deck" situation helping distribute Disastershock resources to Ukrainian refugees is completed.

Principle 8: Highlight successes and express gratitude for contributions

It is important to reward team and member achievements. We typically did this with an email congratulating the individual who had accomplished something important and copying the rest of the team so that the praise was made public. In this situation, the congratulated member usually received additional emails from other members congratulating them also.

Table 27.1 Actions taken on DGRT member recommendations

Recommendation	Action
1 Meaningful ongoing projects	Tip Sheet Project, Reporter's Notebook project, Ways of Coping Phase 2 study, Ambassadors team, Public Health Literacy Internship,
2 Research on usefulness of Disastershock materials	Proposed evaluation of both Disastershock books and Tip Sheets in San Francisco schools
3 Short check-ins	Already implemented, e.g. Rose, Thorn, Bud approach
4 More future lectures	TBA
5 Younger members involved	Launching of Ambassadors program
6 Instagram page/media that is current	TBA
7 Inviting more members from other parts of the world	Expansion of Ambassadors team to India and Taiwan
8 Continuing with Tip Sheet Initiative	Currently being implemented: 22 languages now available
9 Persisting promoting and distributing Disastershock resources	Actively being implemented during the War on Ukraine
10 Creating our own video content	Partly implemented: Reporter's Notebook on Expressive Arts page; Disastershock Ambassadors video (Cal Poly University Humboldt)
11 Creating our own audio content	TBA

Multicultural Considerations

Diversity is essential in maintaining a global humanitarian relief organization. It was through having diverse contacts that the DGVT was able to rapidly develop 26 translations of Disastershock. The languages for which we have now have translations are:

Arabic
Bengali
Cantonese
Czech
Dutch
English
Farsi
Finnish

French
German
Hebrew
Hindi
Hungarian
Indonesian
Italian
iZulu
Japanese
Malayalam
Mandarin
Polish
Portuguese
Romanian
Russian
Spanish
Tagalog
Taiwanese
Tamil
Turkish
Ukrainian
Vietnamese
Yoruba

We anticipate developing many additional translations in the future.

Challenges and solutions

The fact that we are an all-volunteer organization is both a challenge and a solution. When we have difficulty finding a volunteer translator, we do not have the luxury of hiring one. This is an indication that fundraising will be important as a future DGRT task. Alternatively, being an all-volunteer organization ensures that the persons who join us are compassionate and highly motivated to help others. This passion to help others is a driving force in the organization. Consequently, we view future fundraising as not for staff salaries but for emergency funding for developing new translations, and providing hard copies of Disastershock materials to disaster victims.

Conclusion

We are a small, passionate volunteer organization that coalesced around efforts to mitigate the global pandemic. Our energy came from the giving spirit that each member brought to the organization and the willingness to commit time to developing and delivering valuable coping resources to children and families suffering from disaster-related stress. Most of the principles we have outlined here for developing a successful global psychological first aid organization were clear to Shaffer and Gerrard from the beginning: especially Principles 1, 2, 2A, 2B, 3, 4, and 8. The others emerged as we grew the organization. During our first year, the most frequently used phrase we used to describe our experience was "We are building the airplane as we are flying it." This phrase captures nicely the risk-taking and excitement of being in on the ground floor of a deeply meaningful developing team. We hope that what we have learned from our success will be of benefit to you as you build your psychological first aid organization and experience the excitement of flying it as you go!

Resources

https://www.disastershock.com/
This is the website of the Disastershock Global Response Team. It contains many resources for helping children, families, and schools affected by disaster-related stress.
Gerrard, B., Carter, M. J., & Ribera, D.(Eds.) (2019). *School-based family counseling: An interdisciplinary practitioner's guide.* Routledge.
This book gives a comprehensive overview of the practice of school-based family counseling.
Gerrard, B., Selimos, E. & Morrison, S. (Eds.) (2022). *School-based family counseling with refugees and immigrants.* Routledge.
As the title suggests this book provides the reader with SBFC strategies for collaborating with refugees and immigrants.

Reference

Blake, R. R., & McCanse, A. A. (1991). *Leadership dilemmas--grid solutions.* Routledge.

Index

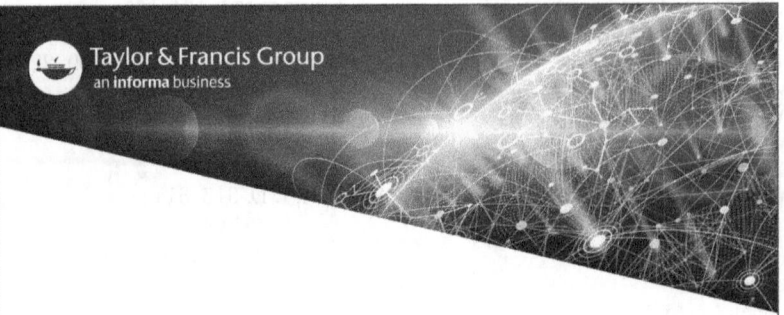

Taylor & Francis Group
an **informa** business

Taylor & Francis eBooks

www.taylorfrancis.com

A single destination for eBooks from Taylor & Francis
with increased functionality and an improved user
experience to meet the needs of our customers.

90,000+ eBooks of award-winning academic content in
Humanities, Social Science, Science, Technology, Engineering,
and Medical written by a global network of editors and authors.

TAYLOR & FRANCIS EBOOKS OFFERS:

A streamlined
experience for
our library
customers

A single point
of discovery
for all of our
eBook content

Improved
search and
discovery of
content at both
book and
chapter level

REQUEST A FREE TRIAL
support@taylorfrancis.com

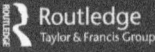 Routledge
Taylor & Francis Group

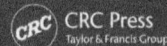 CRC Press
Taylor & Francis Group